Practical Drug Safety from A to Z

A to Z

Barton L. Cobert, MD, FACP, FACG, FFPM
Vice President, Global Regulatory Initiatives
and Pharmacovigilance
Medidata Solutions Worldwide

Pierre Biron, MD
Honorary Professor of Pharmacology
Department of Pharmacology
Université de Montréal

JONES AND BARTLETT PUBLISHERS
Sudbury, Massachusetts
BOSTON   TORONTO   LONDON   SINGAPORE

World Headquarters

Jones and Bartlett Publishers, LLC	Jones and Bartlett Publishers	Jones and Bartlett Publishers
40 Tall Pine Drive	Canada	International
Sudbury, MA 01776	6339 Ormindale Way	Barb House, Barb Mews
978-443-5000	Mississauga, Ontario L5V 1J2	London W6 7PA
info@jbpub.com	Canada	United Kingdom
www.jbpub.com		

Jones and Bartlett's books and products are available through most bookstores and online book-sellers. To contact Jones and Bartlett Publishers directly, call 800-832-0034, fax 978-443-8000, or visit our website, www.jbpub.com.

Substantial discounts on bulk quantities of Jones and Bartlett's publications are available to cor-porations, professional associations, and other qualified organizations. For details and specific discount information, contact the special sales department at Jones and Bartlett via the above contact information or send an email to: specialsales@jbpub.com.

Production Credits

Executive Publisher: Christopher Davis	Manufacturing Buyer: Therese Connell
Production Director: Amy Rose	Composition: ATLIS Graphics
Production Editor: Daniel Stone	Cover Design: Kristin E. Ohlin
Associate Editor: Kathy Richardson	Printing and Binding: Malloy, Inc.
Associate Marketing Manager: Rebecca Wasley	Cover Printing: Malloy, Inc.
Associate Marketing Manager: Ilana Gordon	

Library of Congress Cataloging-in-Publication Data
Cobert, Barton L.
    Practical drug safety from A to Z / Barton Cobert, Pierre Biron.
        p. ; cm.
    Based on: Pharmacovigilance from A to Z / Barton L. Cobert, Pierre Biron. c2002.
    ISBN-13: 978-0-7637-4527-1
    ISBN-10: 0-7637-4527-8
    1. Pharmacoepidemiology—Handbooks, manuals, etc.   2. Drugs—Side effects—Handbooks, manuals, etc.   3. Drugs—Safety measures—Handbooks, manuals, etc.
I. Biron, Pierre.   II. Cobert, Barton L. Pharmacovigilance from A to Z.   III. Title.
    [DNLM: 1. Pharmaceutical Preparations—adverse effects—Handbooks.   2. Drug Toxicity—Handbooks.   3. Pharmacoepidemiology—Handbooks.   4. Product Surveillance, Postmarketing—Handbooks. QZ 39 C655pa 2008]
    RM302.5.C634 2008
    615'.7042—dc22

                                                                                    2007047351

The authors, editor, and publisher have made every effort to provide accurate information. However, they are not responsible for errors, omissions, or for any outcomes related to the use of the contents of this book and take no responsibility for the use of the products and procedures described. Treatments and side effects described in this book may not be applicable to all people; likewise, some people may require a dose or experience a side effect that is not described herein. Drugs and medical devices are discussed that may have limited availability controlled by the Food and Drug Administration (FDA) for use only in a research study or clinical trial. Research, clinical practice, and government regulations often change the accepted standard in this field. When consideration is being given to use of any drug in the clinical setting, the health care provider or reader is responsible for determining FDA status of the drug, reading the package insert, and reviewing prescribing infor-mation for the most up-to-date recommendations on dose, precautions, and contraindications, and determining the appropriate usage for the product. This is especially important in the case of drugs that are new or seldom used.

Printed in the United States of America
12 11 10 09 08   10 9 8 7 6 5 4 3 2 1

Dedication

To my daughter Emilie with all my love.

Barton Cobert

To my wife Ninon, who gracefully accepted to share an academician's life and to let me spend half of my retirement days in front of a computer.

Pierre Biron

Contents

About the Authors

Barton Cobert, MD, FACP, FACG, FFPM

Dr. Cobert is Vice President of Regulatory Initiatives and Pharmacovigilance at Medidata Solutions Worldwide. Prior to joining Medidata, Dr. Cobert was Global Head of Drug Safety & Pharmacovigilance at Novartis Consumer Health. Dr. Cobert has extensive experience in the pharmaceutical industry.

Dr. Cobert is a gastroenterologist with board certification in Internal Medicine and Gastroenterology. He completed his medical school internship, residency, and fellowship at the New York University School of Medicine (Bellevue Hospital) in Manhattan. He did post-doctoral work in liver disease at the French National Institute of Health & Research (INSERM) in Paris, France.

After practicing gastroenterology in New York City, Dr. Cobert joined the pharmaceutical industry in 1981 at American Home Products (now Wyeth), where he ran clinical research trials. He later joined Hoechst Roussel Pharmaceuticals (now Sanofi-Aventis).

In 1992 Dr. Cobert joined the Schering-Plough Research Institute in New Jersey in the regulatory department and a year later became Global Head of Drug Safety and Pharmacovigilance, a position he held until his retirement in 2004. He was the business lead for the development of an in-house drug safety database ("CAVIAR"), and he also developed and directed the safety/risk management department of over 150 people.

Dr. Cobert has broad experience in drug and device safety and risk management, clinical research, regulatory affairs, quality, software development, and clinical medicine.

Dr. Cobert has been active in many international organizations and was a participant in the International Conference on Harmonization (ICH) from its outset in 1989 working first in the GCP and clinical trial areas and then in drug safety where he co-chaired an Expert Working Group on PSURs and was a member of the E2B (electronic transmission of safety data) Expert Working Group representing PhRMA.

Dr. Cobert has published two textbooks on Drug Safety. The first, *Pharmacovigilance from A to Z* co-authored with Pierre Biron, published in 2002 and the second in 2007, entitled *Manual of Drug Safety and Pharmacovigilance.* Dr. Cobert has multiple publications in peer-reviewed journals and has been a speaker and trainer at many conferences around the world on drug safety, risk management, and quality.

Dr. Cobert is on staff at the New York University School of Medicine and the University of Medicine and Dentistry of New Jersey. He is a fellow of the American College of Physicians, the American College of Gastroenterology, and the Faculty of Pharmaceutical Medicine (UK).

Pierre Biron, MD

Dr. Biron studied medicine at the Université de Montréal where he obtained his MD degree. He received an MSc degree in Investigative Medicine at McGill University in Montreal, completed by postgraduate studies at the Rockefeller University in New York City, and at University Hospitals in Paris.

Dr. Biron joined the Department of Pharmacology at the Université de Montréal where, for three decades he taught undergraduate and graduate medical students. Dr. Biron's first 20 years were spent in basic, clinical, and observational research. Dr. Biron's last 10 years were devoted to drug safety by singlehandedly setting up a university-based regional pharmacovigilance center and writing his first pharmacovigilance dictionary.

Now Honorary Professor of Pharmacology, Dr. Biron focuses on the clinical trials and pharmacovigilance scene and is concerned by the effects on patients' safety of the relationships between industry, regulators, academics, and prescribers.

Introduction

Much to our surprise, the explosion in the issues and controversies in the field of drug safety/pharmacovigilance in North America, Europe, and elsewhere has not brought about a corresponding increase in the number of textbooks and manuals covering this field.

We have revised and rewritten our earlier publication (*Pharmacovigilance from A to Z*) which appeared in 2002, expanded its coverage, and oriented its content to make it a much more practical and useful book. It is aimed at drug safety professionals working in the pharmaceutical and allied industries, regulatory agencies, clinical research organizations, students and their teachers in medicine, nursing, and pharmacy, those who make decisions regarding drug therapy, whether in public health, industry, or clinical practice.

It should be particularly useful to those who will have to deal with the new FDA Revitalization Act requirements and obligations that will happen over the next few years in the United States. Similar changes will come about in one form or another in Europe, Canada, Japan, and elsewhere as the field of pharmacovigilance finally begins to develop the needed techniques and technology to take advantage of the enormous amount of data sitting in governmental and commercial databases around the world.

This book should be on the shelf (or on the PC) of anyone in the field and especially those preparing for courses, seminars, and conferences on drug safety. In fact we sincerely hope it will foster the teaching of pharmacovigilance in medical and pharmacy schools and encourage the publication of much-needed updated textbooks in drug-induced diseases.

It should also serve as a quick and useful reference to quickly look up unfamiliar terms. In particular, as this book does not have an index, we strongly recommend using the CD-ROM version of the book with the Adobe® search tool to find all the occurrences of a term or phrase throughout the whole book.

Notice

This book is not meant to be used in the practice of medicine or for the prescription of medicines or drugs. The medications described do not necessarily have specific approval by the FDA or any other health authority for use in the diseases, patients, and at the dosages discussed. The FDA approved labeling (the package insert) in the US and the local labeling for countries outside the US should be consulted. Because standards for usage change, it is advisable to keep abreast of revised recommendations, particularly those concerning new drugs.

This book is not intended to express opinions about the value of specific products or about their comparative value within a drug class, even when a specific product is used to provide examples of adverse reactions. The content of the book is not meant to be used in choosing one product or another in medical practice. As with all medications, the official, approved product labeling should be consulted before prescription or use.

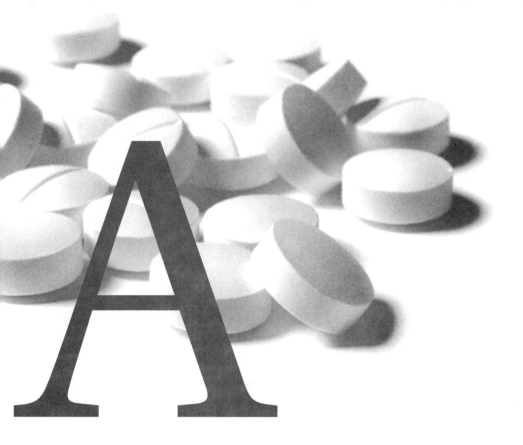

Nothing in this book is meant to advise on legal liability or responsibility. In all such situations, legal counsel should be sought.

"THE AGENCY"

Refers to the FDA in the field of drug regulation. The expression is also used to designate the Central Intelligence Agency (CIA) in the field of justice.

ABBREVIATED NEW DRUG APPLICATION (ANDA)

A submission to the FDA's Center for Drug Evaluation and Research, Office of Generic Drugs, for the review and approval of a generic drug product. The equivalent for generic products of an NDA for a new chemical entity. See http://www.fda.gov/cder/regulatory/applications/anda.htm.

ABCD TABLE

See Two by Two Table.

ABCDE SYSTEM

Hurwitz and Wade (1969) proposed four categories or mechanisms of adverse events: side effect, excess effect, allergy (hypersensitivity), and idiosyncrasy.

The first two categories have been combined under Type A and the second two mechanisms under Type B, a classification in current use.

- Type A reactions are also known as pharmacologically predictable, dose-related reactions. They include an exaggeration of the desired effect and the so-called "side effects," which represent the stimulation of undesired target/receptors.
- Type B reactions are also known as pharmacologically unpredictable reactions. They include allergic (hypersensitivity) effects, which are not dose related, and other idiosyncratic effects.

Three more categories have been proposed:

- Type C (for chronic) reactions are ADRs due to products administered for long periods of time in patients with chronic diseases. They are usually discovered by structured epidemiologic studies. For example, postmenopausal hormone replacement therapy ADRs were discovered in long-term epidemiologic studies.
- Type D (for delay) reactions are ADRs whose latency (the time period after the last dose to the onset of the ADR) is long and makes causality difficult to ascertain. Examples: amiodarone ADRs and teratogenic products.
- Type E (for end of use) reactions are those with a rebound or withdrawal effect.

Deswarte later proposed eight categories: overdose, side effect, secondary effect (indirect), interaction, intolerance, idiosyncrasy (primary toxicity), allergy, and pseudoallergy (anaphylactoid)

Authors' note: In practice these categories are rarely used and these systems are somewhat confusing or even contradictory to current usage. For example, "side effect" is now considered a lay term that is to be avoided in the medical literature. "Overdose" is not an ADR but a possible cause in some patients, especially those reported to Poison Control Centers. Nonetheless, MedDRA does recognize "overdose" as an AE/ADR for coding purposes.

ABPI

See Association of the British Pharmaceutical Industry.

ABSOLUTE RISK

In the drug safety context, the probability of occurrence of an adverse event in patients exposed to a drug. It can be expressed in a single cohort as a rate of incidence: 1 in 10, 10%, or 0.1. When exposed and unexposed cohorts are compared, it may be expressed as a risk difference or as a relative risk (ratio of two absolute risks).

See Risk and Absolute Risk Reduction.

ABSOLUTE RISK REDUCTION (ARR)

The difference in an event rate between the control group and the treated group when the outcome measure of benefit is a risk reduction. This variable should be presented in all drug trial reports and even incorporated in the abstract in addition to the relative risk reduction. For example, if the control group had an event rate of 7.3% and the treated group had an event rate of 3.3%, then the absolute risk reduction for this event is 7.3% − 3.3% = 4%. Thus for 100 patients treated with this drug, four bad outcomes would be avoided. The inverse of the ARR gives the NNTB (Number Needed to Benefit); 25 patients in this example.

ABUSE

Persistent or sporadic, intentional, excessive use of a drug, accompanied by harmful physical, psychological, and/or behavioral effects. It is by itself an abnormal behavior, and in some cases may be induced by the pharmacological effects of the drug (a Type A effect). It occurs in susceptible individuals. May also be described as out of control, compulsive consumption despite negative consequences. The drugs in question are usually psychoactive but not always. An anorexic person could overuse diuretics to lose weight and thus risk severe electrolyte imbalance.

Authors' note: Depending upon the drug(s) in question, abuse may or may not be illegal. Medication abuse may be due to the patient and/or the prescriber. The word "abuse" should not be used to describe increasing the dose of cancer chemotherapy where the oncologist "pushes" higher doses of various agents beyond the approved labeling in an attempt to eradicate the tumor (often in the context of a clinical trial).

ACADEMIA

In the drug safety context, it refers to medical, pharmacy, nursing, other health science schools and their involvement in pharmacovigilance. Some clinical pharmacy and clinical pharmacology departments teach the rudiments of pharmacovigilance, but too many do not. A few universities offer postgraduate courses in pharmacoepidemiology and related matters.

Authors' note: The teaching of drug safety does not occupy the place it deserves during initial and continuing medical education nor is the general public made aware in most countries of the need for pharmacovigilance.

ACCEPTABILITY OF AN ADR

An ADR is considered acceptable depending upon the beneficial effect and the patient population being treated. For example, drug-induced hair loss or low white blood cell counts are acceptable in the treatment of cancer where the drug may be lifesaving, but are not acceptable in treating a benign disease (e.g., head cold or allergies).

Authors' note: An ADR becomes acceptable when the expected benefit is greater than the likelihood that the ADR will occur. This is a medical judgment made by the regulatory authorities when approving a new drug, by the physician when prescribing the drug, and by the patient when taking it. It is based on the frequency and severity of the ADR(s), the expected benefit, and the severity of the disease.

ACCEPTABLE RISK

The level of probability of having an adverse event that society, the FDA and other health agencies, the treating physician, and/or the patient will accept. The acceptable risk varies from country to country (triazolam is banned in the UK but is allowed in the US as a sleep aid), situation to situation, and patient to patient.

ACCOUNTABILITY

In the context of pharmacovigilance, this refers to the responsibility of each stakeholder and provider in the development, research, and use of drugs to ensure that they are used in a rational, efficacious, benevolent, and safe manner. There are complex and multiple interdependencies and responsibilities in this chain falling on all parties involved to varying degrees: pharmaceutical companies, legislators, health authorities, medical educators, editors of medical journals, prescribers, sellers, dispensers, and users. The goal of all of the people and organizations involved is to avoid ADRs due to negligence, imprudence, and errors or "irregularities" when these ADRs are preventable.

ACKNOWLEDGMENT LETTER FOR AN AE REPORT

All pharmacovigilance centers (governmental, industrial, or academic) should reply promptly to every person who notifies them of an adverse event. This reply may be a letter, phone call, fax, or email and should thank the sender for the information, acknowledge its receipt, and ask for further information if needed to clarify the case. Additional information should be requested when the information is insufficient or certain lab tests are needed for validation of the event (e.g., cardiograms, X-ray or scan reports, etc.), the case represents a particularly important signal, or if the event is very severe medically and may alter the benefit/risk analysis if confirmed.

ACTIONS TAKEN WHEN A SIGNAL IS POSITIVE

1. **At the Public Health Level**
   When a signal is felt to be confirmed following a pharmacovigilance investigation, the governmental health authorities and the manufacturer will take various measures to reduce inevitable and unacceptable risk in order to make continued use of the product safer.

2. **Regulatory Measures**
   Regulatory measures or actions taken affecting the status of the drug, which are taken during or after a pharmacovigilance investigation with the goal of preventing further ADRs that are judged unacceptable for the public health. Such measures can be taken either separately or together by the manufacturer and the health authorities. Actions taken by the manufacturer may be either voluntary or obligatory. In most cases, action is taken only after a signal is confirmed. However, if a new ADR appears to be clearly unacceptable and/or too frequent to allow the risk of waiting for confirmation from a request for intensified AE reporting or from clinical trials, urgent temporary regulatory measures can be taken.

3. **Label Changes**
   Changes in medical information are usually included in the product labeling for the healthcare professional as well as for the patient (Patient Information Leaflet). Sometimes information is even put on the packaging, such as by attaching a sticker to the bottle.
   Possible labeling actions include:

   - Major changes: withdrawal of an indication, addition of contraindications, new precautions or warnings. These changes

produce alterations in the package insert (official labeling) and possibly on the packaging or bottle. These changes can include:
- A reduction in the recommended dose.
- The removal of one or more indications.
- An absolute or relative restriction on the population being treated.
- A new warning or contraindication for patients with certain medical conditions, diseases, or for patients using other specific drugs or classes of drugs (drug interaction).
- Making the product a secondary or tertiary treatment rather than a first-line treatment.
- Recommendation of concomitant treatment with another drug to prevent or correct the problem produced by the drug.
- Recommendation of periodic lab test or clinical observation (e.g., ALT for hepatotoxic products, ECGs for cardiotoxic products, etc.).

- Limitation of Access to the Drug
  - Alteration of availability: categorizing it as a controlled drug or limiting its prescription in hospitals.
  - Limitation on the prescribers (i.e., reserved only to specialists) for the initial prescription or for renewals.
  - Limitation on methods of prescription: no automatic renewals, no telephone prescriptions.
  - Limitation to place of dispensation: moving a drug from OTC to "behind the counter" (requiring pharmacist consultation).
  - Obligatory laboratory testing (e.g., negative pregnancy test before, during, and for some months after stopping treatment).
  - Written justification of the indication by the prescriber.
  - Informed consent signed by the patient and, possibly, the prescriber or pharmacist.
  - Withdrawal (weaning) of patients under treatment.
  - Requirement of other measures while taking the drug; e.g., two methods of contraception for teratogenic medications.

- Modification of the Product Itself
  - Change in the active entity.
  - Removal or substitution of one of the active ingredients in a combination product (e.g., the removal of pseudoephedrine from cough and cold products).
  - Removal of one of the dosage strengths available (usually the highest dose).
  - Change or removal of excipients.

- Modification of the quantity in the bottle or box.
- Change in packaging.
- Change in an accompanying device.
- Change in storage or preparation (e.g., allow a refrigerated product to return to room temperature before injecting).
- Withdrawal from the Market
  - Withdrawal of a particular active ingredient, a specific product, a specific formulation.
  - Temporary or definitive suspension of sales.
  - Cessation of manufacture and distribution.
  - Withdrawal of stocks to the wholesaler, pharmacist, or patient level depending upon the severity of the problem.
  - Withdrawal of the drug from individual patients under medical care.
- Methods of Communication of the Changes
  - The labeling in the official monograph (labeling, package insert, summary of product characteristics, etc.).
  - The labeling in the packaging documentation.
  - The labeling on the sticker of the box or bottle.
  - A Dear Doctor, Dear Pharmacist, or Dear Healthcare Professional letter or email.
  - Direct notification by the manufacturer's sales representatives to the prescribing physicians.
  - A pharmacovigilance bulletin either in writing, on the Internet, or both.
  - An article in a scientific or professional periodical.
  - A press release to the media and on the Internet.
  - An alert notification from one health authority to another (e.g., a WHO Uppsala alert to worldwide health agencies).
  - In rare instances, direct use of mass media to alert the general public of a critical safety issue.

ACTIVE INGREDIENT (MOIETY)

The chemical or molecular entity in a drug that produces the pharmacologic effect (and usually, but not always, the ADRs). As opposed to the inactive ingredients, fillers, or excipients, which are usually not thought of as producing efficacy or ADRs.

Authors' note: Inactive ingredients in high doses may indeed produce effects (e.g., diarrhea when lactose is used as a filler). Drug safety personnel should always keep in mind the possibility that an AE/ADR is due not to the active ingredient(s) but to fillers or manufacturing quality problems.

ACTIVE QUERY

In pharmacovigilance, active query refers to directed follow-up on a spontaneous case report, carried out by health authorities or drug safety groups in pharmaceutical companies, in order to obtain more complete information about the patient's problem. Such queries should be direct and specific (e.g., "Please send hospitalization and outcome information regarding the myocardial infarction the patient experienced on April 22, 2007").

As a part of a drug safety investigation triggered by an alert signal, active query refers to searches done in a drug safety database to extract the relevant information.

Authors' note: Queries of the database should be done by someone very familiar with the database, its structure, and computer query language (SQL), as well as drug safety—in other words, a "super-user"—in order to be sure the query captures all relevant cases. For example, the query "Provide a line listing of all patients who took drug X and had chest pain or myocardial infarctions" requires a search in the database using all appropriate MedDRA codes to capture chest pain or myocardial infarction but not other cardiac diseases or diagnoses.

ACTIVE SURVEILLANCE

Refers to systems or situations in which AEs/ADRs are purposely sought. It is the opposite of "passive surveillance," in which health authorities and pharmaceutical companies wait for healthcare professionals, patients, or consumers to make the effort to contact the authority or company to report an AE or ADR.

Active surveillance is at its peak in clinical research trials, where the investigator questions the patients in the study on whether they have had AEs since the last visit.

Forms of active surveillance in the postmarketing setting include:

- A health authority's request to all physicians to report, for example, episodes of torsades de pointes seen with a particular drug or class of drugs. This is also known as prompted reporting or stimulated reporting.
- A request in a PSUR by the rapporteur to more closely follow a particular AE or ADR that is a potential or weak signal.
- A company-sponsored follow-up of a cohort of, say, 10,000 patients taking drug X looking for a particular AE or AEs.

ACTUAL MEDICATION ERROR

See Medication Error.

ADDENDUM REPORT FOR PSUR

In response to a special request by regulators or in the situation where an international birthdate is being harmonized globally, this term refers to reports covering a period outside the routine PSUR reporting cycle (e.g., if the reports are based on the local approval date in that country rather than on the IBD). It updates the most recently completed PSUR. It is prepared in the usual PSUR format.

An addendum report is used when it is not possible to synchronize PSURs for all authorities requiring submissions. The addendum report is an update to the most recently completed PSUR. It should be used when there is data for more than 3 months for a 6-month PSUR, and more than 6 months for a longer PSUR. It is not intended as an in-depth report (which will be done in the next regularly scheduled PSUR). It should contain an introduction, any changes to the core safety information (CSI), significant regulatory actions on safety, line listings, and/or summary tabulations and a conclusion.

ADDICTION

In the pharmacological context, the compulsive need for or use of a drug that becomes habit-forming and that produces tolerance with continued use and withdrawal symptoms upon cessation. This may occur with "street drugs" (e.g., cocaine), medicinals such as narcotics (e.g., morphine), or societal drugs (e.g., nicotine). The dependence may be physical or psychological.

ADDICTIVE DRUGS CLASSIFICATION

A mechanistic classification of addictive drugs was recently proposed:

Class I: Activation of $G_{i/o}$-coupled receptors, such as morphine and other opioids, cannabinoids.
Class II: Binding to ionotropic receptors and ion channels, such as nicotine, benzodiazepines, ethanol.
Class III: Binding to transporters of biogenic amines, such as cocaine, and amphetamine and its derivatives.

(Source: Luscher 2006)

ADME

Absorption, distribution, metabolism, and elimination of a drug. Study of ADME is in the field of pharmacokinetics as (opposed to pharmacodynamics). In the clinical development of a drug, these areas are thoroughly investigated in phase I trials and usually completed in phase II.

THE AUSTRALIAN ADVERSE DRUG REACTIONS BULLETIN (ADRAC)

A respected publication on drug safety from the Australian Therapeutic Goods Administration (TGA) produced six times a year. A free subscription is available at: www.tga.gov.au/adr/adrac-bulletin-subscribe.asp.

ADROIT

See Adverse Drug Reactions On-Line Information Tracking.

ADVERSE DRUG EXPERIENCE (ADE)

Any adverse event associated with the use of a drug in humans, whether or not considered drug related, including the following: an adverse event occurring in the course of the use of a drug product in professional practice; an adverse event occurring from drug overdose, whether accidental or intentional; an adverse event occurring from drug abuse; an adverse event occurring from drug withdrawal; and any failure of expected pharmacological action. (FDA 21CFR314.80)

ADVERSE DRUG REACTION (ADR) AKA ADVERSE REACTION (AR)

"An appreciably harmful or unpleasant reaction, resulting from an intervention related to the use of a medicinal product, which predicts hazard from future administration and warrants prevention or specific treatment, or alteration of the dosage regimen, or withdrawal of the product." (Uppsala Monitoring Centre)

In the preapproval (i.e., not yet marketed, experimental) phase of a product, the definition is:

"All noxious and unintended responses to a medicinal product related to any dose should be considered adverse drug reactions." This means "that a causal relationship between a medicinal product and an adverse event is at least a reasonable possibility, i.e., the relationship cannot be ruled out." (ICH E2A)

For postapproval (i.e., marketed) products, the definition is:

"A response to a drug which is noxious and unintended and which occurs at doses normally used in man for prophylaxis, diagnosis, or therapy of disease or for modification of physiological function." (ICH E2A) This definition has also been proposed for adoption by FDA (proposed regulations of March 14, 2003).

ADVERSE DRUG REACTIONS ON-LINE INFORMATION TRACKING (ADROIT)

The spontaneous ADR reports database of the Medicines Control Agency (MCA) in the UK. It contains details of reports of suspected ADRs that have been reported to the MCA since 1964 via the Yellow

Card Scheme of the UK Committee on Safety of Medicines (CSM). This has been replaced by a new database called Sentinel at the UK Health Authority (now called the MHRA, Medicine and Healthcare Products Regulatory Agency).

ADVERSE EVENT REPORTING SYSTEM (AERS) DATABASE

The FDA's electronic database designed to support the FDA's post-marketing safety surveillance program for all approved drug and therapeutic biologic products. Incremental zipped files in either ASCII or SGML formats are available from the FDA's website for downloading. See http://www.fda.gov/cder/aers/default.htm.

Also, a commercial database is available from the Oracle Corporation for AE event handling. It is not associated with the FDA's AERS database. See http://www.oracle.com/industries/life_sciences/aers45_datasheet.pdf.

ADVERSE EVENT (AE)

"Any untoward medical occurrence in a patient or clinical investigation subject administered a pharmaceutical product and which does not necessarily have to have a causal relationship with this treatment." (ICH E2A)

"Any unfavorable and unintended sign (including an abnormal laboratory finding, for example), symptom, or disease temporally associated with the use of any dose of a medicinal product, whether or not considered related to the medicinal product." (ICH E2A)

ADVERSE EVENT DICTIONARY

See Data Dictionary.

AEGIS

See AIDS Education Global Information System.

Also refers to an unrelated pharmaceutical company by this name.

AFSSAPS

Acronym for the French drug agency. *See* Agence Française de Sécurité Sanitaire des Produits de Santé.

AGE, DRUG'S

Refers to the time on the market of a drug product.

Authors' note: Drugs, like people, have natural lifespans. They are "young" when newly introduced and age over the course of years as

other products are introduced that are (or are perceived to be) supe-
rior, producing lowered usage of the drug. Some drugs are short-
lived (e.g., chlorthiazide, which has largely been replaced by
hydrochlorthiazide), whereas others live for many years (e.g., as-
pirin). The drug may or may not remain on the market. This is usu-
ally a choice of the manufacturer.

In regard to drug safety, the safety profile of a drug is much better
known after several years on the market.

AGE, PATIENT'S

One of the "minimum information" characteristics that can be used
to identify a patient in an individual case safety report. A critical
piece of knowledge in drug safety and pharmacovigilance in the
analysis of an AE in an individual patient as well as in epidemiology. *See* Minimum Information for Reportability.

Authors' note: The age of the patient must be taken into account
when completing an AE/ADR report form because it facilitates the
identification of the patient, the analysis of the case, and the assess-
ment of causality. For example, a report of myocardial infarction in
a 65-year-old (who might also have other risk factors for coronary
disease) would not, in general, be considered unusual and might
not be ascribed to an ADR. However, in a 20-year-old with no risk
factors, a drug cause may be much higher in the list of causal
considerations.

AGENCE FRANÇAISE DE SÉCURITÉ SANITAIRE DES PRODUITS DE SANTÉ (AFSSAPS)

The French drug agency. Their website in English is http://agmed.
sante.gouv.fr/ang/indang.htm.

AGGREGATE REPORT

A report on a drug product that summarizes and analyzes multiple
AEs, signals, clinical trials, frequency analyses, etc. There are sev-
eral types in general use around the world, including the US NDA
Periodic Report and IND Annual Report, the Periodic Safety Update
Report (PSUR). They are in contrast to the Individual Case Safety
Report (ICSR), which describes a single patient's AEs. In many phar-
maceutical companies there is a separate group within the Drug
Safety Department that specializes in writing these reports.

AGRANULOCYTOSIS

A frequently used term in hematovigilance, because it is more likely
to be an ADR rather than a "spontaneous" event. It designates an
isolated severe usually symptomatic neutropenia, which affects

the white blood cell granulocyte line. The criteria for diagnosis have been defined as:

- an acute, severe, and isolated neutropenia defined as a poly-morphonuclear neutrophil count less than 500 μL/L (0.5 x10^9/L),
- without anemia (hemoglobin greater than 100g/L), and
- without thrombocytopenia (platelet count greater than 100 million/L).

AIDS EDUCATION GLOBAL INFORMATION SYSTEM (AEGIS)

A very large database containing information on AIDS, including sections on drug treatments, interactions, clinical trials, etc. (http://www.aegis.com)

AIDS TEST FOR BLOOD, FDA APPROVAL

The approval of this test in 1985 was the Agency's first major action to protect patients from infected donors.

Authors' note: A landmark in the history of hemovigilance in the US, for improving the safety of blood products.

ALANINE AMINOTRANSFERASE (ALT) ALAT AKA SERUM GLUTAMIC
PYRUVATE TRANSAMINASE (SGPT)

A so-called "liver function test" (LFT). An enzyme found primarily in the liver, but also found in smaller amounts in the kidneys, heart, muscles, and pancreas. ALT formerly was called serum glutamic pyruvate transaminase (SGPT). It is found in the blood (serum) in low levels in normal individuals and is increased when there is damage to the other organs noted above (e.g., myocardial infarction). Most serum elevations are due to liver damage.

Other tests of liver damage include aspartate aminotransferase (AST), alkaline phosphatase, gamma glutamyl transpeptidase, lactate dehydrogenase (LDH), and bilirubin. If several of these are elevated at the same time, the likelihood of their source being the liver (and hence liver damage) is higher.

Authors' note: The liver is a frequent target for drug toxicity; as a result the measurement of liver function tests is a very common screen for such drug toxicity. Most clinical laboratories offer a "liver screen" looking at these enzymes as well as hepatitis antigens and antibodies.

ALT/AP RATIO

See Liver Function Tests.

ALERT

1. Older synonym for signal or a signal warranting a safety investigation. The term is generally not used any longer in this context. *See* Signal.
2. A solicitation to the medical profession or public by a health authority to send in particular AE reports (e.g., all ventricular arrhythmias seen with NSAIDs) or to watch a certain drug. It is a form of active surveillance.
3. A notice to the medical profession and the public about a particular public health issue or problem associated with a product. For example: "December 12, 2006. FDA orders unapproved quinine drugs from the market and cautions consumers about 'off-label' use of quinine to treat leg cramps." (Published on FDA's CDER home page http://www.fda.gov/cder/.)
4. An expedited ("alert") 7- or 15-day report sent to a health authority.

ALERT REPORT

A common term for a 7- or 15-day expedited report sent to the FDA or other health authorities. *See* Expedited Report.

ALGORITHM, CAUSALITY

An algorithm is a step-by-step, detailed instruction on how to perform a task or reach a conclusion. It may be in diagrammatic form and may have multiple steps and decision points.

Over 30 algorithms have been developed for both manual and computerized causality assessment of individual AE case reports. One of the earliest algorithms was developed by Prof. J. Venulet in 1980 and updated in 1986. Based on a recent study by an expert panel in which various algorithms were compared, the authors concluded that full agreement with the WHO method was not found for any level of causality, but full agreement among experts using their clinical intuition was not found, either. Making an etiologic (causality) diagnosis is part of the art of medicine. Safety experts in industry and agencies must master the principles of causality assessment of case reports based on bibliographical, chronological, and clinical criteria.

ALLERGIC REACTION

A hypersensitivity reaction in humans or animals to an allergen (a sensitizing substance such as a drug, bee sting, or food). It may be seen in some people and not others. On the initial exposure, the body's reaction may be mild but subsequent exposures may produce increasingly intense responses, and the time to onset is characteristically shorter. Such reactions may be mild or severe and occasionally may be fatal.

ALLERGY, DRUG

A noxious immunologic response to a drug. Not all drug AEs/ARs are immunologic or allergic. The allergic reaction may be mild (skin rash) or severe (anaphylaxis). The reaction may be to a specific drug or to a class of drugs (e.g., penicillins, dyes used in radiology).

Drug allergy is also called hypersensitivity and it represents a Type B adverse reaction due to an immunologic reaction of the host. A classification scheme proposed by Gell and Coombs has been in use since 1975:

- *Type 1 Immediate:* The antigen attaches to a specific IgE antibody on the surface of the mast cell, producing the release of inflammatory mediators. There are several types: atopic reactions (such as atopic asthma or atopic dermatitis) and urticarial reactions, angioedema, and anaphylaxis, of which anaphylactic shock is the most severe. In anaphylactoid reactions, such as those due to radiologic contrast agents or NSAIDs, the drug in question produces the release of inflammatory mediators without involving an antigen–antibody reaction.
- *Type 2 Cytotoxic:* An antibody reacts with a cellular antigen. The cytotoxic reaction arises frequently in hematovigilance. Examples include hemolytic anemia due to penicillin and thrombocytopenia due to quinidine.
- *Type 3 Immune Complex:* The prototype is serum sickness.
- *Type 4 Delayed:* The prototype is contact dermatitis.

ALWAYS EXPEDITED REPORT

A group of adverse events that the FDA proposed in 2003 to be reportable as 15-day expedited reports whether labeled/listed or not. They include congenital anomalies, acute respiratory failure, ventricular fibrillation, torsades de pointes, malignant hypertension, seizures, agranulocytosis, aplastic anemia, toxic epidermal necrolysis, liver necrosis, acute liver failure, anaphylaxis, acute renal failure, sclerosing syndromes, pulmonary hypertension, pulmonary fibrosis, transmission of an infectious agent by a marketed drug/biologic, and endotoxin shock, plus any future terms the FDA adds to the list. This list is similar to the list of "critical terms" used by the UMC, the WHO's monitoring center in Uppsala, Sweden.

Authors' note: Though not officially put into the regulations by the FDA, this list is used by some companies as if it were. Some companies maintain additional lists of events that are always serious.

AMA

American Medical Association

ANAPHYLAXIS/ANAPHYLACTIC REACTION

An immune reaction to an allergen that binds to IgE, producing the release of vasoactive mediators from basophils and mast cells. This in turn produces a variety of symptoms (mild to severe), such as skin rash, urticaria, pruritus, edema, nasal congestion, tearing, coughing, airway obstruction, and bronchospasm. Such reactions may be caused by drugs, bee stings, food, and other triggers.

ANAPHYLACTOID REACTION

An ADR is said to be anaphylactoid or pseudoallergic when its mechanism of action does not involve the antibodies of the host but nevertheless does involve the direct liberation of inflammatory mediators from mast cells (histamine and others). The clinical presentation is that of an immunoallergic reaction. It can be localized or generalized. Fatal anaphylactoid shock can occur in anaphylactoid reactions as well as in classic immunologically mediated anaphylactic reactions. Two examples:

- Vancomycin: An intravenous antibiotic that can produce the "red neck syndrome," an ADR associated with high-dose therapy and with rapid infusion rates.
- Radiocontrast Agents and NSAIDs: Iodinated contrast agents and NSAIDS (in particular, ASA) can produce urticaria, angioedema, nasal congestion, and asthma, and very rarely can be fatal.

ANATOMIC, THERAPEUTIC, CHEMICAL CLASSIFICATION (ATC, NORDIC ATC)

A classification system for drugs used mainly in Europe. Drugs are divided into five different groups:

1st level, anatomical main group: A—alimentary tract and metabolism
2nd level, therapeutic subgroup: A10—drugs used in diabetes
3rd level, pharmacological subgroup: A10B—oral blood glucose-lowering drugs
4th level, chemical subgroup: A10BA—biguanides
5th level, chemical substance: A10BA02—metformin

See the WHO Collaborating Centre Drug Statistics Methodology website: http://www.whocc.no/atcddd/.

ANECDOTE, ANECDOTAL EVIDENCE

In drug safety, a story or case description of an adverse drug reaction often with little or no documentation, or insufficient evidence suggesting causality, as opposed to a well-documented case or case series providing strong evidence for causality. Usually used pejoratively, as in "All we have is anecdotal evidence for pancreatitis in patients using drug XX."

See also Orphan ADR.

ANGIOEDEMA

Angioedema is localized edema found in the deep layers of the skin and is indicative of a severe stage of an immediate type of drug allergy. This term is frequently used in dermatovigilance and allergy surveillance. Its seriousness depends on its anatomic site. There is an immediate, life-threatening risk of airway obstruction when the larynx or glottis are involved. Angioedema may be due to an anaphylactic reaction in which bronchospasm and shock can be life threatening if untreated. The face, eyes, and lips are most often involved. Emergency treatment with epinephrine is required.

Authors' note: Visceral (abdominal) angioedema associated with ACE inhibitors can be difficult to diagnose for two reasons, besides its rarity: (a) The intestine is not an expected site for angioedema and a high level of suspicion is needed, along with confirmation by abdominal scanning, and (b) the time lag in the appearance of the ADR is quite variable and is often very long—sometimes measurable in years of continuing treatment.

ANIMAL PHARMACOLOGY AND TOXICOLOGY

Studies done on animals (usually several different species) to characterize a drug's properties before testing begins on humans. Studies look at the drug's toxicology, reproductive effects in males and females, ADME, carcinogenicity and, where animal models exist, efficacy.

ANONYMIZED DATA

Safety data or clinical trial data in which the identity of the patient and the reporter are removed to protect the privacy of the individuals. Sometimes it is sufficient just to remove demographic information (such as age, sex, initials, address, and country). In other cases additional data may also need to be removed (the name of the hospital, the dates of treatment, etc).

ANONYMIZED SINGLE PATIENT CASE REPORT

An ADR report (e.g., MedWatch or CIOMS I form, E2B transmission) where all information that might identify the patient or reporter has been removed.

ANTICIPATORY NAUSEA AND VOMITING

This is an interesting phenomenon that occurs in patients who have had cancer chemotherapy with nausea and vomiting in the past. Some of these patients develop nausea and vomiting before the next dose is to be given. Thus we have the adverse drug reaction occurring before the actual taking of the drug(s), providing an illustration of the nocebo effect. It is felt to be an example of classical Pavlovian conditioning.

APPLICATION SITE REACTION

An adverse reaction such as one affecting the skin, eye, mucosa, muscle, or articular cavity. The application may be topical (e.g., a cream or ointment) or invasive (e.g., subcutaneous, intramuscular, or intravenous). A form of a localized, *in situ*, reaction.

APPROVABLE LETTER

Approvable letter means a written communication to an applicant from the FDA stating that the agency will approve the application or abbreviated application if specific additional information or material is submitted or specific conditions are met. It suggests that the benefit:risk relationship is acceptable. An approvable letter does not constitute approval of any part of an application or abbreviated application and does not permit marketing of the drug that is the subject of the application or abbreviated application. (21CFR314.3)

APPROVAL LETTER

Approval letter means a written communication to an applicant from the FDA approving an application or an abbreviated application. (21CFR314.3) This means the benefit:risk relationship is acceptable (unless there are certain conditions requested in the letter in regard to safety or labeling).

APPROVAL, FDA

The acceptance by the FDA for marketing of a drug after review of its NDA or ANDA dossier. The product must show an acceptable benefit:risk relationship. It means that the drug may be marketed (sold) in the US for a particular indication, in a particular group of subjects, and at a specified dose or dose range using a particular formulation.

ARCHIVING/ARCHIVES

The storage of all documents relating to the safety of a drug for a period of time in a format that is rapidly and easily accessible should it be needed for analysis by the pharmaceutical company, health authority, or other bodies. Storage may be as paper or in other media (e.g., electronic, microfilm) or both. Attention must be paid to protection of the data from fire, water, insects, and other damage. The requirements for data protection and privacy must also be met. If the storage medium becomes outmoded (e.g., 3-1/2" floppy discs), the data must be transferred to accessible media. Although various health authorities (and lawyers) set timeframes for data retention (e.g., 15 years), many companies or health authorities will retain data "forever."

ASSOCIATION OF THE BRITISH PHARMACEUTICAL INDUSTRY (ABPI)

The trade association for the more than 75 companies in the UK producing prescription medicines. Its member companies research, develop, manufacture, and supply more than 80 percent of the medicines prescribed through the National Health Service (NHS) and produce a compendium of UK drug labeling. See their website: http://www.abpi.org.uk/.

ASSOCIATE, DRUG SAFETY

Also known as a Drug Safety Specialist, Scientist, or Technician. A health professional trained to receive, complete, code, and enter into the safety database clinical trial or spontaneous safety reports submitted by clinical trial investigators, health professionals, or consumers to the National or Regional Center of an agency or to a pharmaceutical company.

Authors' note: These terms are not fully standardized. In some companies the term Drug Safety Associate is applied to a nonmedical professional who does initial data entry. The medical professional is called a Drug Safety Scientist or Specialist.

ATTRIBUTABILITY

See Causality.

ATTRIBUTABLE RISK

See Risk Difference.

AUDIT OR INSPECTION

A systematic and independent examination of activities and documents related to suspected adverse drug reaction reports to determine whether the evaluated activities were conducted and the data were recorded, analyzed, and accurately reported according to relevant manuals, standard operating procedures, good pharmacovigilance practice, and regulatory requirements. Such inspections may be done by a health authority (e.g., EMEA, FDA, MHRA), internal company auditors, or third parties.

For information on audits by the UK see http://www.mhra. gov.uk/home/idcplg?IdcService=SS_GET_PAGE&nodeId=827& selectedSection=Inspection%20process%20and%20findings.

For information on audits by the EMEA see http://www.emea. europa.eu/Inspections/PhVInspcoord.html.

For information on audits by the FDA see http://www.fda.gov/ cder/aers/chapter53.htm (Inspection Manual).

AUSTRALIAN DRUG REACTION ADVISORY COMMITTEE (ADRAC)

A subcommittee of the Australian Drug Evaluation Committee (ADEC) formed in 1970 to advise the Therapeutic Goods Administration (TGA) on the safety of medicines. It is composed of independent medical experts in areas of importance to the evaluation of medicine safety. See http://www.tga.gov.au/adr/adrac.htm.

AUSTRALIAN ADVERSE DRUG REACTIONS BULLETIN

National bulletin of Australian pharmacovigilance prepared by the Australian Drug Reactions Advisory Committee (ADRAC). It is available online at http://www.tga.gov.au/adr/aadrb.htm and is regularly reviewed in *Reactions Weekly*, published by Adis. Several important signals first appeared in this highly respected bulletin.

AUSTRALIAN PRESCRIBER

An independently published quarterly on pharmacotherapy distributed without charge. Although subsidized by the Australian health authority, its editors have consistently maintained an independent point of view. It is a member of The International Society of Drug Bulletins, whose editors are known for their uprightness. See www.australianprescriber.com

AUTO NARRATIVES

A computer program that is able to generate narrative descriptions or summaries of an AE case based on key words or fields in a safety database.

Authors' note: The narratives generated may sometimes produce curious results. All such narratives should be reviewed by a medical professional.

AUTO ENCODER

A computer program that is able to take a verbatim medical term or sentence and choose the "best" AE code or codes (usually MedDRA).

Authors' note: The codes chosen may not always be the best codes for the case, particularly if there are many choices and there is not a direct "hit" in MedDRA (PT or LLT) for the verbatim term. All coding should be reviewed by a medical professional.

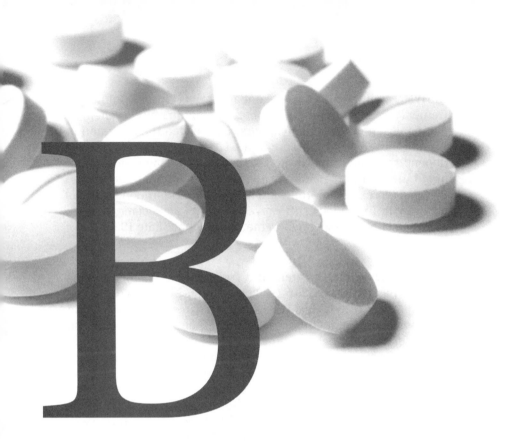

BASELINE RISK, BACKGROUND RISK

The rate of incidence of an adverse event (AE) in a specified population not exposed to a suspect drug. When the rate of an AE in a population exposed is measured, it may be divided by the baseline rate to obtain the relative risk; when the baseline rate is substracted from it, one obtains the risk difference.

An example of baseline risk, relative risk, and risk difference: Zimeldine was the first SSRI antidepressant efficacious in clinical trials, but its development ended when shown associated with the Guillain-Barre syndrome, a serious neurological condition. Whereas the baseline risk of this syndrome was 20 cases per million patient-years, it rose to 580 per million in patients exposed to zimeldine. The relative risk is 29 (580 over 20) and the risk difference is 560 (580 minus 20) cases per million. (Source of example: Martinez 1997.)

BAYESIAN CONFIDENCE PROGAGATION NEURAL NETWORK (BCPNN)

A data mining methodology for uncovering new safety signals by exploring correlations between suspect drugs and ADRs in Vigibase, the WHO spontaneous report database at the Uppsala Monitoring Center (UMC) containing more than 3.5 million reports sent in by National Centers. A statistical parameter called the Information Component (IC) is a measure of the strength of the quantitative dependency between drug and ADR; it does not give information about the qualitative causality of a drug–ADR combination. If the IC value increases over time and its lower 95% confidence limit is positive, the likelihood of a positive quantitative association is high, although clinical assessment remains essential. (Bate 1998)

BAYH–DOLE ACT (1980)

The Bayh–Dole Act, or Patent and Trademark Law Amendments Act, was passed in the US in 1980 (35USC200-212 and 37CFR401). Among other provisions, it gave universities the right to hold patents for discoveries from research that they performed that also had federal government funding. Previously, government agencies had been hesitant about letting universities and small businesses obtain or license government-held or -sponsored patents. This act encouraged universities and small businesses to move discoveries into the marketplace and produced several new and useful medicines and devices developed in university settings. http://www.cogr.edu/docs/Bayh_Dole.pdf#search='bayhdole%20act

Authors' note: The downside is a situation of possible conflict of interest when the same university scientists are called upon to teach topics related to those products. In another more subtle sense, it has redirected some university research from the more theoretical to the applied, industrial research and development in the hope of making large amounts of money. Some advocacy groups believe that such arrangements may lower the vigilance of academics toward the negative effects of products in development. Several patent-related lawsuits have arisen following passage of this act.

BEHIND THE COUNTER

See Nonprescription Product.

BENDECTIN™

The saga of Bendectin™ is a landmark false alarm in the history of pharmacovigilance. The product was a fixed combination of three active ingredients used for the treatment of nausea and vomiting during pregnancy: 1) doxylamine, an H1 antihistamine that acts as an antinausea and antivomiting agent; 2) pyridoxine, also called vitamin B6; and 3) dicycloverin (which was removed from the product shortly before market withdrawal of Bendectin™).

This product was incorrectly suspected of causing congenital abnormalities but nevertheless numerous lawsuits still occurred. Several case-control studies exonerated this product. It had been on the market for about 27 years and had been taken by some 33 million pregnant women in the United States, representing 20%–40% of all pregnant women.

It was voluntarily withdrawn from the US market and never returned, even after its exoneration. It did, however, return to the market in Canada when a local laboratory was authorized to sell a product containing doxylamine and pyridoxine under the name of Diclectin™, without negative consequences.

BENEFIT

A positive and desirable effect produced by a drug. Since the comparison of risk to benefit is the cornerstone of pharmacovigilance, a review of the various types of benefits attainable from a medication must be considered:

- Corrective of overdose: antidotes, antagonists
- Diagnostic: contrast agents, radioisotopes, allergens
- Cure: antibiotics, antivirals, gene therapies
- Prophylaxis: Prevention of cardiovascular events by lipid-lowering drugs, antihypertensives, antiaggregants, anticoagulants, etc.
- Substitution or replacement therapies: hormones (e.g., insulin), electrolytes (e.g., potassium), blood products
- Symptomatic therapies: analgesics, antiemetics
- Facilitation of interventions: anesthetics for surgery, immunosuppressors to prevent rejection of a graft.

In prophylactic pharmacotherapy one must always make the distinction between a "pharmacologic effect" on intermediate criteria (surrogate endpoint, marker) used in many clinical trials and a true therapeutic (clinical) benefit, which can often be found only in large, long-term, costly, and more rarely performed clinical trials.

For instance, cholesterol levels in a short-term trial are surrogate endpoints, whereas myocardial infarcts, cerebrovascular accidents, and cardiovascular death are clinical outcome measures.

BENEFIT–RISK ASSESSMENT (AKA BENEFIT–RISK BALANCE, RATIO, OR EVALUATION)

This assessment is a crucial determinant of the marketing authorization of a new drug or a new indication. It is both quantitative and qualitative and requires weighing all the evidence for and against the use of the drug.

The CIOMS IV Working Group published an extensive review of the methodology of making this assessment. The risk evaluation looks at the background information; the weight of evidence for the suspected risk (incidence, etc.); detailed presentations and analyses of data on the new suspected risk; probable and possible explanations, preventability, predictability, and reversibility of the new risk; the issue as it relates to alternative therapies and no therapy; a review of the complete safety of the drug, focusing on selected subsets of serious AEs (e.g., the three most common and three most medically serious adverse reactions); similar profiles for alternate drugs, when possible; an estimate of the excess incidence of any adverse reactions known to be common to the alternatives; and, when there are significant adverse reactions that are not common to the drugs compared, a review of the important differences between the drugs. See www.cioms.ch/.

In some situations, quantitative evaluations may be useful and required. As a fictitious example of a new indication, let us consider low-dose aspirin in 1000 people with a previous heart attack (i.e., for secondary prevention). In one year of treatment there would be 20 fewer heart attacks but 3 more gastrointestinal bleeds (the margin is ~7x). The benefit:risk analysis is favorable. Let us also consider the indication of an oral anticoagulant in 1000 people with nonvalvular atrial fibrillation with a moderate to high risk of stroke: in one year of treatment there would be 44 fewer vascular events but 9 more major bleeding events (the margin is ~5x). The benefit:risk analysis is favorable again, but somewhat less so since poor dosage control may lead to greater bleeding risk or lesser thrombotic protection, thus reducing the margin. (Source of example: Bandolier review, www.jr2.ox.ac.uk/bandolier/band86/b86-2.html.)

Authors' note: A reasonable margin must be required; for example, a product or indication that would prevent three heart attacks but induce one major hemorrhage may not carry conviction. Often the data are variable from one study to another (e.g., meta-analyses) and thus comparisons are difficult. The statistical term "ratio" should be avoided because the benefit:risk balance is not a quantitative relationship of two magnitudes of the same dimension. See Ratio. The pessimist refers to the "risk: benefit analysis."

BfArM

The German health authority. *See* Bundesinstitut für Arzneimittel und Medizinprodukte.

BIAS

Biases are "systematic errors" occurring in observational and experimental studies, in contrast to "random errors" resulting unavoidably from sampling variability and "confounders" linked to both the treatment and the outcome. Epidemiologists and trialists must try to control biases as much as possible by proper design and surveillance during the study; otherwise they must resort to appropriate statistical adjustments. The main systematic errors are called susceptibility and protopathic biases by epidemiologists.

Susceptibility bias results when the compared groups have an inequality of prognosis when entering a study. For example, menopausal women exposed to replacement hormones were found to have slightly fewer coronary events than the unexposed after an observational study. But following an experimental trial that randomized equally the levels of socioeconomic status and quality of medical care, the treated group was not found to benefit from this apparent protective effect.

Protopathic bias results when the indication for treatment is linked to an outcome. For example, when a depressed patient receives an antidepressant and develops suicidal ideas, is the outcome suicidality caused by the depression that led to the antidepressant, or is it a rare and paradoxical ADR of the drug? As another example, when the level of beta-2 agonist used for bronchodilation is associated with more asthmatic deaths, are these deaths the result of asthma severity or a rare, serious ADR?

BIG PHARMA AND DRUG SAFETY

The dozen or so large "full-service" companies with revenues in the billions of dollars. These companies are multinational, with headquarters primarily in the United States or Europe but with some located in Japan and elsewhere. They usually have scientists doing drug discovery to come up with new patentable drugs that will hopefully become "blockbusters" (drugs with sales of over a billion dollars a year, by some definitions). They do their own preclinical studies (pharmacology and toxicity) and clinical trials (phases I–IV).

Big Pharma companies have large marketing and sales divisions with thousands of "representatives," "sales reps," or "detailers." A Big Pharma company does much of its own manufacturing in factories throughout the world. There are large departments to handle regulatory issues, legal issues, and patents.

There is a large drug safety department which is often, but not always, located in the corporate headquarters. This is the major center for tracking drug safety with receipt of some or all of the individual case safety reports for data entry, as well as preparation of MedWatch, CIOMS I forms, E2B transmissions, New Drug Application (NDA) periodic reports, Investigational New Drug

Application (IND) annual reports, Periodic Safety Update Reports (PSURs), annual clinical trial reports, and other aggregate reports. There also are on-site drug safety departments in most or all subsidiaries or affiliates to receive local safety reports (in the local language) and make submissions (sometimes in English, sometimes in the local language). These subsidiaries may have a separate physician serving as safety officer or may have the medical director (often the only medical doctor in the local company) also serve as the safety physician. The subsidiaries often serve as "pass through" points for adverse events (AEs) to be sent to central or regional data centers for data entry into the safety database. In some situations where the corporate headquarters are located in a smaller country, one of the "subsidiaries" will become the dominant center for drug safety (e.g., in the European Union or the United States). There is a tendency for safety departments to now be located in major English-speaking countries, such as the United States or the United Kingdom. There is also a trend to outsource ("outservice") some functions—even safety—to CROs around the world.

BIOAVAILABILITY STUDY

A clinical trial in which a substance or its active moiety is delivered from a pharmaceutical form and becomes available in the general circulation. "Absolute bioavailability" of a given dosage form may be studied against a form that has 100% bioavailability (e.g., oral solution or intravenous). "Relative bioavailability" studies are done when a dosage form is compared to the same dosage form or some other nonintravenous form (e.g., oral tablet vs. oral capsule). These studies may be done in animals or humans.

Plasma levels over time after dosing are summarized by the area under the curve (AUC) statistical parameter. Generic products have to undergo bioavailability studies and have to be shown as bioavailable as the branded form before their marketing authorization; they are then considered "bioequivalent." Insufficient bioavailability of a product may lead to lack of efficacy and excessive bioavailability may lead to dose-related ADRs.

See http://www.emea.eu.int/pdfs/human/ewp/140198en.pdf.

BIODIVERSITY AMONG HUMANS

In drug safety, the phenomenon that certain drugs work differently in different populations. For example, ACE inhibitors and beta blockers for hypertension are felt to be less effective in African-Americans than in Caucasians. In such cases, higher doses may be needed to attain the same therapeutic effect, thus increasing the dose-related AEs.

Japanese males were found to have lower σ-alcohol dehydrogenase activity than Caucasians, with no difference in the other gastric isozymes.

BIOEQUIVALENCE STUDY

A clinical trial of two medicinal products to determine if their bioavailabilities in blood and target tissues after administration in the same molar dose are similar to such a degree that their effects, with respect to efficacy and safety, are expected to be essentially the same. See EMEA's "Note for Guidance on the Investigation of Bioavailability and Bioequivalence 2001." http://www.emea.eu.int/pdfs/human/ewp/140198en.pdf.

The FDA in 2003 has defined bioequivalence as "the absence of a significant difference in the rate and extent to which the active ingredient or active moiety in pharmaceutical equivalents or pharmaceutical alternatives becomes available at the site of drug action when administered at the same molar dose under similar conditions in an appropriately designed study." (FDA 2003)

BIOETHICS

The field involved in the study of the ethics and morality in the area of healthcare products and their delivery, as well as other biologic issues. It may be defined narrowly or broadly. In the field of drug safety, it revolves around whether physicians use drugs only in the best interests of their patients; whether drug companies develop drugs properly and receive, evaluate, and report all safety issues in a rapid and correct way in which the patients' interests are paramount; and whether health agencies also act in the best interests of public health.

BIOLOGICS, BIOLOGIC PRODUCTS

"Biologics, in contrast to drugs that are chemically synthesized, are derived from living sources (such as humans, animals, and microorganisms). Most biologics are complex mixtures that are not easily identified or characterized, and many biologics are manufactured using biotechnology. Biological products often represent the cutting-edge of biomedical research and, in time, may offer the most effective means to treat a variety of medical illnesses and conditions that presently have no other treatments available." See http://www.fda.gov/cber/about.htm.

Biologic products include vaccines and allergenic products, blood products (including blood grouping reagents and donor screening tests for bloodborne pathogens), cellular and gene therapies, and xenotransplantation. The term "biovigilance" has been suggested to describe their surveillance.

BIOLOGIC LICENSE APPLICATION (BLA)

A request for permission to introduce, or deliver for introduction, a biologic product into interstate commerce in the US. It is usually submitted by the manufacturer (called the applicant). It includes form FDA 356h (cover sheet), applicant information, product and manufacturing information, preclinical studies, clinical studies, and labeling. It uses the internationally accepted Common Technical Document (CTD), which can be submitted electronically. (21 CFR 601.2)

BIRTH DEFECT

Synonym: Congenital anomaly. Any abnormal physical, genetic, nongenetic, or biochemical trait present at birth. A birth defect may be minor, producing little or no problem, or major, producing disability and even death. In the context of drug safety reporting, a birth defect (whether major or minor) is always considered "serious" and if it is not contained in the product labeling (SmPC monograph, etc.) it must be reported as a 15-day expedited report in most areas. The surveillance of birth defects is called teratovigilance.

BLACK BOX WARNING

A black box warning is the strongest type of warning that the FDA can require in the product labeling for a drug. It is used to warn prescribers about ADRs that can cause serious injury or death. It is usually displayed prominently at the beginning of the labeling with a dense black line around the warning to call the reader's attention to it.

BLACK TRIANGLE

Black triangle products are new drugs and vaccines that are being intensively monitored by the UK health authorities (such as MHRA and CHM) in order to confirm the benefit:risk profile of the product. A black triangle is assigned to a new product if the drug is a new active substance or is assigned to an older product if the drug is a new combination of active substances; is administered via a new route of administration or drug delivery system; or has a significant new indication, which may alter the established benefit:risk profile of that drug.

There is no standard time for a product to retain black triangle status. An assessment is usually made following two years of post-marketing experience and the black triangle symbol is not removed until the safety of the drug is well established.

http://www.mhra.gov.uk/home/idcplg?IdcService=SS_GET_PAGE&nodeId=748

BLINDED STUDY/TRIAL

Generally referred to in the context of prospective randomized clinical trials. Such a trial or study involves two or more groups of patients with a disease receiving different treatments. For example, one group may get drug A and the other group may get drug B or a placebo. The test may be single-blinded (the patient does not know if he or she gets A or B) or double-blinded (neither the patient nor the investigator knows what the treatment assignment is). This control measure is used in randomized controlled trials to avoid biases, neutralize both the placebo effects and the nocebo effects, and ensure unbiased symptom evaluations and objective measures by the research team.

BLINDING AND UNBLINDING IND REPORTS

In general, health authorities do not want to receive 7- or 15-day expedited reports that are blinded in the course of clinical trials. Thus when there is a 7- or 15-day reportable case (death or life threatening for a 7-day report and serious for a 15-day report, plus unlabeled, possibly related reactions), the sponsor should, in general, unblind the specific patient (but not the whole study) and indicate the treatment on the MedWatch or CIOMS I report submitted to the health authorities. The sponsor may attempt to limit the unblinding only to the drug safety department and the health authority, but this is often difficult in practice as the investigator(s) and ethical committees/investigational review boards must also be notified. In April 2007, the FDA issued a new guidance on reporting to IRBs and included comments on unblinding noting the lack of usefulness of blinded reports.

BLOOD LEVELS (OF DRUGS)

In clinical medicine: The plasma (or serum) level of a drug and/or its metabolites is a part of the surveillance of patients in pharmacotherapy, particularly when there is a very narrow therapeutic window. This is also known as *therapeutic drug monitoring*. The goal is to obtain plasma levels sufficiently high to obtain the desired pharmacologic effect while avoiding levels that are too high and that would be toxic. Therapeutic drug monitoring is thus a means of *preventing* dose-dependent adverse drug reactions rather than a means of detecting such reactions.

In causality determinations: When an ADR is tied to a supratherapeutic dose or to a frank overdose, the plasma level of the drug or its metabolites can turn out to be very useful in many cases. It is used routinely in anti-poison centers and during autopsies done for forensic reasons. Ideally, the blood is drawn just as the undesirable reaction is beginning.

BLOOD SAFETY SURVEILLANCE

Also called hemovigilance; the postmarketing surveillance of blood and blood products (e.g., platelets, albumin). At the FDA, this generally falls under the province of CBER rather than CDER. Not to be confused with hematovigilance, the surveillance of ADRs on the blood cells and blood forming organs.

BLUE CARD

Name given to the printed reporting form of the Australian pharmacovigilance program.

BOILERPLATE

Refers to the use of standardized sentences, phrases, clauses, etc., in protocols, SOPs, and safety exchange agreements. They are universally accepted and rarely change. Examples include the definitions of "serious" or "adverse event."

Authors' note: The dangers in boilerplate are that 1) when they do change people rarely notice or make changes in the boilerplate so that older versions persist, and 2) they are rarely read, as everyone presumes they know what is contained in the boilerplate.

BRADFORD HILL CRITERIA

Developed by Austin Bradford Hill, a British statistician and epidemiologist, to explain the factors needed to ascribe causality of an event. His criteria are modified somewhat and summarized here in the context of drug safety:

1. **Temporal Relationship, the Chronological Criteria**
   It is logically necessary that exposure always precede the outcome in time. If drug A is believed to cause an AE, then it is clear that drug A must be taken before the AE. A short time to onset usually argues in favor of causality. (Note: See anticipatory nausea & vomiting)

2. Strength of the Relationship

This is defined by the size of the association as measured by appropriate statistical tests between the independent variable and the dependent variable. For example, if statistical analysis shows a strong correlation between intake of drug A and sudden death, then this is evidence for causality. The stronger the relationship, the more likely it is that causality exists. Correlation and relative risk are a measure of strength.

3. Dose–response Relationship

If a clear dose–response relationship is present (i.e., if a higher dose of a drug produces a more frequent or more severe AE), then this is strong evidence for a causal relationship.

4. Consistency

Across different settings, methods, and populations, if a drug class consistently leads to a muscular lesion (e.g., rhabdomyolysis) in men and women, in younger or older patients of several countries, and in observational and experimental studies, this is strong evidence of causality.

5. Plausibility

Causality is more likely if there is a rational basis for imagining a mechanism of action for the treatment and a mechanism for the physiopathological response. An insulin dose that one suspects of causing loss of consciousness (syncope) would be a plausible association, because a blood sugar level that is too low may produce fainting and syncope.

6. Are Alternate Explanations Available?

One must consider other—and possibly more likely and logical—causes of an AE in addition to the suspect drug. A myocardial infarction in an older, overweight, hypertensive diabetic smoker with a cardiac family history may be pathogenic rather than iatrogenic.

7. Experiment

The AE can be prevented or improved or worsened/reproduced by an appropriate change in treatment or regimen. An example of this would be a positive dechallenge or a positive rechallenge.

8. Specificity

This condition is fulfilled when a single causative agent produces a single specific effect. It is rarely found because numerous adverse events have multiple and additive causes. An example of specificity would be cancer of the vagina seen in young daughters born of mothers exposed to DES during pregnancy and phocomelia in newborns whose mother took thalidomide. It also applies to AEs occurring at the site of application of a medical product.

9. Coherence

The association should be compatible with existing medical science and the current state of knowledge concerning the treatment and the condition being treated.

BRANDED GENERIC DRUG

A product marketed by a drug company (or its subsidiary) other than the innovator and sold under a trade name other than the product's generic approved name. See the FDA's white paper on drug prices: http://www.fda.gov/oc/whitepapers/drugprices.html.

BREAST FEEDING

See Lactation.

BRIDGING REPORT FOR PSUR

A concise document integrating the information presented in two or more PSURs to cover a specified period over which a single report is requested or required by regulatory authorities. The report should not contain any new data but should provide a brief summary bridging two or more PSURs. The format should be identical to that of the usual PSUR. See http://www.fda.gov/CDER/GUIDANCE/5524fnl.htm.

BRITISH NATIONAL FORMULARY (BNF)

A pharmacotherapy guide published by the Royal Pharmaceutical Society and edited by independent experts. See http://www.bnf.org/bnf/.

BROWSER

In the context of drug safety, software that is used to search for the appropriate coding terms in MedDRA. Since MedDRA has over 80,000 terms it is not feasible to search for the best code for an AE by manually looking up terms in a manual of MedDRA codes. The software allows for rapid searching of codes. Some browsers allow "autocoding," in which a sentence containing AEs or medical terms is entered into the browser and possible codes for each AE or medical term are returned.

BULLETIN, ADR

National pharmacovigilance centers regularly publish bulletins to inform prescribers of newly reported signals and new restrictions of use related to safety of health products:

- In the USA, the FDA and its subdivisions CDER, MedWatch, AERS, VAERS, and CBER maintain updated websites on the safety of drugs, biologics, vaccines, devices, food supplements, etc.
- In Australia, the Therapeutic Goods Administration publishes the ADRAC Bulletin online at www.tga.gov.au/adr/aadrb.htm.
- In Canada, MedEffect publishes a Canadian Adverse Reaction Newsletter online at http://www.hc-sc.gc.ca/dhp-mps.medeff.
- In the UK, the CSM publishes Current Problems online at http://www.mhra.gov.uk.

BULLOUS ERUPTION

A category of cutaneous disease, including erythema multiforme, Stevens–Johnson syndrome, and toxic epidermal necrolysis (Lyell's syndrome). Whereas the first one is the least severe and often due to a nondrug etiology, the last two pathologies are much more severe and are generally drug induced.

BUNDESINSTITUT FÜR ARZNEIMITTEL UND MEDIZINPRODUKTE (BfArM)

The name of the German drug agency. (In English: Federal Institute for Drugs and Medical Devices.) The agency is expected to be reorganized soon and renamed.

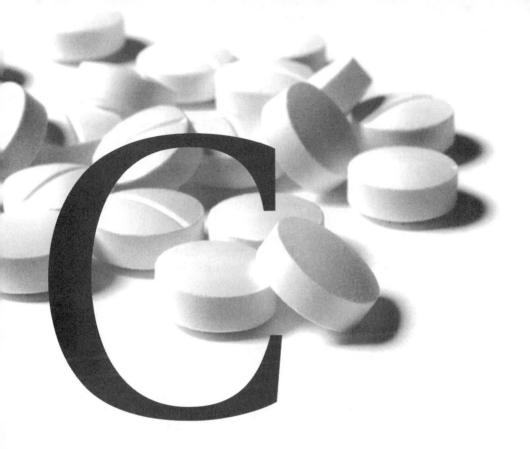

CALENDAR DAYS

The number of days between two dates, such as AE receipt date and AE submission date to health authorities, as calculated by counting on a calendar. Some authorities consider the initial receipt day as day "zero" and others consider it as day "one." Calendar days are different from "working days," which exclude holidays and weekends.

Authors' note: Using working days had proven to be difficult in practice in the world of global drug safety, as holidays (nonworking days) in one country are working days in other countries. Following ICH and CIOMS recommendations, most authorities and companies now use calendar days rather than working days.

CALL CENTER

Also called a phone center. A centralized telephone bank staffed by people to receive reports of AEs, product quality complaints, queries, and so forth, from the general public and healthcare professionals. They may also do marketing activities such as reimbursements and dispensing of coupons.

The call centers have classically been national, not crossing international boundaries. The phone number is usually toll free (e.g., an "800 number"), and may be found in the package labeling for the healthcare professional or patient. It may also appear on the box or bottle.

The staff at the center may be nonmedical, medical professionals, or a mix. If the initial person the caller encounters is nonmedical and the call involves medical issues, it may be transferred right away ("hot" or "warm" transfer) to a medical professional. Alternatively, the nonmedical staff may respond using preapproved scripts. Product-specific information may not deviate from the approved labeling (i.e., no off-label indications are supported).

Authors' note: There is now a tendency to outsource and/or "off shore" call centers to countries such as India that have lower costs, many available medical personnel, and good English language skills.

CALL FOR INFORMATION OR CALL TO REPORT

A request from a health authority (rarely from a pharmaceutical company) to the general public or medical personnel in a country or region for specific information relating to a drug or AE. For example, a call from the health authority for practitioners to report all cases of torsades de pointes associated with antihistamine use.

Authors' note: This is one of many possible responses to a signal and is thus a form of prompted reporting focused on a drug and an AE, usually a new, suspected ADR. When such a request prompts the reporting of cases—particularly strong and well-documented cases—the signal may be largely validated. When the request does not elicit new cases, this does not prove the signal to be false but does weaken the evidence linking a suspect product.

CARCINOGENICITY

The capacity of a drug to cause cancer or increase the risk of developing cancer. Carcinogenicity studies in at least two species of animals are a normal part of the preclinical toxicology of a drug in development.

CARDIAC ARRHYTHMIA SUPPRESSION TRIALS (CAST I AND II)

A trial begun in the late 80s that turned out to be a landmark in the detection of paradoxical ADRs. It was initially designed to evaluate the efficacy and safety of arrhythmia suppression therapy in patients with asymptomatic or mildly symptomatic premature ventricular beats after myocardial infarction with the hope of reducing cardiac mortality. Patients were randomized to receive placebo or treatment with encainide, flecainide, or moricizine. After less than one year of follow-up the encainide and flecainide arms of the trial were stopped due to increased cardiac mortality and nonfatal cardiac arrests (resistant to electrical cardioversion) compared to placebo, the opposite of what was expected. The protocol was modified and the study continued as CAST II and compared moricizine to placebo. The CAST II study was also stopped early due to excess mortality and nonfatal cardiac arrests in the moricizine arm compared to placebo. The working hypothesis of decreased mortality with treatment was refuted. See http://www.nhlbi.nih.gov/resources/deca/descriptions/cast.htm and *NEJM* 1989; 321:406–12, *NEJM* 1992; 327:227–33

Authors' note: The CAST trials demonstrate:

- *why it is critically important to carefully track AEs during clinical trials, even with well-known marketed drugs;*
- *why it is important to do careful interim safety analyses during trials;*
- *why using surrogate endpoints (premature ventricular beats) does not replace clinical endpoints (cardiac mortality); and*
- *why large-scale randomized controlled trials using clinical outcome measures must be done to scientifically prove medical hypotheses which, in theory, appear logical, rational, useful, safe, and efficacious.*

CASCADE EFFECT

Also called "secondary" effects or "chaining." An adverse event due to a preceding adverse event.

For example, if a patient becomes dizzy and falls (perhaps due to a drug he or she is taking), breaking his or her shoulder and abrading the skin, the primary event is dizziness and the cascade effects would be the fall, the shoulder fracture, and the skin abrasions.

A similar example would be a patient who becomes anemic (primary ADR) from a drug affecting red blood cell production, and then suffers a hypoxic event (a myocardial infarction), which is a secondary ADR.

Authors' note: An ongoing controversy in drug coding is whether secondary events should be coded or not in reports entered into the safety database and reported to health authorities. Some argue that the secondary event is not really appropriate for coding, as the drug did not truly produce that event directly. However, others note that it is still important for the patient and healthcare professional to know about cascade effects—especially ones that are not obvious or frequently thought of.

In the second example, coding anemia is obligatory, as it is the primary event/reaction, but coding the infarction is less clearly appropriate.

CASE ASSESSMENT

Also known as "Case Review." The evaluation of an AE case in a pharmaceutical company or health agency including:

- the initial determination of whether the case contains the four minimal elements to be a valid case,
- whether the case is serious or not,
- whether the events are labeled/listed or not,
- whether the events are felt to be related to the drug (for clinical trial cases),
- the quality review against source documents, and
- the medical review by a physician to see if the medical context and coding of the case are correctly done.

CASE CLOSURE

Also known as "Case Completion" or "Case Locking." In the databasing of an AE case, the point at which the information is deemed to be finished and nothing further will be added to that version of the case.

Authors' note: Most pharmaceutical companies will mandate by SOP case closure at a particular time (e.g., calendar day 10 after initial receipt) in order to avoid having the potential for a late expedited 15-day report. Any subsequent case information will be entered into the case in the database as a new version and submitted as a follow-up report.

CASE COMPLETION

See Case Closure.

CASE-CONTROL STUDY

A type of epidemiologic study that determines the chance (or "odds" or "probability") of having taken the suspect drug in question in a group of patients already suffering from an AE and compares that with the chance of having taken the drug in a group of patients who did not suffer from the AE. In other words, a study of a group of cases with the AE and another group of cases without the AE to see how many in each group took the drug in question.

Logically speaking, it is a retrospective study with the epidemiologist looking backward. This form of inquiry is more sensitive and less costly for confirmation and quantification of an ADR than, for example, a prospective study such as an observational cohort or a clinical trial. After spontaneous reporting, it remains the most sensitive tool for the detection of signals. Case-control studies are best summarized by the odds ratio, an approximation of relative risk, valid under certain conditions such as the rarity of the adverse event. However, the absolute risk cannot be derived.

CASE HISTORY

The medical story of the patient who had the AE. It includes the recent AE, reasons for taking the drug (indication) and concomitant diseases, exposure to the suspect product and concomitant medications, appropriate medical history (risk factors for the suspected ADR and alternative etiologies), as well as the course of the event after the AE occurred.

CASE LOCKING

See Case Closure.

CASE NUMBER

Also known as "case control number," "control number," or "manufacturer's number." The unique number assigned to a patient who has one or more AEs reported to a health authority or pharmaceutical company. This number must be stored in the safety database and transmitted to health authorities.

Authors' note: Issues arise because each case may have multiple case numbers. For example, a case originating in a pharmaceutical company's affiliate abroad would be assigned a local case number there. The case is then sent to company headquarters for entry into the safety database where it is assigned a company number. The case is then submitted to the FDA where it receives an FDA number, to the EMEA where it receives another number, and to multiple other company affiliates and health authorities, each of which may assign local case numbers. This poses potential problems in terms of duplicate report avoidance and the handling of follow-up information that the company might receive.

CASE REPORT

The medical description of a patient who experienced an AE.

The FDA, in its March 2005 guidance on "Good Pharmacovigilance Practices and Pharmacoepidemiologic Assessment," recommends that sponsors make a reasonable attempt to get complete information for case assessment during initial and follow-up contacts. Companies should use trained healthcare practitioners. If the report is from a consumer, it should be followed up with contact with the healthcare practitioner. The most aggressive efforts should be directed at serious AEs, particularly those not previously known to occur with the drug (i.e., unexpected SAEs). The EU rules also require medical follow-ups to obtain complete data. See http://www.fda.gov/Cder/guidance/6359OCC.htm.

CASE REPORT COMPLETENESS

Completeness is achieved from a medical viewpoint when an ADR case report contains enough information to form a judgment about the case in regard to seriousness, expectedness and, for clinical trial cases, causality. The information is then used for regulatory reporting, signal detection, and so forth.

When the causality assessment is important (though difficult to determine), a complete case report should ideally include:

Reporter
- Name, profession, medical specialty, medical license number, address, telephone, fax, email address

  Comment: The identification of the reporter is not a part of the case information but rather is a part of the validation of the case.

Report
- Date of report, initial or follow-up, who else has been notified (i.e., health authority, manufacturer), case control number or identification number assigned by health authority, company, and any other relevant information.
- Will the patient (and reporter if other than the patient) allow the authorities to transmit the information elsewhere?

  Comment: The first item helps to avoid duplicate reporting and allows follow-up reports to be tied to the initial report.

Patient Identification and Demography
- Sex, age, birthdate, initials.

  Comment: The age and sex may be risk factors for the ADR. Note that patient privacy must be respected.
- Case or chart number (office/hospital), weight, height, race, occupation.

  Comment: The case number is necessary to correctly record follow-up information when requested and received from the clinician, when the course or outcome of the event is final, or when additional testing or visits to the physician are required. Weight is mainly useful at the "extremes of life" (babies and the elderly) when the pharmacokinetics and dose are risk factors for an ADR. Height is useful only if the calculation of the degree of obesity is done and is a risk factor. In babies, height is useful to follow the growth of the child. Race and ethnicity may be useful in regard to alternate etiologies which might produce a problem or increased susceptibility (e.g., sickle cell and thalassemia) or increased susceptibility to the ADR (e.g., the neurologic syndrome seen in Japan with the antidiarrheal clioquinol). Occupation may also be useful if workplace exposure to stress or toxins is an issue.

- Parity, date of last menstrual period (to calculate the beginning of the pregnancy)

   Comment: This information is useful in teratovigilance and in assisted pregnancy.

Patient's Prior ADR History

- Previous use of the suspect product followed by the AE/ADR in question? If yes, this is a positive prechallenge and the details of this occurrence should be included.
- Previous use of the suspect product without reaction? If this is the case, this is a negative prechallenge.
- Same reaction with a different suspect product? If yes, this can be a case of a cross reaction or "cross intolerance."
- Same adverse event without exposure to a drug product? If yes, this represents an argument in favor of an alternate etiology for the current AE.

Chronology of the AE/ADR

- Time until appearance, time to onset
  - Time from the first dose or from the last dose (as applicable).
  - Time from a single, unique dose (if applicable).
  - Dates of the critical doses (first/last/unique/augmented). (*See* Critical Dose Date.)
- Dechallenge
  - Cessation or reduction of the suspect product? (No, unknown, or yes.)
  - If yes, date of cessation or reduction. Abatement of the reaction? "Yes" means the dechallenge is positive, "no" means a negative dechallenge.
  - Date of the beginning of the improvement, date of complete disappearance, calculation of the time to disappearance.
- Rechallenge
  - Reintroduction of the suspect product? If yes, date of restarting.
  - Increase in dose of the suspect product? If yes, date of reintroduction.

- Reappearance of the reaction? Yes (positive rechallenge) or no (negative rechallenge). If yes, date of reappearance and calculation of the time to reappearance.

Medical condition and past medical history
- Examination for alternative etiologies (hypotheses)
  - Current illness (i.e., the indication for the use of the suspect product), new illness, underlying, subclinical, intercurrent, concurrent, latent.
  - Concomitant medications: indication, name, dose, start and stop dates.
    Comment: The indication for each concomitant product helps in understanding the global medical condition of the patient. The medical reviewer may decide to consider a concomitant medication to be a suspect medication or to be involved in a drug–drug interaction.
- In looking for *risk factors* for an ADR:
  - Check those related to the use of the suspect product:
    Excessive dose (if the pharmacologic effect is excessive)
    Excessive duration of treatment
    Administration too rapid
    Incorrect administration
    Comment: Blood level of the suspect product may be useful in case of suspected overdose.
  - Check those related to the underlying status of the patient
    Organ dysfunction: renal or hepatic insufficiency, other
    Genetic predisposition (enzyme deficiency, etc.)
    Nutritional issues (alcohol, dehydration, obesity, fasting)
    Physiologic state: pregnant, nursing mother, newborn, post-operative
    Drug–drug interaction
    Allergies: previous history
    Medical device issues (hemodialysis, stents, etc.)

Suspect Product
Trade name, generic name, manufacturer, formulation (capsule, gel cap, suspension, solution, etc.), route of administration, single dose unit, daily dose, prn dose, following prescribed and labeled instructions or not (check compliance), total cumulative dose taken, total duration of treatment, blood level in case of autopsy, massive overdose and/or narrow therapeutic index/window.

Adverse Event
- Medical term or syndrome or major manifestations, medical coding (MedDRA), start date, date of beginning of improve-

ment or date of ending of the AE, calculation of total duration of the reaction and, if applicable, details of treatment given for the AE (corrective treatment).
- Laboratory tests: for each pertinent result indicate:
  - Date, units, type of test, result, normal values.
- For repeated analyses, indicate details for lab tests done:
  - Before the first dose (reference value).
  - First abnormal result (to calculate the time to appearance).
  - The most abnormal result (to evaluate the severity).
  - The last abnormal result (to calculate the duration of the reaction).
  - The first improved result (to calculate the time to disappearance).
  - First normal results.

Outcome and Evolution
- Classification as serious or nonserious according to the regulatory criteria in force.
- Outcome of the reaction in the case report: recovered, not recovered, unknown.
- Details of the disability, hospitalization, death.
- Description of the treatment required to prevent disability, hospitalization, or death.
- *In the case of death:* circumstances, autopsy results, reported causes of death, date of death.
- *For hospitalization:* copy of the discharge summary.

Authors' note: Completeness is sometimes confused with validity. Validity may mean that the four minimum requirements for identification (see Minimum Information for Reportability) are provided, but it may also mean that a consumer report is verified by a medical professional. A case may be complete but not validated (not verified by a medical professional); conversely, a case may be validated but incomplete (more information would be needed).

CASE REVIEW
See Case Assessment.

CASE SERIES
Multiple reports of the same or similar AEs from different patients used in signal identification and work up.

Individual case safety reports on patients (the cases) with a suspected adverse drug reaction reported spontaneously or during a trial, a cohort, or a case-control study. No control group is involved.

After an initial postmarketing spontaneous case report is found, additional cases should be sought in the sponsor's database, the FDA AERS database, the Uppsala database, published literature, and other databases. Cases should be evaluated and followed up for additional information where needed and where possible for signal evaluation.

CAUSALITY

1) *A process:* Determining that a drug produced an AE and that the AE would not have occurred if the drug had not been taken. Also called causality assessment or "imputation." If the AE is suspected to be caused by the drug then it is considered an ADR.
2) *A result:* The result of the process of determining the relationship or link between the drug and the AE. Various rank scales exist describing the confidence in the judgment so made: not related, unlikely, possible, probable, definite. *See* Adverse Event, Adverse Drug Reaction, and Causality Determination.

CAUSALITY ALGORITHM

See Algorithm, Causality.

CAUSALITY DETERMINATION

The analysis of whether a particular AE in a particular patient was due to a particular drug. This is required for individual case safety reports for expedited clinical trial cases but not for postmarketing expedited cases where all cases are presumed by definition to be "possibly related." Case causality determination is particularly difficult in real time, especially for the first report of a particular AE. Only after multiple reports or a case series might the retrospective determination of causality become clearer.

Authors' note: The causality determination in an individual case may be impossible if there is inadequate, incomplete, or contradictory information. Even when there is full information, it may be very hard to come to a definitive conclusion in an individual case due to background noise, comedications, and other confounders. Many algorithms have been devised to determine causality, with none appearing to be particularly better than the others. The gold standard is usually held to be review by one or more physicians experienced in drug safety, with clinical acumen, common sense, and an open mind. The task is eased by the accumulation of case reports; consistency in temporal and clinical characteristics across cases is strong evidence for causality.

It may be necessary to resort to clinical trials or observational studies in order to determine the relationship between a particular AE and a drug.

CAUSALITY, CASE

See Causality Determination.

CAUSALITY, EPIDEMIOLOGICAL

The determination that a particular AE is due to a drug as established by epidemiologic studies in addition to or instead of using individual cases and case series to make such a determination.

CAUSALITY, LEGAL (CIVIL AND CRIMINAL)

A determination in a court of law that a particular AE was caused by a particular drug. It may or may not be the same as the case causality and/or epidemiologic causality.

CAUSALITY, REGULATORY

A determination made for reporting purposes of whether an AE is related to use of a particular drug in a specific patient.

In the spontaneous postmarketing AE situation, all AEs are presumed to have some level of causality due to the drug. It is reasoned (originally by the CIOMS I Working Group in 1990) that the physician, by making the report to the manufacturer, is indicating that there is some level of causality possible in the report, that the drug is somewhat suspected of causing the event—irrespective of the level of this suspicion. Thus for regulatory reporting, neither the sponsor nor the reporter's opinion on causality is needed or used for expedited 15-day reporting of serious AEs.

In the clinical trial setting, however, the investigator and the manufacturer (sponsor) each generally make real-time independent causality assessments that are used for determining whether a case is considered an expedited 7- or 15-day report. If one or both feel that an AE case has some level of causality due to the drug, the case is considered for regulatory causality and reporting to be "related" or "possibly related."

CBER

See Center for Biologics Evaluation and Research.

CCSI

See Company Core Safety Information.

CDC

See Centers for Disease Control and Prevention.

CDER

See Center for Drug Evaluation and Research.

CDRH

See Center for Devices and Radiological Health.

CDS

See Core Data Sheet.

CENTER FOR BIOLOGICS EVALUATION AND RESEARCH (FDA)

Called CBER (pronounced "see-burr"). The FDA division that is charged with regulating biologics and related products including blood, vaccines, tissue, allergenics, and biological therapeutics. Many of their safety duties were transferred to the Center for Drug Evaluation and Research (see this term) several years ago. See http://www.fda.gov/cber/.

CENTER FOR DEVICES AND RADIOLOGICAL HEALTH (FDA)

Called CDRH. The part of the FDA that is charged with regulating devices. CDRH's involvement with safety is as follows:

CDRH may order a manufacturer to conduct postmarketing surveillance of certain medical devices using the following criteria:

- Failure of the device would be reasonably likely to have serious adverse health consequences.
- The device is intended to be implanted in the human body for more than 1 year.
- The device is intended to be used to support or sustain life and to be used outside a user facility.

Postmarketing surveillance means the active, systematic, and scientifically valid collection, analysis, and interpretation of data or other information about a marketed device. The data can reveal unforeseen adverse events, the actual rate of anticipated adverse events, or other information necessary to protect the public health. See http://www.fda.gov/cdrh/devadvice/352.html#introduction.

Authors' note: Device product problems must be reported even before any adverse event is produced by the defect in question. The situation is comparable to that of automobiles, when a quality problem is found that could lead to accidents and injuries. The problem must be reported, and sometimes acted upon by a car recall, before accidents occur.

CENTERS FOR DISEASE CONTROL (CDC)

The CDC is one of the 13 major operating components of the Department of Health and Human Services (HHS). They are not primarily involved in drug safety or pharmacovigilance but do interact with the FDA on certain matters where there are common interests. The main office is located in Atlanta, Georgia. They are well known for tracking of epidemics, pandemics and acute health issues as well as providing health information for travelers. See http://www.cdc.gov: Their mission is to promote health and quality of life by preventing and controlling disease, injury, and disability. The CDC seeks to accomplish its mission by working with partners throughout the nation and the world to:

- monitor health
- detect and investigate health problems
- conduct research to enhance prevention
- develop and advocate sound public health policies
- implement prevention strategies
- promote healthy behaviors
- foster safe and healthful environments
- provide leadership and training.

They publish the well-known *Morbidity and Mortality Weekly Report* (MMWR). See http://www.cdc.gov/tobacco/data_statistics/MMWR/2006/

There are seven national centers:

- Environmental Health and Injury Prevention
  - *National Center for Injury Prevention and Control (NCIPC)*—prevents death and disability from nonoccupational injuries, including those that are unintentional and those that result from violence.
  - *National Center for Environmental Health (NCEH)*—provides national leadership in preventing and controlling disease and death resulting from the interactions between people and their environment.
- Global Health
  - *Coordinating Office for Global Health (COGH)*—provides national leadership, coordination, and support for CDC's global health activities in collaboration with CDC's global health partners.

- Health Promotion
  - *National Center on Birth Defects and Developmental Disabilities (NCBDDD)*—provides national leadership for preventing birth defects and developmental disabilities and for improving the health and wellness of people with disabilities.
  - *National Center for Chronic Disease Prevention and Health Promotion (NCCDPHP)*—prevents premature death and disability from chronic diseases and promotes healthy personal behaviors.
  - *Office of Genomics and Disease Prevention*—provides national leadership in fostering understanding of human genomic discoveries and how they can be used to improve health and prevent disease.
- Infectious Diseases
  - *National Center for Infectious Diseases (NCID)*—prevents illness, disability, and death caused by infectious diseases in the United States and around the world.
  - *National Immunization Program (NIP)*—prevents disease, disability, and death from vaccine-preventable diseases in children and adults.
  - *National Center for HIV, STD, and TB Prevention (NCHSTP)*—provides national leadership in preventing and controlling human immunodeficiency virus infection, sexually transmitted diseases, and tuberculosis.
- Public Health Information, Health Marketing, and Health Statistics
  - *National Center for Public Health Informatics (NCPHI)*—provides national leadership in the application of information technology in the pursuit of public health.
  - *National Center for Health Marketing (NCHM)*—provides national leadership in health marketing science and in its application to impact public health.
  - *National Center for Health Statistics (NCHS)*—provides statistical information that guides actions and policies to improve the health of the American people
- Terrorism Preparedness and Emergency Response
  - *Coordinating Office for Terrorism Preparedness and Emergency Response (COPTER)*—provides national leadership to protect health and enhance the potential for full, satisfying, and productive living across the lifespan of all people in all communities related to community preparedness and response.

- Workplace Health and Safety
  - *National Institute for Occupational Safety and Health (NIOSH)*—ensures safety and health for all people in the workplace through research and prevention.

CENTER FOR DRUG EVALUATION AND RESEARCH (FDA)

Called CDER (pronounced "see-derr"). The FDA division charged with regulating drug products (prescription, OTC, and generics). See http://www.fda.gov/cder.

The FDA's view of drug safety is summarized in an FAQ on their website (http://www.fda.gov/cder/about/faq/default.htm):

"Q6: Once the FDA approves a drug, does this mean that the product is perfectly safe?

A: No drug product is "perfectly" safe. Every single drug that affects the body will have some side effects. Since the FDA considers both the benefits and risks of all medications before approval, side effects are generally not serious. For every drug the FDA approves, the benefits are balanced against its risks. In addition, the FDA makes sure the labeling (package insert) outlines the benefits and risks reported in the tested population. You and your healthcare provider should decide together if the benefits outweigh the risks for YOU. Talking about your medicines with your healthcare provider is just as important and good for your health as a complete check-up and taking your medicine as directed."

The Office of the CDER Center Director has under it the Office of Surveillance and Epidemiology and the Office of Safety Policy and Communication Staff. The Office of Surveillance and Epidemiology has under it three divisions: 1) Drug Risk Evaluation, 2) Surveillance, Research, and Communication Support, and 3) Medication Errors and Technical Support.

The Office of Safety Policy and Communication Staff has the MedWatch group and the Drug Safety Oversight Board. The Office of New Drugs has many offices and divisions under it with specific specialties (e.g., gastroenterology, pulmonary products, etc.), which are also involved at times in safety evaluations.

There is an advisory committee of outside experts on Drug Safety and Risk Management as well as other advisory committees that meet periodically to review data and advise the FDA on various issues, including drug approvals and policy issues. See http://www.fda.gov/oc/advisory/acdrugs.html.

CENTERS FOR EDUCATION AND RESEARCH IN THERAPEUTICS (CERTS)

Per their website, this institution is a research program administered by the Agency for Healthcare Research and Quality (AHRQ), in consultation with the FDA and the Department of Health and Human Services (HHS). The mission of the CERTS is to conduct research and provide education that will advance the optimal use of drugs, medical devices, and biological products to develop knowledge, manage risk, improve medical practice, and inform policymakers. There are 11 centers throughout the US. They have done studies and research in such drug safety-related areas as drug–drug interactions, the cytochrome P450 system, AEs with chronic glucocorticoid use, and medication errors. See their website: http://www.certs.hhs.gov/index.html.

CENTRAL APPROVAL OR AUTHORIZATION

Also called Centralized Approval or Authorization. The most common mechanism to obtain marketing authorization for a product within the European Union. This route (compared to national or mutual recognition authorization) allows marketing of the product within the entire EU of 27 member states.

CENTRE FOR ADVERSE REACTIONS MONITORING (CARM)

New Zealand's national monitoring center for adverse reactions, located at the University of Otago. It collects and evaluates spontaneous reports of adverse reactions to medicines, vaccines, herbal products, and dietary supplements from health professionals in New Zealand. Currently the CARM database holds over 50,000 reports, provides New Zealand-specific information on adverse reactions to these products, and serves to support clinical decision-making when unusual symptoms are thought to be therapy related. See http://carm.otago.ac.nz/index.asp?link=carm.

CHALLENGE

In drug safety, the drug administration (a certain dose at a given time) suspected of causing the AE being looked at in a case report. It may have occurred during routine medical practice or during a clinical trial.

Authors' note: Medical allergists use this term to describe the reintroduction of a test dose of a suspected allergen, a maneuver called rechallenge in pharmacovigilance.

CHANNELING BIAS

Also called channeling effect. A type of selection bias in which a clinician prescribes a drug based on the patient's expected prognosis. Thus a drug might be selected or avoided in a patient depending upon the severity of his disease, comedications, and/or

other medical problems. This introduces difficulty in clinical trials and treatment comparisons. It may be done consciously or
subconsciously.

CHIEF SAFETY OFFICER

In a pharmaceutical company, a senior-level physician who is responsible for the final decision on medical safety issues for the corporation. This job includes decisions on product withdrawals,
stopping clinical trials, amending protocols, changing product labeling, and so forth, for safety reasons. He or she may also chair
the Corporate Safety Committee (see this term). *See also* Qualified
Person for Pharmacovigilance.

CHILDREN AND AES

In general, children are not studied during the development phases
of new drugs in spite of the need for this and the encouragement
of the FDA and other health authorities. Efficacy, safety, and dosing in children are generally not known for many drugs. Clinicians
thus tend to extrapolate from adult data which does not always
apply as children are not just "small adults." In particular, use in
neonates and very young children may differ due to differences in
absorption, distribution, metabolism, and excretion.

CHI-SQUARED TEST

A statistical test of the fit between a theoretical frequency distribution and the actual frequency distribution of categorical (yes/no)
data. It may also be used to determine whether two groups have the
same proportion of observations for a common characteristic. This
test may be used in certain analyses of AEs/ADRs but it does not
take into account the severity of the adverse events. Ranking scales
and continuous variables provide more information.

CHRONOLOGIC CAUSALITY CRITERIA

The use of certain time-related observations in determining the
causality of an AE. These include the dates of administration and
the dates of the AE, as well as the time to onset, the time to offset,
etc.

*Authors' note: The use of these measurements is key in causality
analysis whether done by algorithm or global introspection. For example, the time of onset of an AE after ingestion is examined in light
of the drug's absorption, distribution, metabolism, and excretion. A
drug with a half-life of minutes would not be likely to produce an AE
that occurs many hours after ingestion. A drug that has been used for*

only a few days would be unlikely to produce cancer of the colon, which takes years to develop.

CIOMS (COUNCIL FOR INTERNATIONAL ORGANIZATIONS OF MEDICAL SCIENCES)

CIOMS is an international, non-governmental, non-profit organization established jointly by WHO (World Health Organization) and United Nations Educational, Scientific and Cultural Organization (UNESCO) in 1949. The membership of CIOMS includes 48 international member organizations, representing many of the biomedical disciplines, and 18 national members, mainly representing national academies of sciences and medical research councils. The main objectives of CIOMS are:

- To facilitate and promote international activities in the field of biomedical sciences, especially when the participation of several international associations and national institutions is deemed necessary.
- To maintain collaborative relations with the United Nations and its specialized agencies, in particular with WHO and UNESCO.
- To serve the scientific interests of the international biomedical community in general.

Starting in the early 1980s, CIOMS Working Groups composed of experts from industry and governments have been examining key issues in drug safety. They have issued six Working Group reports, several of which have served as seminal documents in drug safety. See the listings for CIOMS Report I through VI. CIOMS is based in Geneva, Switzerland. See their website: http://www.cioms.ch/.

CIOMS I FORM

A standard format form for submission of individual case safety reports to health authorities. This form (which is very similar to the US MedWatch form) contains the basic information on the patient, the reporter, the drug, the AE(s), the course, and outcome. See http://www.cioms.ch/cioms.pdf. See Appendix 4 for a copy of the CIOMS I form.

CIOMS I REPORT: INTERNATIONAL REPORTING OF ADVERSE DRUG REACTIONS (1990)

The output from the CIOMS I Working Group of 1990. Their goal was "to develop an internationally acceptable reporting method whereby manufacturers could report post-marketing AEs/ADRs rapidly, efficiently and effectively to regulators." The report established several conventions that have largely been adopted, including the following:

- The concept and format of a report ("a CIOMS I report") from the manufacturer receiving the event to the regulators.
- "Reactions" are different from "events." "Reactions" are reports of clinical occurrences that have been judged by a physician or healthcare worker as having a "reasonable possibility" that the report has been caused by a drug. "Events" have not had a causality evaluation made and, thus, may or may not be related to or associated with the drug.
- No particular method of assessing causality is recommended. Manufacturers should not separate out those spontaneous reports that they receive into those that seem to be drug related and those not felt to be drug related. The reporting physician, by making the report to the manufacturer, is indicating that there is some level of causality possible in the report. This is a "suspected reaction." This has become a fundamental concept in most spontaneous reporting systems around the world wherein all spontaneous reports are to be considered possibly related to the drug; that is they are "reactions" not "events."
- Because labels for marketed drugs differ from country to country, it is recommended that all reactions be collected at one point and then submitted to local authorities on a country-by-country basis based on whether the reactions are labeled locally or not.
- Four minimum requirements for a valid report are defined: an identifiable source (reporter), a patient (even if not precisely identified by name), a suspect drug, and a suspect reaction.
- All reports are to be sent to health authorities as soon as received and no later than 15 working days after receipt to create a common worldwide deadline. This concept has been adopted, but the 15 working days has been changed to 15 calendar days due to differences in the designation of "working days" and nonworking days (holidays) around the world. The reporting clock starts the date the report is first received by anyone anywhere in the company.
- The CIOMS I form for reporting individual case reports to authorities was created.
- Reporting of reactions is to be in English.

CIOMS II LINE LISTING

See Line Listing.

CIOMS II REPORT: INTERNATIONAL REPORTING OF PERIODIC DRUG-SAFETY UPDATE SUMMARIES (1992)

The output from the CIOMS II Working Group of 1992. Their goal was to create a standard for Periodic Safety Update Reports (PSURs) of AEs/ADRs received by manufacturers on marketed drugs. This standard, with modifications from the ICH and other organizations, has been widely adopted. The document defined several key terms:

- *CIOMS Reportable Cases or Reports:* "serious, medically substantiated, unlabeled ADRs with the four elements (reporter, patient, reaction, suspect drug)."
- *Core Data Sheet (CDS):* A document prepared by the manufacturer containing all relevant safety information, including adverse drug reactions (ADRs). This is the reference for "listed" and "unlisted." Note that this concept, which has been widely accepted, has since gotten more complex and one must distinguish "labeled" (in the SPC, US PI, or other national labeling) from "listed" (contained in the Core Safety Information).
- *International Birth Date (IBD):* The date that the first regulatory authority anywhere in the world has approved a drug for marketing.
- *Data Lock-Point (Cut-Off Date):* The closing date for information to be included in a particular safety update.
- *Serious:* Fatal, life-threatening, involves or prolongs inpatient hospitalization.

The sections of the PSUR were defined to include the following:

1. Introduction
2. CDS (Core Data Sheet)
3. Drug's licensing (i.e., marketing approval) status
4. Review of regulatory actions taken for safety, if any
5. Patient exposure
6. Individual case histories (including a "CIOMS line listing")
7. Studies
8. Overall safety evaluation
9. Important data received after the data lock-point

Other fundamental concepts were established:

- Reports should be semiannual and not cumulative (unless cumulative information is needed to put a safety issue into context).
- The same report goes to all regulatory authorities on the same date irrespective of the local (national) approval date of the drug.
- Reactions reported should be from studies (published and unpublished), spontaneous reports, published case reports, cases

received from regulatory authorities, and other manufacturers. Duplicate reports should be eliminated.

- The manufacturer should do a "concise critical analysis and opinion in English by a person responsible for monitoring and assessing drug safety."

CIOMS III REPORT: GUIDELINES FOR PREPARING CORE CLINICAL SAFETY INFORMATION ON DRUGS (1995), INCLUDING NEW PROPOSALS FOR INVESTIGATOR'S BROCHURES (1998/1999)

The output from the CIOMS III Working Group of 1995 with a revision in 1998/1999. The Core Safety Information document (a subset of the Core Data Sheet-CDS) was introduced. It contains basic safety information:

- The CSI is the core safety information that should appear in all countries' labeling for that drug. Additional information could be added at the national level, but the core information should be included in all countries' labels. The CSI (and national labels) are guides for health care professionals and contain the most relevant information needed for the drug's use.
- Marketing considerations should not play a role in the preparation of the CSI.
- The CSI was proposed primarily as a medical document and not as a legal or regulatory document.
- Every drug should have a CSI prepared and updated by the manufacturer.
- AEs due to excipients should be included.
- AEs that have no well-established relationship to therapy should not be included.
- The CSI should include important information that physicians are not generally expected to know.
- As soon as relevant safety information becomes sufficiently well established, it should be included. The specific time when it is included occurs when the safety information crosses the "threshold for inclusion." This is defined as the time when "it is judged that it will influence physicians' decisions on therapy."
- Thirty-nine factors were proposed that can be ranked and weighed for an ADR for a particular drug to see whether the information has crossed the threshold. The threshold should be lower if the condition being treated is relatively trivial, the drug is used to prevent rather than to treat disease, the drug is widely used, or the ADR is irreversible.
- Hypersensitivity reactions should be noted early.

- Substantial evidence is required to remove or downgrade safety information.
- Ten general principles were proposed:
  1. In general, statements that an adverse reaction does not occur or has not yet been reported should not be made.
  2. As a general rule, clinical descriptions of specific cases should not be part of the CSI.
  3. If the mechanism is known, it should be stated, but speculation about the mechanism should be avoided.
  4. As a general rule, secondary cascade effects or sequelae should not be listed.
  5. A description of events expected as a result of progression of the underlying treated disease should not be included in the CSI.
  6. Unlicensed or "off-label" use should be mentioned only in the context of a medically important safety problem.
  7. The wording used in the CSI to describe adverse reactions should be chosen carefully and responsibly to maximize the prescriber's understanding. For example, if the ADR is part of a syndrome, this should be made clear.
  8. The terms used should be specific and medically informative.
  9. The use of modifiers or adjectives should be avoided unless they add useful important information.
  10. A special attribute (e.g., sex, race) known to be associated with an increased risk should be specified.
- Where possible, AE/ADR frequencies should be provided, although this is admittedly very difficult with spontaneous safety data. A classification was proposed:
- Very common: ≥1/10 (≥10%)
- Common (frequent): ≥1/100 and <1/10 (≥1% and <10%)
- Uncommon (infrequent): ≥1/1,000 and <1/100 (≥0.1% and <1%)
- Rare: ≥1/10,000 and <1/1000 (≥0.01% and <0.1%)
- Very rare: <1/10,000 (<0.01%)

CIOMS IV REPORT: BENEFIT-RISK BALANCE FOR MARKETED DRUGS: EVALUATING SAFETY SIGNALS

The output from the CIOMS IV Working Group of 1998. "It examines the theoretical and practical aspects of how to determine whether a potentially major, new safety signal signifies a shift, calling for significant action in the established relationship between benefits and risks; it also provides guidance for deciding what options for action should be considered and on the process of decision-making should such action be required."

The report looks at the general concepts of benefit-risk analysis and discusses the factors influencing assessment, including stakeholders and constituencies, the nature of the problem (risk), the indication for drug use, the population under treatment, time constraints, available data and resources, and economic issues.

The report recommends a standard format and content for a benefit-risk report:

- Introduction.
- Brief specification/description of the drug and where marketed.
- Indications for use, by country, if there are differences.
- Identification of one or more alternative therapies or modalities, including surgery.
- A very brief description of the suspected or established major safety problem.
- Benefit evaluation.
- Epidemiology and natural history of the target disease(s).
- Purpose of treatment (cure, prophylaxis, etc.).
- Summary of efficacy and general tolerance data compared with other medical treatments, surgical treatment, or other interventions and no treatment.
- Risk evaluation.
- Background.
- Weight of evidence for the suspected risk (incidence, etc.).
- Detailed presentations and analyses of data on the new suspected risk.
- Probable and possible explanations.
- Preventability, predictability, and reversibility of the new risk.
- The issue as it relates to alternative therapies and no therapy.
- Review of the complete safety of the drug; when appropriate, focus on selected subsets of serious AEs (e.g., the three most common and three most medically serious adverse reactions).
- Provide similar profiles for alternate drugs.
- When possible, estimate the excess incidence of any adverse reactions known to be common to the alternatives.
- When there are significant adverse reactions that are not common to the drugs compared, highlight important differences between the drugs.
- Benefit-risk evaluation.
- Summarize the benefits as related to the seriousness of the target disease and the purpose and effectiveness of treatment.

- Summarize the dominant risks (seriousness/severity, duration, incidence).
- Summarize the benefit-risk relationship.
- Provide a summary assessment and conclusion.
- Options analysis.
- List all appropriate options for action.
- Describe the pros and cons and likely consequences (impact analysis) of each option under consideration.
- If relevant, outline plans or suggestions for a study that could provide timely and important additional information.
- If feasible, indicate the quality and quantity of any future evidence that would signal the need for a reevaluation of the benefit-risk relationship.
- Suggest how the consequences of the recommended action should be monitored and assessed.

CIOMS V REPORT: CURRENT CHALLENGES IN PHARMACOVIGILANCE: PRAGMATIC APPROACHES (2001)

The output from the CIOMS V Working Group of 2001. This is a very large report covering a multitude of areas in drug safety. Some of the highlights include:

Individual Case Safety Reports

New types of individual case safety reports are now appearing, including Internet reports, solicited reports from patient support programs, surveys, epidemiologic studies, disease registries, regulatory and other databases, and licensor and licensee interactions.

Consumer reports should be scrutinized and should receive appropriate attention and be included in PSURs.

Literature Reports

Literature reports should be sought in at least two internationally recognized literature databases realizing, however, that publications may be a source of false information and signals.

Broadcast and lay media should not ordinarily be monitored.

If the product source or brand is not specified, a company should assume it was its product.

If there is a contractual agreement between two or more companies (e.g., for comarketing), the contract should specify the responsibility for literature searches and reporting.

English should be the standard language for literature report translations.

The clock starts when a case is recognized to have the four minimum criteria for reportability (reporter, patient, drug, event).

The Internet

A procedure should be in place to ensure daily screening of a company's or regulator's website(s) to identify potential case reports, but companies and regulators do not need to routinely monitor the Internet beyond their own sites for AEs.

Solicited Reports

Solicited reports should be regarded as distinct from spontaneous unsolicited reports. They should be processed separately and so identified in expedited and periodic reporting.

For regulatory reporting, solicited reports should be handled in the same way as study reports. Causality assessments are needed.

Clinical Trials and Studies

Quality-of-life studies should be handled like clinical trial data.

Epidemiologic studies should have the same reporting rules for suspected ADR cases as clinical trials.

For epidemiologic studies, unless there is specific attribution in an individual case, expedited reporting is generally not appropriate.

If relevant, studies should be summarized in PSURs.

Expedited reports from comparator drug data should be forwarded to the relevant manufacturer(s) for their regulatory reporting.

Registries and Databases

A registry is not a study. Cases should be treated as solicited reports (causality assessment required).

It is unnecessary for a company to attempt to routinely collect ADRs from regulatory databases.

Licenser–Licensee Interactions

When companies codevelop, comarket, or copromote products, it is critical that explicit contractual agreements specify processes for exchange of safety information, including timelines and regulatory reporting responsibilities.

The time frame for expedited regulatory reporting should normally be no longer than 15 calendar days from the first receipt of a valid case by any of the partners.

Case Evaluation

The company or regulatory authority staff can propose alternate clinical terms and interpretations of the case from those of the reporter, but the reporter's original terms must also be reported.

When a case is reported by a consumer, his or her clinical description should be retained even if confirmatory information from a healthcare professional is obtained.

There is an important distinction between a suspected ADR and an "incidental" event. An incidental event is one that occurs in reasonable clinical temporal association with the use of the drug product, but is not the intended subject of the spontaneous report (i.e., it did not prompt the contact with the company or regulator). There is also no implicit or explicit expression of possible drug causality by the reporter or the company's safety review staff. They should be included as part of the medical history and not be the subject of expedited reporting. Incidental events should be captured in the company database.

When cases do not meet the minimum criteria (patient, reporter, event, drug) even after follow-up, the case should be kept in the database as an "incomplete case."

The regulatory reporting clock starts in the European Union at the first contact with a healthcare professional, but in the United States and Canada it starts when the case is initially reported to the company, even by a consumer.

One or more of the following automatically qualify a patient as identifiable: age, age category (e.g., teenager), sex, initials, date of birth, name, or patient number. Even in the absence of such qualifying descriptors, a report referring to a definite number of patients should be regarded as a case as long as the other criteria for validity are met. For example, "Two patients experienced..." but not "a few patients experienced...."

Criteria for Seriousness

Hospitalization refers to admission as an inpatient and not to an examination and/or treatment as an outpatient.

All congenital anomalies and birth defects, without regard to their nature or severity, should be considered serious.

There is a lack of objective standards for "life threatening" and "medical judgment" as seriousness criteria; both require individual professional evaluation that invariably introduces a lack of reproducibility.

Within a company the tools, lists, and decision-making processes should be harmonized globally.

Expectedness

The terminology associated with expectedness depends on which reference safety document is being used and for what purpose: "Listed" or "unlisted" refers to the ADRs contained in the CSI for a marketed product or within the development CSI (DCSI) in the investigator's brochure. "Labeled" or "unlabeled" refers to the ADRs contained in official product safety information for marketed products (e.g., Summary of Product Characteristics in the European Union, the Package Insert in the United States, or the Product Monograph in Canada) in each country.

Determining whether a reported reaction is expected or not is a two-step process: first, is the reaction term already included in the CSI? Second, is the ADR different regarding its nature, severity, specificity, or outcome?

Expectedness should be strictly based on inclusion of a drug associated experience in the ADR section of the CSI. Special types of reactions, such as those occurring under conditions of overdose, drug interaction, or pregnancy, should also be included in this section. Disorders mentioned in "contraindications" or "precautions" as reasons for not treating with the drug are not expected ADRs unless they also appear in the ADR section.

If an ADR has been reported only in association with an overdose, it should be considered unexpected if it occurs at a normal dose.

For a marketed drug CSI, events cited in data from clinical trials are not considered expected unless they are included in the ADR section.

Class labeling does not count as "expected" unless the event in question is included in the ADR section.

Lack of expected efficacy is not relevant to whether an AE is expected or not.

Unless the CSI specifies a fatal outcome for an ADR, the case is unexpected as long as there was an association between the reaction and the fatality.

Case Follow-Up Approaches
Highest priority for follow-up are cases that are serious and unexpected followed by serious, expected and nonserious, unexpected.

Cases "of special interest" (e.g., ADRs under active surveillance at the request of the regulators) also deserve high priority, as well as any cases that might lead to a labeling change.

For any cases with legal implications, the company's legal department should be involved.

Note: When the case is serious and if the ADR has not resolved at the time of the initial report, it is important to continue follow-up until the outcome has been established or the condition stabilized.

How long to follow up on such cases requires judgment.

It is recommended that collaboration with other companies be done if more than one company's drug is suspected as a causal agent in a case.

Follow-up for unexpected deaths and life-threatening cases should be done within 24 hours.

If a reporter fails to respond to the first follow-up attempt, reminder letters should be sent as follows:

- A single follow-up letter for any nonserious expected case.
- For all other cases, a second follow-up letter should be sent no later than four weeks after the first letter.

In general, when the reporter fails to respond or is incompletely cooperative, the two follow-up letters should reflect sufficient due diligence.

Role of Narratives

A company case narrative is different from the reporter's clinical description of a case, though the reporter's comments should be an integral part of the company narrative. The reporter's verbatim words should be included for the adverse reactions.

Alternate causes to that given by the reporter should be described and identified as a company opinion.

The same evaluation should be supplied to all regulators.

Narratives should be prepared for all serious (expected and unexpected) and nonserious unexpected cases but not for nonserious expected cases.

Narratives should be written in the third person past tense. All relevant information should be in a logical time sequence.

In general, abbreviations (except laboratory parameters and units) and acronyms should not be used.

Time to onset of an event from the start of treatment should be given in the most appropriate time units (e.g., hours), but actual dates can be used if helpful to the reader.

If detailed supplementary records are important to a case (e.g., autopsy report), their availability should be mentioned in the narrative.

Information may be supplied by more than one person (e.g., initial reporter and supplementary information from a specialist); all sources should be specified.

When there is conflicting information provided from different sources, this should be mentioned and the sources identified.

If it is suspected that an ADR resulted from misprescribing or other medication error, judgmental comments should not be included in the narrative due to legal implications. Only the facts should be stated.

The narrative should have eight sections that serve as a comprehensive stand-alone "medical story":

1. Source of the report and patient demography.
2. Medical and drug history.
3. Suspect drug(s), timing and conditions surrounding the onset of the reaction(s).
4. The progression of the event(s) and its outcome in the patient.
5. If the outcome is fatal, the relevant details.
6. Rechallenge information, if applicable.
7. The original reporter's clinical assessment.
8. The narrative preparer's medical evaluation and comment.

PSURs: Content Modification

For reports covering long time periods (e.g., five years), it is more practical to use the CSI current at the time of PSUR preparation.

Clinical trial data should be supplied only if they suggest a signal or are relevant to a possible change in the benefit-risk relationship.

For 5-year reports, follow-up information on cases described in the previous report should be provided only for cases associated with new or ongoing safety issues.

Inclusion of literature reports should be selective and cover publications relevant to safety findings, independent of listedness.

For PSURs with large numbers of cases, discussion and analysis for the overall safety evaluation should be by system organ class rather than by listedness or seriousness.

An abbreviated PSUR saves time and resources if little or no new safety information is generated during the time period covered. Criteria for an abbreviated report:

- No serious unlisted cases.
- Few (e.g., 10) serious listed cases.
- No significant regulatory actions for safety.
- No major changes to the CSI.
- No findings that lead to a new action.

PSURs: Bridging Report

A summary bridging report is a concise document that provides no new information and integrates two or more previously prepared PSURs to cover a specified period.

Its format follows that of a regular PSUR, but the content should consist of summary highlights of the reports being summarized.

PSURs: Addendum Report

This report is prepared on special request of the regulators to satisfy regulators who require reports covering a period outside the routine PSUR reporting cycle (e.g., if the reports are based on the local approval date in that country rather than on the IBD).

It updates the most recently completed PSUR.

It follows the usual PSUR format.

PSURs: Miscellaneous Proposals

A brief (e.g., one-page) stand-alone overview (executive summary) should be provided.

Manufacturers should be allowed to select the IBDs for their old products to facilitate synchronization of PSURs.

If there is no CSI for an old product, the most suitable local labeling should be considered for use.

The evaluation of cases in a PSUR should focus on unlisted ADRs with analyses organized primarily by system organ class (body system).

Discussion of serious unlisted cases should include cumulative data.

Complicated PSURs and those with extensive new data may require more than 60 days to prepare adequately and the regulators should be flexible.

The possibility of "resetting" the PSUR clock (from annual to semiannual reports as the result of a new indication or dosage form) should be allowed by the regulators.

PSURs: Population Data

Detailed calculations on exposure (the denominator) are ordinarily unnecessary, especially given the unreliability of the numerator; rough estimates usually suffice, but the method and units used should be explained clearly.

Drug exposure data are approximate and usually represent an overestimate.

For special situations, such as when dealing with an important safety signal, attempts should be made to obtain exposure information covering the relevant covariates (e.g., age, gender, race, indication, dosing details).

CIOMS VI REPORT: MANAGEMENT OF SAFETY INFORMATION FROM CLINICAL TRIALS (2005)

The output from the CIOMS VI Working Group of 2005. This is a very large report covering clinical trial safety issues. Some of the highlights include:

General Concepts

These concepts apply to trials in phases I through IV.

Any study that is not scientifically sound should be considered unethical.

Informed consent is the cornerstone of human subject research, but there are situations in which it is either not possible or not appropriate.

Systematic Approach to Managing Safety Data

Sponsors must have in place a well-defined process to readily identify, evaluate, and minimize potential safety risks. The process should start before the first phase I study. A formal development risk management plan should be developed.

A dedicated safety management team should be formed for each development program to review safety information on a regular basis—at least quarterly—and the team should consider changes to the investigator's brochure, informed consent, and protocol as needed.

When licensing partners are involved, a joint safety committee should be created with clear roles and responsibilities. This should ideally be defined in the initial contract. A project management function should be set up to ensure scheduling, tracking, and timelines.

All pertinent data must be readily available from the clinical trial and safety databases as well as preclinical toxicology, mutagenicity, pharmacokinetic, pharmacodynamic, and drug interaction data. Epidemiology should be incorporated into the planning process.

Certain toxicities should be considered for all new drugs, including abnormalities of cardiac conduction, hepatotoxicity, drug interactions, immunogenicity, bone marrow toxicity, and reactive metabolite formation.

Data Collection and Management

The investigator should report (immediately if judged critical) to the sponsor any information that is considered to be important in regard to safety even if the protocol does not call for it. The sponsor must carefully train the investigative site in this matter.

The collection of "excessive" data can have a negative impact on data quality. Case report form fields should collect only those data that can be analyzed and presented in tabular form. All other data should be collected as text comments.

Safety monitoring in phase IV studies may not require the same intensity as for phases I–III trials, but the same principles and practices should apply.

If a company provides any support for an independent trial it does not sponsor (investigator-initiated studies/trials), the company should still obtain at a minimum all serious suspected adverse reactions. The company should do its own causality assessment and, if appropriate, report it to the health authorities even if the investigator has already done so.

In the early phases of drug development, it is often necessary to collect more comprehensive safety data than in postmarketing studies. Some studies may require longer follow-up.

Phase I data are especially important because these data are collected in healthy volunteers and are critical to the future development of the drug.

There is no definitive way to determine causality of a particular AE. That is, its attribution to the drug or to a background finding with only a temporal association cannot be definitively done. Thus the following is recommended: All AEs, both serious and nonserious, are collected whether believed to be related or not. This applies to the experimental product, placebo, no treatment, and active comparators. Similarly, studies initiated during the immediate postapproval period should continue this practice. Once the safety profile is judged to be well understood, it may be possible to collect less data (e.g., nonserious AEs believed not to be due to the drug).

The use of herbal and other nontraditional treatments should be sought when data are being collected in all studies.

Although causality assessments based on aggregate data or case series are usually more meaningful than those based on individual cases, the investigator causality assessment should be done and may play a role in the early detection of significant safety events, especially rare ones.

The investigator should be asked to use a "simple binary decision" for drug causality of serious AEs: related or not related, reasonable possibility or no reasonable possibility, and so on. The use of the words "unknown" or "cannot be ruled out" should be avoided.

Causality for nonserious AEs should not be requested from investigators routinely.

Where appropriate, the investigator should supply a diagnosis rather than signs and symptoms. However, when a diagnosis is supplied for a serious AE, the accompanying signs and symptoms should be recorded.

Before starting a study, AEs of special interest and anticipated AEs (if known) should be communicated to the investigator.

Medically serious clinical events that are recorded in a trial as clinical efficacy outcomes or endpoints should be reviewed by the sponsor and data monitoring committee even though they are not considered AEs.

It is preferable to frame questions to patients in general terms rather than suggesting that the study treatment was responsible for reported AEs. Although a "laundry list" of AEs should not be read to the patient, patients should be alerted to known issues of medically important suspected or established AEs to alert the investigator as soon as possible.

Data collection should start from the time of the signing of the informed consent.

Safety data event collection should continue after the last dose of the drug for at least an additional five half-lives of the experimental product.

General Rules for Data Quality

Cases should be as fully documented as possible. There should be diligent follow-up of each case. The reporter's verbatim terms should be captured and retained. If the reporter's terms are considered inaccurate or inconsistent with standard medical terminology, attempts should be made to clarify them. If disagreement continues, the sponsor should code the AE terms according to its judgment but identify them as distinct from the reporter's terms and reasons for differences noted.

Primary analyses of the data should be done using the reporter's terms. Additional analyses may be done using the sponsor's terms. Any differences must be noted and explained.

Individual case safety reports should be categorized and assessed by the sponsor using trained individuals with broad experience. Investigators should obtain specialist consultation for clinically important events that fall outside their expertise.

AE tables may display both the reported investigator's verbatim term and the sponsor's terms.

The sponsor (as well as health authorities) may wish to consider the use of a listing of event terms that are always regarded as serious and important.

Such events then routinely trigger special attention and evaluation.

Cases should not be "overcoded" using more terms than minimally necessary to ensure retrieval of the cases. Similarly, cases should not be "undercoded" where the terms chosen downgrade the severity or importance of events.

Risk Identification and Evaluation

Sponsors should develop a system to assess, evaluate, and act on safety information on a continuous basis during drug development to ensure the earliest possible identification of safety concerns to allow risk minimization.

The integrity of the studies should not be compromised by the safety monitoring and analysis.

Safety Data Management

Safety data should be handled using consistent standards and criteria with care and precision.

Safety evaluations must be individualized for each product because there are no standard approaches to evaluating or measuring "an acceptable level of risk."

Review of Safety Information

Safety data analysis should involve both individual case reports and well as aggregate data. Individual cases should be reviewed within specified time frames and aggregate data on a periodic basis.

The evaluation should be done in the context of the patient population, the indication studied, the natural history of the disease, and currently available therapies.

Causality determinations should be done for all reported cases. The investigator causality assessment should be taken into account.

AEs of special interest should be identified in the protocol and handled as if they are serious even if they do not meet the regulatory definition of serious.

Non-serious AEs should be reviewed to see whether there are events of special interest with particular attention paid to those associated with study discontinuation.

Safety review of all data should be done frequently: Ad hoc for serious and special interest AEs. Routine periodic review of all data whose frequency varies from trial to trial or program to program. Reviews triggered by specific trial or program milestones. At the time of study completion and unblinding.

Analysis and Evaluation

Subgroup analysis, though possibly limited by small sample size, should be done for dose, duration, gender, age, concomitant medications, and concurrent diseases.

Data pooling should include studies that are of similar design. This can include all controlled studies, placebo-controlled studies, studies with any positive control, studies with a particular positive control, and particular indications.

If the duration of treatment varies widely among participants, data on the effect of treatment duration should be analyzed.

Statistical Approaches

The techniques for use of statistics for analyzing safety data are less well developed than for efficacy.

Statistical association (probability values) alone may or may not be of clinical value. Examination of both statistical and clinical significance must involve a partnership between the statistical and clinical experts.

It may be necessary to acknowledge when the data are insufficient to draw conclusions on safety: "absence of evidence is not evidence of absence."

Regulatory Reporting and Communications of Safety
The group endorses ICH Guideline E2A and recommends the harmonization of criteria for expedited reporting whereby such reporting to authorities should include only suspected ADRs that are both serious and unexpected.

Only under exceptional circumstances should other cases (i.e., expected cases) be submitted as expedited reports. If reporting without regard to causality is required, it should be done on a periodic basis with clearly defined timelines and format.

The regulators should adopt the phrase "a reasonable possibility of a causal relationship" and not use the ICH E2A phrase of "a causal relationship cannot be ruled out" in regard to suspected ADRs.

Once a drug is marketed, the company Core Safety Information document should be used as the reference safety document for determining expectedness for regulatory reporting of phase IV trials. For new indication trials the DCSI document should be used. The two documents should be aligned as much as possible.

As with spontaneous reports, reportability for case reports from trials should be determined at the event level. That is, a case would be expedited if there is a suspected adverse reaction that is serious and unexpected.

Suspected ADRs that are serious and unexpected and thus are expedited reports should, in general, be unblinded. There may be certain circumstances where this should not occur, however (e.g., serious AEs that are also efficacy endpoints). Such exceptions should be agreed on by the regulatory authorities and be clearly described in the investigator brochure and the protocol.

Unblinded placebo cases should not be reported to regulatory authorities as expedited cases. Unblinded (and open label) comparator drug cases should be reported to the regulatory authorities and/or the company owning the comparator on an expedited basis whether expected or not.

Seven-day reports should be limited to cases from clinical trials and not spontaneous reports. This should apply both in countries where the drug is approved and where it is only under clinical study.

The sponsor should develop clear standard operating procedures for the expedited or prompt reporting of other safety issues with special attention to when the clock starts for non-clinical safety issues that might have implications for human subjects:

- A higher incidence of a serious AE for the drug compared with the comparator or the background rate in the general population.
- An increased frequency of a previously recognized serious adverse reaction.
- A significant drug interaction in a pharmacokinetic study.
- AEs that are deemed not to be drug related but are considered study related.

Contrary to established regulations, the working group recommends that routine expedited cases reported to investigators and investigational review boards and ethics committees (as opposed to reports to regulatory authorities) be eliminated and replaced with regular updates of the evolving benefit-risk profile highlighting new safety information.

For unapproved products, the reports to investigators and IRBs should include a line listing of unblinded clinical trial cases that were expedited to regulatory agencies during this time period, a copy of the current DCSI with an explanation of changes, and a brief summary of the emerging safety profile. Quarterly updates are the "default" with other frequencies as appropriate.

For approved products, the reports to investigators and IRBs should be quarterly if the product is in phase III trials. For well-established products, a less frequent interval would be acceptable. At some point, only investigators and IRBs would need to be updated for significant new information. For phase IV investigators and IRBs, only changes to the CCSI would be needed.

The reports, whether for approved or unapproved products, should include in the line listings only unblinded expedited reports from trials and include only interval data (i.e., changes since the last update). A summary of the emerging safety profile should be included with cumulative data as needed. MedDRA should be used. The listings should not include spontaneous reports, which should be described in narrative form in the update.

Should a significant safety issue be identified (i.e., an issue that has a significant impact on the course of the clinical trial or program or warrants immediate update of the informed consent), the sponsor should promptly notify the regulatory authorities, investigators, IRBs, and, if relevant, data safety monitoring committees.

A safety management team should review all safety data on a regular basis: quarterly before approval and coordinate with the

PSUR schedule postapproval. Ad-hoc meetings would occur as needed to address urgent safety issues and signals. They would review the overall evolving safety profile to make changes to the DCSI, informed consent, and protocol as needed.

A single Development Safety Update Report (DSUR) should be submitted to regulators annually. The format and content would be defined and would cover the drug product, not just a single study.

For marketed products with well-established safety profiles and for which most trials are in phase IV in the approved indications, the PSUR would replace the DSUR.

Sponsors should incorporate the DCSI into every investigator brochure, either as a special section of the investigator brochure or as an attachment. The sponsor should clearly identify the events for which the company believes there is sufficient evidence to suspect a drug relationship. These events would be considered expected ("listed") for regulatory reporting criteria.

The investigator brochure and DCSI should be reviewed and updated at least annually.

If the developer or manufacturer of a product is not the sponsor of a particular trial but rather supports an external clinical or non-clinical investigator sponsored study, a provision of any agreement should be the prompt reporting to the company of all serious suspected ADRs in humans or significant findings in animals.

As with the CCSI for marketed drugs (see CIOMS III/VI), the same threshold criteria should be applied to the DCSI and informed consent in preapproval drugs.

Informed consent should be renewed with the subjects whenever there is new information that could affect the subjects' willingness to participate in the trial. In certain circumstances, a more immediate communication may be appropriate.

CIOMS VII WORKING GROUP

An ongoing CIOMS Working Group set up to establish specifics for the format and content of the DSUR and establish links to the PSURs that will be written after the marketing of the drug.

CLAIMS DATABASE

An insurance database (either public or private) that includes bills ("claims") linked to specific medical, hospital, or pharmaceutical services provided. These databases can be used for pharmacoepidemiologic studies: pharmacovigilance, pharmacoeconomic, drug utilization review, etc. Examples of such databases include Medicaid (US, public), Kaiser (US, private), Health Insurance of

Canadian provinces (CA, public). These databases may or may not contain actual medical records. If not, they can be linked electronically to medical databases containing these patients' medical information. However, the medical data, whether in the claims database or in a linked database, may be of varying completeness (e.g., only in-patient information, no information on OTC medications, no source documents available, etc.).

The results obtained from a study done in a database must be interpreted carefully, taking into account the selected and secondary nature of the data.

CLASS ACTION LAWSUIT

Primarily in the United States, litigation filed by one or more people on behalf of a larger group of people (including themselves) who allege that they have suffered the same or similar injuries. In drug safety, these lawsuits may be filed on behalf of thousands of patients who claim that a drug produced a particular injury.

CLASS EFFECT

A concept that has been used in many ways. In drug safety this is generally meant to be a group of "related" drugs (related by chemical structure, indications for use, mechanism of action, etc.) that produce the same or similar adverse events. This concept is applied to drug labeling for safety issues. For example, all NSAIDs may have a "class labeling" saying that they produce a "class effect" of gastrointestinal hemorrhage.

Authors' note: Although this concept is felt by many to be somewhat vague and even misleading, in the safety world this has proved to be quite practical and useful in labeling. It is worthwhile to warn clinicians that a group of antibiotics may promote gastrointestinal overgrowth or that NSAIDs may produce bleeding. Class labeling is not, however, considered to be "labeled/listed" for the purposes of regulatory reporting assessment unless the event is also mentioned in the AE section of the labeling. Once the AE is established for a particular drug it moves out of the "class labeling" and into the AE/ADR section of the labeling and is now considered expected.

CLASS LABELING

See Class Effect.

CLIN-ALERT

Begun in 1962, *Clin Alert* was the first pharmacovigilance bulletin ever published. It summarizes clinical ADRs and is published twice monthly.

This newsletter provides pharmacists, physicians, and other healthcare professionals with comprehensive summaries of adverse drug reactions, drug interactions, and market withdrawals from over 100 key medical and research journals from around the world. Its primary focus is drug–drug interactions, but it also explores food–drug interactions, medication errors, and dietary supplements. Reports include:

- The primary drug suspected (including common trade names, dosages, and duration of therapy).
- The adverse drug reaction/interaction.
- Relevant laboratory data.
- Management of the reaction.
- Any relevant pre-existing condition.
- Potential legal repercussions.
- Complete journal citation including reprint information.

Also features *First Report*—a notice of the first documented report of an adverse clinical event.

See the website http://cla.sagepub.com/.

CLINICAL END POINT

A medically meaningful outcome measure used to determine the effect of an intervention (e.g., myocardial infarctions after hyperlipidemia therapy, survival after antineoplastic treatment) in contrast to a surrogate endpoint or marker (e.g., cholesterol and triglyceride blood levels or tumor size, respectively). *See* Surrogate Marker.

CLINICAL EPIDEMIOLOGY

See also Pharmacoepidemiology. "The science and method of studying optimal decisions in clinical medicine" (Jenicek), encompassing clinical pharmacology and pharmacoepidemiology. It represents the application of medical knowledge to decisions taken in medical practice.

Authors' note: The determination of causality in an ADR case report provides an example of applying both epidemiologic and pharmacoepidemiologic knowledge to a particular patient.

CLINICAL PHARMACOLOGY

A medical science applied to interactions between drugs and the human organism. Includes pharmacodynamics (effect of drug on the organism) and pharmacokinetics (handling of the drug by the body). This interface between pharmacology and human physiology is mainly based on controlled clinical trials in humans done during phases I, II, and III of a drug's development. This term is also used to indicate clinical trials done in man as opposed to those done in animals.

CLINICAL RESEARCH ORGANIZATION (CRO)

Also known as Contract Research Organization. Companies that handle some or all clinical and regulatory functions that pharmaceutical companies do, including phases I–IV studies, regulatory submissions, safety data, and IND and NDA preparations. Some CROs specialize purely in safety functions rather than the classic role in setting up and running clinical studies. These companies may collect, database, and report adverse events from marketed drugs for a pharmaceutical company that does not wish to handle this function and outsources it. In particular, these CROs function during "crisis" situations (e.g., drug recalls), when the pharmaceutical company's internal resources are overwhelmed.

CLINICAL RESEARCH UNIT (CRU)

In- or outpatient services established by a university or other organization to perform phases I, II, III, and IV clinical studies and trials. When functioning as sponsors, the CRU takes on all sponsor responsibilities as outlined in the regulations (and local institutional policies) for the study, as if it were a pharmaceutical company or a large consortium running trials (e.g., cancer trials, National Institutes of Health, etc.). When functioning as a study site for a pharmaceutical company, its safety functions revolve primarily on sending AEs (particularly serious ones) to the sponsor and notifying the IRB of serious cases.

Authors' note: CRUs may be non-profit-making institutions that are part of a larger entity, such as a university, or they may be profit-making commercial companies. No matter which they are, they must all follow the same rules.

CLINICAL STUDY/TRIAL

A research program in which humans are given one (or sometimes more than one) product such as a drug, device, or biologic, to examine the effects (both efficacy and safety) produced. There is usually a control group receiving a different product or no product, against which the effects are compared. Such studies are rigidly regulated by health authorities, governments, universities, and other organizations.

Authors' note: Some people refer to studies as those programs done in nondiseased normal people and trials in people (patients) with a disease, though this usage is inconsistent.

CLIOQUINOL

An example of market withdrawal for safety reasons with a very long delay between the discovery of the first significant ADR and the market withdrawal. Clioquinol was an amebicide used to treat diarrhea that produced subacute myelo-optic neuropathy with ensuing paralysis and blindness. Clioquinol was first commercialized in 1934 with the first report of this AE in 1935. However, it was not withdrawn from the market until 1979. An estimated 11,000 people were victims of this ADR in Japan between 1955 and 1970.

CLOCK START DATE

For regulatory reporting purposes, the day that a report of an AE is first received by a manufacturer, sponsor, pharmaceutical company, etc. It is used in calculating the 7- and 15-day reporting time requirements for serious adverse events to health authorities.

Authors' note: Although seemingly straightforward, this concept is not as simple as it seems. For example, the clock starts for 15-day reporting when a case is deemed to be serious and has all four minimum requirements for a valid AE. Thus if a case is initially received as a nonserious case and becomes serious after receipt of follow-up information, the 15-day clock starts on the day the seriousness was determined, not the date of the nonserious receipt.

The clock start date occurs when anyone in the company (or its agents) first receives the case, not when it first arrives in the drug safety unit.

In some countries there is a "day 0" (the day the case is first received), thus making 15-day expedited reports into "16-day reports."

COCHRANE COLLABORATION

The Cochrane Collaboration is an independent, international not-for-profit organization, dedicated to making up-to-date, accurate, impartial information about the effects of health care readily available worldwide. It produces and disseminates narrative systematic reviews and meta-analyses of healthcare interventions and promotes the search for evidence in the form of clinical trials and other studies of interventions. The Cochrane Collaboration was founded in 1993 and named for the British epidemiologist Archie Cochrane. The major product of the Collaboration is the Cochrane Database of Systematic Reviews, which is published quarterly as part of the Cochrane Library. A new appendix (Appendix 6b) of their Handbook for reviewers provides recommendations for including adverse effects in Cochrane reviews. Their website is www.cochrane.org.

Authors' note: A trusted source for pharmacoepidemiologists. It is well worth perusing their site even if one is not well versed in epidemiology.

CODE OF FEDERAL REGULATIONS (CFR)

In the US, a compilation of all final regulations, issued by federal agencies (including the FDA) and Presidential Executive Orders. It is published annually by the US government and is divided into 50 sections called "titles." For example, the regulations that govern INDs are in 21CFR312 and NDAs 21CFR314. The complete code is available online at http://www.gpoaccess.gov/cfr/index.html.

CODING

The use of a controlled and standardized vocabulary of adverse event terms and drug names. Standardized coding is done for consistency and to allow for retrieval of the data in a systematic and complete way when doing database searches, reporting to health authorities, signaling, preparing drug labels, etc.

CODING ACCURACY

The use of the most correct and appropriate term in entering an AE case into a safety database. In particular, this usually refers to the use of MedDRA for AEs and medical history and to the WHO Drug Dictionary for drug name and formulation coding. Case series retrieval and signaling cannot be accurately performed if coding is not consistent and correct. Companies and health agencies may have special "coders" whose job is to review codes and ensure their accuracy and consistency.

Authors' note: Coding can be notoriously difficult. With drugs, the exact same trade name may (unfortunately) contain totally different ingredients in different countries, making accurate coding extremely difficult. In MedDRA, with some 81,000 plus terms, coding choices can be perplexing. Should one code "skin rash on face and neck" or just "rash"? Should one code "low blood glucose" or "hypoglycemia"? Various conventions have been developed to get around these problems. However, coding still remains inconsistent. When doing a database search, it is always wise to cast a wide net and search on multiple related terms.

CODING CONVENTION

An agreed-upon method of coding or classifying an AE, a disease, a drug, etc. in order to obtain standardization and consistency in coding and to allow for complete retrieval of data at a later time. Conventions may be created by government agencies (e.g., the

FDA), CIOMS, the MSSO, a pharmaceutical company, and so forth. Examples include the use of the term "myocardial infarction" to also include "heart attack" and "myocardial infarct," or the use of "flu-like syndrome" to include fever, myalgia, malaise, etc.

CODING SYMBOLS FOR THESAURUS OF ADVERSE REACTION TERMS

See COSTART.

CODING DEPARTMENT OR UNIT

A group within a pharmaceutical company (or health authority) that verifies that AE coding (and possibly drug coding) is done in a consistent and standardized manner. This may be a separate group in a company or within the drug safety group, the clinical research group, or the quality group.

COHORT STUDY

In drug safety, a type of epidemiologic study in which two groups of patients are chosen from a database. The first group includes those who took the drug in question for a certain amount of time and the second group includes those who did not take the drug (the control or cohort group). The investigator attempts to choose a control group that is as close demographically to the exposed group as possible.

The patients' records are reviewed and the incidence of the AE in question is calculated for each of the groups. The relative risk, the absolute risk, and the risk difference may then be calculated. (See these terms.) The power to detect rare ADRs lies about midway between clinical trials and case-control studies.

COLLABORATING CENTRE FOR DRUG STATISTICS METHODOLOGY (CCDSM)

Located in Oslo, Norway, the Centre's main tasks are development and maintenance of the ATC/DDD system, including:

- Classifying drugs according to the ATC system.
- Giving priority to the classification of single substances, while combination products available internationally (i.e., important fixed combinations) will be dealt with as far as possible.
- Establishing DDDs (the defined daily dose = the average maintenance dose of a drug's main indication in an adult) for drugs that have been assigned an ATC code.
- Reviewing and revising as necessary the ATC classification system and DDDs.
- Stimulating and influencing the practical use of the ATC system by cooperating with researchers in the drug utilization field.

See http://www.whocc.no/atcddd/.

COMEDICATION, CONCURRENT MEDICATION, COMED, CONMED

In an individual case safety report, a drug given or taken at the same time as the suspect drug(s). By definition, a comedication is felt not to be suspected of causing the AE/ADR in question and not suspected of causing a drug–drug interaction.

Authors' note: It is sometimes difficult to determine whether a drug is a possible cause (suspect drug) or an innocent bystander (comed) in an AE case. Sometimes this determination is based on the known pathology and pharmacodynamics or pharmacokinetics of the drug. In other instances it may be a clinical judgment. One must, however, guard against allowing commercial interests to influence this decision.

It is also important to classify drugs correctly as suspect drugs or not since comeds may not be looked at or included in queries, signal searches, or in preparing reports to health authorities (e.g., PSURs).

COMMISSION ON HUMAN MEDICINES (UK)

The duties of this Commission, which was founded in the UK in October 2005, include:

- Advising Ministers on matters relating to human medicinal products (except homeopathic products and herbal medicines).
- Advising the Licensing Authority in relation to the safety, quality, and efficacy of human medicinal products.
- Considering representations made in relation to the Commission's advice (either in writing or at a hearing) by an applicant or by a license or marketing authorization holder.
- Promoting the collection and investigation of information relating to adverse reactions for human medicines.

The Commission is setting up expert advisory boards somewhat similar to those set up in the US by the FDA. See http://www.mhra.gov.uk/home/idcplg?IdcService=SS_GET_PAGE&nodeId=863.

COMMITTEE FOR MEDICINAL PRODUCTS FOR HUMAN USE (CHMP)

In the European Union, the Committee for Medicinal Products for Human Use is responsible for preparing the EMEA's opinions on all questions concerning medicinal products for human use. The Committee has a member and an alternate from each of the 27 EU member states, as well as Iceland and Norway.

The CHMP is responsible for conducting the initial assessment of medicinal products for which a community-wide (central) marketing authorization is sought. The CHMP is also responsible for several postauthorization and maintenance activities, including the assessment of any modifications or extensions (variations) to the existing marketing authorization.

In the 'mutual-recognition' and 'decentralized' procedures, the CHMP arbitrates in cases where there is a disagreement between member states concerning the marketing authorization of a particular medicinal product (arbitration procedure). The CHMP also acts in referral cases, initiated when there are concerns relating to the protection of public health (community referral procedure).

The CHMP plays a role in EU pharmacovigilance activity by closely monitoring reports of ADRs and, when necessary, making recommendations to the European Commission regarding changes to a product's marketing authorization or the product's suspension/ withdrawal from the market.

The CHMP can issue an 'urgent safety restriction' (USR) to inform healthcare professionals about changes as to how or in what circumstances the medication may be used.

The CHMP publishes a European Public Assessment Report (EPAR), as well as the Summary of Product Characteristics (SPC), labeling and packaging requirements, for every centrally authorized product that is granted a marketing authorization. The EPARs are available online at http://www.emea.europa.eu/htms/human/ epar/eparintro.htm.

These processes ensure that medicinal products have a positive risk-benefit balance in favor of patients and users.

The CHMP provides assistance to companies researching and developing new medicines.

The CHMP prepares scientific and regulatory guidelines for the pharmaceutical industry.

COMMITTEE FOR PROPRIETARY MEDICINAL PRODUCTS (CPMP)

Former name for the committee of the EMEA now known as the Committee for Medicinal Products for Human Use (CHMP).

COMMITTEE ON THE SAFETY OF MEDICINES (UK)

The British government advisory body within the MHRA handling drug safety. See their website: http://www.mhra.gov.uk/home/ idcplg?IdcService=SS_GET_PAGE&nodeId=301.

COMMON TERMINOLOGY CRITERIA FOR ADVERSE EVENTS

A standard created by the US National Cancer Institute to assess the severity of signs, symptoms, and laboratory abnormalities in cancer trials. Each lab abnormality has five grades: mild, moderate, severe, life-threatening, and death, illustrating a useful application of clinimetrics. There are also five categories of attribution (causality): unrelated, unlikely, possible, probable, and definite. See http://ctep.cancer.gov/forms/CTCAEv3.pdf.

Authors' note: The signs and symptoms section is brief compared to MedDRA and is used primarily in certain cancer trials. The laboratory grading (lacking in MedDRA) is, however, often used in the pharmaceutical industry to classify lab abnormalities and determine whether they are serious or not (e.g., grades 3, 4, and 5 or grades 2, 3, 4, and 5 are considered serious). The grading of clinical and laboratory manifestations belongs to clinimetrics, a segment of clinical epidemiology.

COMORBIDITY OR COMORBID CONDITION

Other diseases or conditions in addition to the one of interest in a patient. The Charlson Index (Charlson 1987) is one attempt to quantify comorbidity.

Authors' note: Comorbid conditions are important in drug safety, as they may represent confounders and must be considered as alternative causes of an AE in addition to the drug.

COMPANY CORE DATA SHEET

This document, prepared by the Marketing Authorization holder, is a summary of the key characteristics of the product. It is updated as necessary and accompanies the Periodic Safety Update Reports (PSURs) as described in the ICH E2C proposals. It includes, in addition to pharmacovigilance data, information on indications, dose, pharmacology, etc. This document (in addition to the PSURs) is not always made public, though many companies compile a "product monograph" (see this entry), which is quite similar and contains much if not all of the information in the CCDS. It includes information (particularly in regard to indications) that is not necessarily applicable in all countries where the product is sold.

COMPANY CORE SAFETY INFORMATION (CCSI)

Also called the "Core Safety Information (CSI)." This was defined originally by the CIOMS III Working Group in 1995 for all marketed drugs. The CCSI contains (only) basic safety information and not speculation or safety information that might appear in only one country's labeling for whatever reason. Thus the information in the CCSI represents the minimal safety data that should appear in all countries' labeling for that drug. Additions may be made in local labeling beyond what is in the CCSI if the local health authority or company so chooses.

Marketing considerations should not play a role in the preparation of the CCSI. AEs due to excipients should be included, but those that have no well-established relationship to the drug should not.

COMPARATIVE SAFETY DATA

Information comparing the AE profile of one product against another. Such data, unless derived from actual head-to-head clinical trials, is generally not permitted to be cited in product labeling or advertising and promotion.

COMPASSIONATE USE

Similar terms: expanded access programs, treatment IND programs, emergency use programs, named patient programs. The use by certain patients (usually with severe or end stage disease) of a product that has not yet received marketing authorization or NDA approval. It is done under carefully monitored conditions. The goals are to allow very ill patients to receive potentially life-saving treatments, as well as to collect further safety and efficacy data on the product. *See also* Named Patient Study.

Authors' note: Some advocacy groups are afraid that such studies may also serve as a form of premarketing promotion. This may be so, but these studies do seem to get the drug to patients who otherwise might never receive the treatment.

COMPENDIUM OF PHARMACEUTICALS AND SPECIALTIES

A listing of medications available in Canada. It is similar to the US *Physicians' Desk Reference* (PDR) or the French *Vidal*. It is available in English and French.

COMPETENCY IN PHARMACOVIGILANCE

A hierarchy of competencies among staff responsible for drug safety has been suggested, inspired by the UK Medicines Control Agency. (Edwards et al, Defining the competencies of those conducting pharmacovigilance, *PEDS* 2006; 15: 193–8.)

- Evidence collectors and gatherers are at the first level. They can receive, identify, validate, and sort incoming ADR reports, questions, or complaints; they can enter them in a tracking sheet.
- Evidence processors and distillers are needed to establish priority, classify and code, assess seriousness and expectedness, compare with labeling, enter into database and line listing, check coding, provide feedback to the reporter, and ask for

follow-up; assess quality, severity and causality; comply with expedited report regulations and ensure inhouse quality control; check literature. They identify and assess signals relevant to benefit-risk, and compile periodic reports.

- Risks and benefits evaluators and issue managers are needed to assess any change in benefit-risk, consider options and possible decisions, make decisions about benefit-risk, and communicate them.

COMPLAINTS

A general term used in drug safety to include adverse events and product quality issues raised by patients or healthcare providers. It generally excludes non-medical issues (cost, lack of availability, etc.).

COMPLIANCE

In drug safety, adhering to all internal requirements (standard operating procedures) and external regulatory and legal obligations in regard to safety tracking, handling, and reporting. A pharmaceutical company must always be in full legal and regulatory compliance in all countries where it sells or studies its products.

COMPLIANCE GROUP OR DEPARTMENT

In pharmaceutical companies, a department charged with ensuring that the drug safety group and others involved with safety remain in full compliance with corporate, legal, and regulatory obligations.

CONCENTRATION SITE REACTION

A rare type of localized, *in situ* reaction, often with very long latency (time after last dose). Characterized by its occurrence at the site or organ where the drug gets concentrated in the body. The following examples concern the thyroid, kidneys, brain, and gallbladder, respectively, and are all very rare:

- Radioactive iodine administered for hyperthyroid disease may produce hypothyroidism many years after the iodine is concentrated in the thyroid.
- A drug may be concentrated in the kidney and produce a nephropathy with crystalluria and calculi, leading to renal colic, insufficiency, and failure.
- Concentrations of silver in the brain and plasma at levels over 100 times normal produced coma in a patient with end-stage kidney disease after two weeks of treatment with silver sulfadiazine for second degree burns. At autopsy profoundly elevated levels of silver were found in brain tissue. (Iwasaki 1997)

- A drug can precipitate in the gallbladder as a calcium salt and produce calculi ("pseudolithiasis"), which can be detected on echography. The latency period can be very short or very long. Cholecystectomy is sometimes needed.

CONCOMITANT MEDICATION

See Comedication, Concurrent Medication, Comed, Conmed.

CONFIDENCE INTERVAL (CI)

A measure of the certainty (or uncertainty) of a value (parameter) or values that are obtained by the study of a sample of the population in question rather than of the entire population. It is usually reported as a percent confidence interval with the upper and lower boundaries given. The confidence values used in medical research are usually 95% or 99%. The higher the percentage value, the greater the confidence that the observed parameter (mean, median, correlation, rate, odds ratio, etc.) does not result from random variations of biological and clinical variables. To obtain a narrow confidence interval, one needs a concentrated variable, and/or a valid measurement tool, and/or a large sample.

For example, for an ADR with a likelihood of occurrence of 5 in every 100 patients with a calculated 95% CI of 2 to 8 in over 100 patients, we would have 95% confidence that the true ADR value for the entire population is between 2 and 8.

The narrower the range (boundaries) of the interval, the better. In situations in which the confidence interval range can "cross zero," there is significant doubt about the likelihood that the study result is correct. For example, if the rate of myocardial infarction as an ADR with drug X compared to placebo is 2% with a 95% confidence interval of −5% to +8% (meaning that drug X may be associated with fewer or more infarctions compared to placebo), then one cannot have much confidence that the rate is truly greater in the drug group.

CONFIDENTIALITY OF DATA

See Data Privacy, Privacy.

CONFLICT OF INTEREST

A situation that occurs when a person is in a position of trust that requires exercising judgment on behalf of other people or situations in which competing personal interests may interfere with the impartial exercise of judgment. Such situations should be avoided or at least publicly acknowledged when unavoidable.

In medicine and drug safety, there are many instances of possible conflicts of interest:

- In a pharmaceutical company, the drug safety group has an ethical and legal obligation to report AEs to the government, but such actions might decrease use of the drug and thus decrease company sales, bonuses, etc.
- Practicing physicians or other healthcare professionals who make presentations of a new drug to other physicians and healthcare providers and get paid for them by the manufacturer may be tempted to downplay the ADRs and fail to disclose the fees received.
- A clinical researcher who is urged to enroll as many patients as possible as rapidly as possible must, to remain ethical, put the interests of the patients above those of the study or its sponsor.

CONFOUNDING

In clinical studies, a confounder is a variable associated with both the treatment (independent variable) and the outcome (dependent variable). For example, depression is a reason for prescribing antidepressants and depression is sometimes associated with suicidal ideation. Concluding that antidepressants sometimes cause suicidal ideation is a real methodological challenge. Another example is age, correlated with the incidence of arthritic pain needing NSAIDs, but also correlated with the occurrence of myocardial infarction. Concluding that NSAIDs cause myocardial infarction also needs appropriate statistical analyses.

A confounder may hide or prevent the demonstration of a true association or it may suggest an association in the study that is not correct. Confounders may be known or unknown, and techniques are employed to diminish or eliminate as much as possible such confounders. These techniques include stratification, matching, and randomizing the study.

CONGENITAL ANOMALIES AND BIRTH DEFECTS

A type of AE observed in a newborn whose mother has been exposed to a suspect drug. Irrespective of the severity of the anomaly or defect, it qualifies as a serious AE for regulatory purposes in most countries, and the case report must be treated accordingly.

Authors' note: Not all congenital anomalies and birth defects are due to drugs. Multiple other toxins may produce anomalies and, in many cases, no particular cause is ever found.

CONSISTENCY

In drug safety, the requirement for using the same standards and criteria for various decisions made about a case: determining whether a case is serious or not, AE coding, creation of standard operating procedures, etc.

Authors' note: Consistency is obviously something everyone strives for but does not always attain. It is critical that consistency be maintained (through written SOPs, training, audits, quality review, etc.) in order to obtain the true safety profile of a drug and to protect the public health.

CONSORT GROUP RECOMMENDATIONS FOR AE REPORTING IN CLINICAL TRIALS

Most interventions have unintended and often undesirable effects in addition to intended effects. Readers need information about the harms as well as the benefits of interventions to make rational and balanced decisions. The existence of adverse effects can have a major impact on whether a particular intervention will be deemed acceptable and useful. Not all reported adverse events observed during a trial are necessarily a consequence of the intervention; some may be a consequence of the condition being treated. Randomized, controlled trials offer the best approach for providing safety data as well as efficacy data, although they cannot detect rare adverse effects.

At a minimum, authors should provide estimates of the frequency of the main severe adverse events and reasons for treatment discontinuation separately for each intervention group. When participants experience an adverse event more than once, the data presented should refer to numbers of affected participants; numbers of adverse events may also be of interest. Authors should provide operational definitions for their measures of the severity of adverse events.

Many reports of RCTs provide inadequate information on adverse events. In 192 reports of drug trials, only 39% had adequate reporting of laboratory-determined toxicity. Furthermore, in one volume of a prominent general medical journal in 1998, 58% (30 of 52) of reports (mostly RCTs) did not provide any details on harmful consequences of the interventions. *Source:* Consort 2001.

CONSUMER GROUPS

Also called activist groups, consumer activist groups, and consumer advocacy groups. In regard to drug safety this refers to collections of individuals who usually have used a product themselves (or have had someone in their family use it) and want to protect themselves and others from unsafe products, governmental or corporate abuse, misleading advertising, inefficacy, risks, misleading information, and/or excessive costs. Their actions may include lobbying, suing, or merely publicizing the use or non-use of certain products in certain diseases, sometimes on their websites or blogs.

There are also consumer groups that work to obtain more funding or research on certain diseases (e.g., the Crohn's and Colitis Foundation of America) or to lend support to sufferers.

The most outspoken group in the US concerned with drug safety is the Health Research Group division of Public Citizen, led by Dr. Sidney Wolfe. Their website is www.citizen.org/hrg/. They are the publishers of Worst Pills, Best Pills; the website is www.worstpills.org/.

CONSUMER REPORTS

1) Adverse events sent to health authorities or pharmaceutical companies by patients or normal subjects. In contrast to reports from healthcare professionals. *See* Consumers, AE/ADR Report by.

2) The name of a respected magazine published in the US. It is published by "Consumers Union, an expert, independent non-profit organization whose mission is to work for a fair, just, and safe marketplace for all consumers and to empower consumers to protect themselves. To achieve this mission, we test, inform, and protect. To maintain our independence and impartiality, CU accepts no outside advertising, no free test samples, and has no agenda other than the interests of consumers." They often cover medical and pharmaceutical issues. The publication's website is http://www.consumerreports.org/cro/aboutus/mission/overview/index.htm.

CONSUMERS, AE/ADR REPORT BY

People who consume drugs, whether they are patients or healthy individuals, may report suspected ADRs to the manufacturer and, in some countries, to health authorities.

Authors' note: In drug safety, the differentiation between consumers and healthcare professionals is a critical component (though not the sole one) in determining the validity and credibility of an AE report. For example, properly evaluating reports by patients under psychiatric care needs special expertise in the field. In some jurisdictions, an AE report must be confirmed by a healthcare professional to be valid or reportable.

CONTAINER-RELATED PROBLEMS

Product quality issues related to defects or problems in the container or packaging of a product. There may or may not be an accompanying adverse event when the container problem is reported.

CONTRACT RESEARCH ORGANIZATION (CRO)

See Clinical Research Organization.

CONTRACTOR

A person or company hired from outside the organization to perform specific duties. In drug safety, this may refer to the hiring of outside clerical or medical personnel or even a clinical research organization to process AE cases, prepare safety reports for government submission, conduct drug trials, etc. They may do the work from their own offices or the hiring company's offices.

CONTRACTUAL AGREEMENTS

See Data Exchange Agreements.

CONTRAINDICATION

In drug labeling, a disease, condition, or other reason to not prescribe a drug. There may be "absolute" contraindications in which the drug in question must never be given in any situation whatsoever (e.g., due to drug interactions, allergies, previous ADR in the same patient, etc.) or "relative" contraindications, in which the drug may be given but with the realization that the dangers may be greater than in other patients. Additional precautions may need to be taken, such as more frequent physician visits, periodic electrocardiograms, etc. In such a situation the benefit-risk balance must be very carefully weighed.

CONTROL NUMBER

See Case Number.

CONTROLLED TRIAL

An experimental clinical investigation incorporating measures ("control measures") to control known and unknown biases, confounders, and random errors.

Groups are compared in such a manner that the test drug may be compared to another drug, another intervention (e.g., surgery), or placebo. Several designs are available, such as parallel studies of two or more groups of patients with one group taking one drug and the other taking a different drug or placebo. Alternatively, one group of patients may receive one drug and then "cross over" and receive a different drug, with a comparison made between the two different treatments.

The most reliable form is the randomized controlled trial, which almost always includes double blinding.

CONTROVERSY

In pharmacovigilance, a signal may produce major controversy when

- The signal is difficult to confirm or disprove.
- A very early signal (e.g., one that is based on epidemiologic data of questionable quality) gets significant play and publicity in the lay or medical press before the pharmacovigilance investigation can be performed.
- Confirmation of the signal may produce an addition to the label of a new adverse event, warning, or precaution, leading to decreasing sales or even market withdrawal.
- Unconfirmed signals or "accusations" circulate in the media or on the Internet.

The controversies may be scientific (conflicting or contradictory evidence or interpretations of the evidence), administrative (regulations differing from one country to another), legal (lawsuits pursued by individuals or groups), business (the senior management, usually marketing and sales, demands definitive data before accepting label changes or other risk mitigation actions), and/or media driven.

CONVENTION

See Coding Convention.

CORE DATA SHEET (CDS)

The basic information that a pharmaceutical company must make available to ensure safe and effective use of its product. The safety section of this document is called the Core Safety Information (CSI) or Company Core Safety Information (CCSI). *See* Company Core Safety Information.

CORPORATE PARTNERSHIPS

See Data Exchange Agreements.

CORE SAFETY INFORMATION (CSI)

See Company Core Safety Information.

CORPORATE SAFETY COMMITTEE

In pharmaceutical companies, a committee staffed by senior people empowered to make decisions on safety issues, both routine and urgent. There should be a formal written procedure delineating the mechanism for review and adjudication of signals and safety questions. The committee should meet on a regular basis. For emergency signals, the committee should be able to meet within 24 hours, if not sooner.

The committee should be composed of the chief medical officer; chief safety officer (if not the same person); heads or senior people from drug safety/pharmacovigilance, regulatory affairs, labeling, clinical research, the legal department, preclinical (animal) toxicology/pharmacology, risk management, and epidemiology; and other corporate subject matter experts as needed (e.g., formulations). If the product is marketed outside the home country, the needs of these countries should also be represented on the committee. Marketing, sales, and similar departments should not be represented on this committee.

In health authorities, the committee structure should be constituted in a similar manner with senior medical, toxicology, pharmacology, labeling, risk management, epidemiology, and legal subject matter experts, as well as any other members needed depending on the structure of the health authority.

CORRECTIVE MEASURES (TREATMENT OF THE AE/ADR)

When the clinician observes an AE occurring in a patient being treated with medication, and if he or she suspects that one of the drugs could be causally associated with the problem, the following corrective measures can be taken in the best interests of the patient:

- Definitive cessation of the suspect product.
- Dosage reduction.
- Change in the route of administration.
- Cessation of the suspect product and substitution of:
  - another product with a similar mode of action from the same drug class.
  - another product with the same active ingredient.
  - another product from a different class of drugs.
- Cessation of the product followed by an intentional rechallenge to:
  - confirm of the diagnosis of a drug induced AE, if appropriate.
  - continue the treatment when it is deemed unacceptable to stop it (i.e., the benefit:risk ratio is still in favor of treatment).
- Continuation of the treatment without stopping even briefly because it is deemed unacceptable to stop it (i.e., the benefit:risk analysis is still in favor of treatment).

- Addition of a drug (treatment) to correct the AE/ADR (e.g., a specific or non-specific antagonist).
- Cessation of the product and addition of a corrective treatment of the AE/ADR.

CORRELATION

A statistical measure of the relationship between two variables or sets of data. It refers to the trend of changes between two variables. It is used to estimate the corresponding change in one of the variables when the other changes. The changes may be in the same direction ("positive correlation") or in the opposite direction ("negative correlation").

The correlation coefficient is usually expressed as a decimal number between -1 and $+1$, with a value of -1 meaning complete negative correlation and $+1$ meaning complete positive correlation. Zero means that there is no relationship between the two variables.

COSMETIC

The FDA defines cosmetics as "articles intended to be rubbed, poured, sprinkled, sprayed on, introduced into, or otherwise applied to the human body . . . for cleansing, beautifying, promoting attractiveness, or altering the appearance" [FD&C Act, sec. 201(i)]. Among the products included in this definition are skin moisturizers, perfumes, lipsticks, fingernail polishes, eye and facial makeup preparations, shampoos, permanent waves, hair colors, toothpastes, and deodorants, as well as any material intended for use as a component of a cosmetic product." See http://www.cfsan.fda.gov/~dms/cos-218.html.

In the EU the European Cosmetics Directive, 76/768/EC, defines a cosmetic as "any substance or preparation intended to be placed in contact with the various external parts of the human body (epidermis, hair system, nails, lips, and external genital organs) or with the teeth and the mucous membranes of the oral cavity with a view exclusively or mainly to cleaning them, perfuming them, changing their appearance, and/or correcting body odours and/or protecting them or keeping them in good condition." The term "cosmetovigilance" has been proposed to describe the surveillance of their safety.

COST CENTER

In a company, the designation used by the accounting department for any group that incurs expenses.

Authors' note: The Drug Safety Group, like any other corporate department, spends money to do its job. Unlike other groups (e.g., Sales) it does not make money for the company directly (a "profit center"). The drug safety personnel will make the argument that their group ultimately saves the company money by preventing safety problems from escalating into crises and by staying in full compliance, preventing expensive corrective actions for failure to obey all rules and regulations. Future money saved is, however, unmeasurable and this argument is perceived to be rather weak.

COSTART

An adverse event dictionary developed and used for many years by the FDA. It stands for COding Symbols for Thesaurus of Adverse Reaction Terms. It has become outmoded and has been replaced at the FDA and elsewhere by MedDRA.

COUNCIL DIRECTIVE

In the European Union, legislation from the European Council (the senior committee made of the heads of state or government of the EU member states) or its designee that binds member states to the objectives of the legislation within a certain time period but allows each member state to create its own form of national law to so achieve it. That is, each member state may modify the wording and requirements of the directive as long as the objectives of the directive are met. This is different from a regulation. *See* Council Regulation.

COUNCIL FOR INTERNATIONAL ORGANIZATIONS OF MEDICAL SCIENCES (CIOMS)

See CIOMS.

COUNCIL REGULATION

In the European Union, legislation from the European Council or designee that is directly applicable and binding in all EU member states without the need for any additional national implementation legislation. That is, the regulation as it is published is, word for word, the law in each of the member states. Note that this is somewhat different from the use of the word "regulation" in the United States. *See also* Council Directive.

COURSE OF AN ADVERSE EVENT

The medical narrative description of the adverse event in relation to time, course, and exposure to the suspected drug. Includes the date of occurrence (onset), the duration, the intensity over time (aggravation, attenuation), and the date of disappearance or resolution. Clinical and laboratory values may be relevant, to allow the calculation of the time to onset (first dose of suspect drug until first manifestation of AE) and the time to offset (last dose of suspect drug until end of AE).

COURSE, DRUG

The usual prescribed administration of a drug treatment requiring more than a single dose, in days and dosings. For example, an amoxicilin course usually refers to a 7- to 10-day course of daily dosing; a chemotherapy course might refer to five monthly infusions over 24 hours of an antineoplasic agent.

Authors' note: Some patients do not finish the course as a result of ADRs or other reasons. Non-compliance is a reality that data mining in health databases cannot always detect. In other words, prescription of a drug is not always equivalent to actual exposure.

CPMP

See Committee for Proprietary Medicinal Products (EU).

CPS

See Compendium of Pharmaceuticals and Specialties (CA).

CRISIS, DRUG SAFETY

A situation when an AE or other safety issue attains a level for which immediate action is required by the pharmaceutical company, health authority, and public. It may involve an unexpected ADR that requires an immediate recall of all supplies from the market.

For a company or a health authority, this may also refer to a situation in which it is perceived (rightly or wrongly) that the appropriate actions were not taken in regard to drug safety in a timely manner to protect the public health. This may build up over time as information is uncovered.

CRITICAL DOSE DRUG

Also called a drug with a "narrow therapeutic index or window." A drug "where comparatively small differences in dose or concentration lead to dose- and concentration-dependent, serious therapeutic failures and/or serious adverse drug reactions that may be persistent, irreversible, slowly reversible, or life threatening, that could result in in-patient hospitalization or prolongation of existing hospitalization, persistent or significant disability or incapacity, or death. Examples include oral digoxin and warfarin (anticoagulant), and injected potassium and insulin. Adverse reactions that require significant medical intervention to prevent one of these outcomes are also considered to be serious." (From Health Canada. See www.hc-sc.gc.ca/dhp-mps/prodpharma/applic-demande/guide-ld/bio/critical_dose_critique_e.html.)

CRITICAL DOSE DATE

In an ADR case report, the timing of the dose that matters when interpreting the chronological criteria for causality assessment: first dose, single dose, last dose (rebound, withdrawal reactions; latent reactions), first augmentation (dose related), first dose of interacting drug.

CRITICAL FINDING (AUDITS AND INSPECTIONS)

From the British MHRA: A deficiency in pharmacovigilance systems, practices, or processes that adversely affects the rights, safety, or well-being of patients, or that poses a potential risk to public health or that represents a serious violation of applicable legislation and guidelines. This category is the most severe of the three types of findings: critical, major, and minor. (*See* Major Finding and Minor (or Other) Finding.)

In drug safety: A finding that impacts the validity or usability of data, has a significant subject protection or safety impact, or has a significant and immediate regulatory impact. This category includes the findings of fraud, as well as repeated or deliberate actions such as non-reporting of reportable AEs, misrepresenting or hiding data, etc.

CRITICAL TERM

In the Uppsala Monitoring Centre's Vigibase, their database of worldwide ADR reports, a small number of selected ADR terms are considered "critical." Reports including critical terms warrant special attention because of their possible association with serious disease states and may lead to more decisive actions than reports on other terms.

CROS (CLINICAL/CONTRACT RESEARCH ORGANIZATIONS)

See Clinical Research Organization.

CROSSOVER STUDY

A type of comparative clinical trial in which the patients under study receive successive treatments. For example, one group of patients may first receive treatment A and another group receives treatment B. After a specified period, the patient groups are switched over. These studies are usually randomized for the sequence (AB and BA) and blinded. It is a powerful design because each patient acts as his or her own control and at the same time two parallel groups are being compared. It is less useful when the treatment leaves a detectable residual, carry-over effect, or when the design lengthens the study to the point of increasing the rate of dropouts.

CRU

See Clinical Research Unit.

CSI (CORE SAFETY INFORMATION)

See Company Core Safety Information.

CSM

See Committee on the Safety of Medicines.

COMMITTEE ON THE SAFETY OF MEDICINES (CSM)

In the UK, an independent body that advised the health authority on drugs and medicines. It was replaced in 2005 by the Commission on Human Medicines.

CULTURAL DIFFERENCES IN AE CODING

A report in 1996 noted marked transatlantic differences in the interpretation of seriousness and expectedness. For example, "total blindness for 30 minutes" was believed to be serious by 89% in the EU survey and 44% in the US survey, compared with "mild anaphylaxis," which was believed to be serious by 37% of the EU responders and 98% of the US responders. (Castle 1996)

Authors' note: These results suggest that coding will differ from region to region and emphasizes the need for harmonization and careful training of safety reviewers.

CURRENT GOOD MANUFACTURING PRACTICE (cGMP)

See Good Manufacturing Practice.

CURRENT PROBLEMS IN PHARMACOVIGILANCE

The highly respected British national bulletin of pharmacovigilance of the MHRA and the Commission on Human Medicines sent to all doctors, dentists, pharmacists, and coroners in the United Kingdom, alerting them to problems with medicines and providing advice on the ways medicines may be used more safely. The website has back issues: http://www.mhra.gov.uk/home/idcplg?IdcService=SS_GET_PAGE&nodeId=368. Replaced by *Drug Safety Updates* in 2007.

CUT-OFF DATE

See Data Lock-Point (for PSURs).

CYTOCHROME P450 SYSTEM (CYP OR P450)

Oxidative enzymes found primarily in the liver and largely responsible for drug metabolism. Drugs may alter the activity of CYP isozymes by induction or inhibition, producing drug–drug interactions. There are 18 families of CYP genes in humans.

A drug might inhibit the cytochrome P450 metabolism of another drug, increasing that drug's blood concentration to toxic levels. Alternatively, a drug may induce the enzyme and produce greater metabolism and clearance of another drug, making it less efficacious.

In the early clinical trials (phases I and II) of drugs, studies of enzyme inhibition and induction with drugs representative of one or more classes of CYP systems are usually performed. Drug metabolism belongs to the field of pharmacokinetics, the study of drug handling by the body.

Authors' note: Foods (e.g., grapefruit juice) and other substances may also inhibit or induce CYP enzymes.

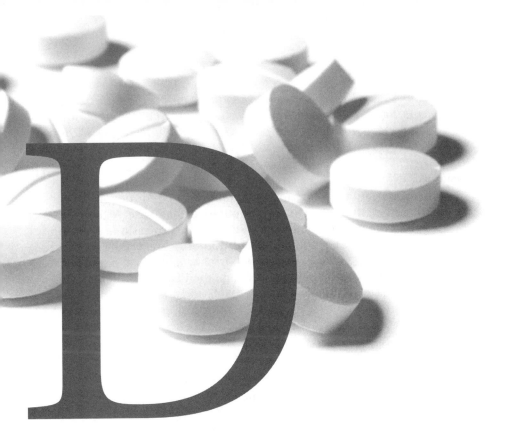

DAILYMED DATABASE

A database maintained by the US National Library of Medicine of the National Institutes of Health. It includes the FDA-approved labeling (package insert) for over 1800 drugs marketed in the US. See the website to access the database: http://dailymed.nlm.nih.gov/dailymed/about.cfm.

DATABASE, DRUG SAFETY

A dedicated informatics system (hardware, software and procedures) to receive, store, and report on drug safety data. In practice this usually refers to software that is used for individual case safety reports and aggregate reports (PSURs, NDA periodic reports, IND annual reports, etc.). Companies and health agencies either develop these databases themselves or purchase them from third parties. There are several commercial databases now in use, including ArisG by ArisGlobal, Argus by Relsys Inc., Clintrace by Phase Forward, Inc., and AERS by Oracle Inc.

Authors' note: These databases are difficult to develop and maintain and the tendency now is to purchase commercial databases

*rather than develop them. They require significant hardware, net-
working and software maintenance with frequent updates to its
components, including add-ons such as dictionaries (e.g., MedDRA,
WHO-Drug). They must be fully tested and validated.*

DATA COLLECTION

In drug safety, this refers to the obtaining of AE information and the
entering of these data into a computerized database. ADR reports
come from patients, consumers, healthcare professionals, poison
control centers, government health authorities (e.g., the FDA), and
other sources. They are collected by pharmaceutical companies,
government health authorities (e.g., the FDA), university-based
programs (e.g., teratovigilance centers), and non-governmental organizations. The WHO Uppsala Monitoring Center collects reports
already submitted to the national drug agencies.

DATA DICTIONARY

In drug safety this refers to two primary types of dictionaries:

1) A dictionary of standard codes applied to AEs, medical and surgical history, etc. The main dictionary now in use is MedDRA
(see this term). Two other dictionaries in use are WHO Adverse
Reaction Terminology (WHO-ART) and SNOMED. (See these
terms.) Other dictionaries have become outmoded.
2) A dictionary of drug names and formulations. There is one
major such dictionary used: the WHO Drug Dictionary
Enhanced. See their website: http://www.umc-products.com.

The EMEA is compiling a dictionary of drugs marketed primarily
in the European Union. It is known as the EudraVigilance
Medicinal Product Dictionary. See http://eudravigilance.emea.
europa.eu/human/evMpd01.asp.

*Authors' note: Some pharmaceutical companies use the WHO
Drug Dictionary and then either purchase the updates from WHO or
update the dictionary themselves as they see fit. This then creates a
unique company dictionary which is divergent from the WHO dictionary used by WHO and other companies.*

DATA DUMP

In drug safety, the transfer or the printing out of a dataset on a drug.
It is usually done quickly without complex querying or analysis.
For example: "I need to see all the AEs on drug X in our database,"
or "Just give me a data dump of all the AEs in a line listing."

DATA ENTRY

In drug safety, the electronic transfer or the manual keying in of AE data from source documents into the safety database. The latter is done by data entry personnel or by medical professionals depending on the company or agency.

DATA EXCHANGE AGREEMENTS

Also known as safety data exchange agreements, and safety exchange agreements. A written document signed by two or more pharmaceutical companies, CROs, distributors, etc., in which the mechanism of the exchange of all needed safety data, including serious and non-serious AEs, PSURs, NDA periodic reports, communications with regulatory agencies on safety matters, literature reports, and clinical trial information, is defined.

Authors' note: This is a complex and critical matter that must be put in place so that all parties studying, selling, and distributing the drug are able to remain in full regulatory compliance.

DATA IMPORT/EXPORT (DATABASES)

Moving safety data from one database to another such as from one company's to another's or from an old ("legacy") database to a new database. This can be very complex and requires significant planning, input, and work from information technology personnel. For safety data, moving individual case safety reports using the E2B mechanism is the most straightforward method if both parties (databases) are able to export and import (respectively) these files. Issues of different versions of MedDRA and different drug dictionaries need to be resolved. If E2B is not available, other import/export techniques must be specified and used by the information technology personnel. All imported and exported data should be validated and fully compliant with regulatory requirements.

DATA LOCK-POINT (FOR PSURs, NDA PERIODIC REPORTS, AND SO FORTH)

The date at which data in a safety database are "frozen" for analysis. That is, no additional data will be used in the report that is being prepared based on the data. Any new information will be presented in a follow-up report or the next version of the report.

For example, for a Periodic Safety Update Report covering January 1, 2007, to June 30, 2007, the data lock-point will be June 30, 2007. All data received after that time will be reported in the following PSUR. Another example: for a 15-day expedited report, all initial data and follow-up data received through day 11 will be incorporated into the expedited report. Any data received after day 11 will be reported in the follow-up expedited report.

This allows the reviewers and medical analysts to come to conclusions with sufficient time for review and approval by others involved in the analysis and reporting process.

DATA MANAGEMENT COMMITTEE

Also called safety data management committee, safety review committee, data and safety monitoring board, and data monitoring committees. *See* Data Monitoring Committees.

DATA MINING

The analysis and discovery of relationships in databases that were not previously evident or known. In drug safety, various techniques are available to display, analyze, and sort data to discover signals in large AE databases. Techniques include Bayesian analysis and proportionality methods (also called disproportionality methods).

Bayesian methodology includes the analysis of the causality of an ADR using conditional probabilities that are, in turn, modified with each new piece of information obtained, successively altering the preceding causalities to come up with a final causality.

Proportionality methods (such as proportional reporting ratios) rely on the proportion of a particular AE or series of AEs for a specific drug compared with the same AE or series of AEs for other drugs either in the same database or in a larger database.

Authors' note: Currently these methods are of interest and are being examined by health authorities, pharmaceutical companies, and academic institutions, but have not quite yet reached the point of being a major resource. Their greatest use is as a screening tool to uncover otherwise weak or non-obvious signals from large masses of data.

Data mining in the FDA AERS database needs to be made easier. The FOI version available on the Web is presented in a difficult-to-use manner. Pharmacoepidemiologists need a public, user-friendly, timely, narrative-containing, and redacted (where necessary to protect privacy) spontaneous reports database.

DATA MONITORING COMMITTEE

As defined by the FDA in its guidance (http://www.fda.gov/cber/gdlns/clindatmon.pdf): "A DMC is a group of individuals with pertinent expertise that reviews on a regular basis accumulating data from an ongoing clinical trial. The DMC advises the sponsor regarding the continuing safety of current participants and those yet to be recruited, as well as the continuing validity and scientific merit of the trial." They are not required in all studies but only those in which there is believed to be the need for additional patient safety, efficacy, and scientific validity monitoring such as "a trial that is large, of long duration, and multi-center." The committees should contain at least three members and include clinicians experienced in clinical trials as well as, in some cases, ethicists, toxicologists, epidemiologists, laboratory scientists, and even nonscientists. It is separate from the IRB.

The DMC is usually set up to receive both aggregate blinded data and unblinded data. It may also receive postmarketing data if relevant. The DMC should have the capacity to do interim analyses and to indicate to the sponsor that the study should continue or be stopped. Most analyses are for safety rather than efficacy.

The EU has published a similar guidance: http://www.emea.eu.int/pdfs/human/ewp/587203en.pdf.

DATA POOLING

The combination of data from multiple sources to improve the usefulness and, hopefully, the accuracy of the data. In drug safety, when looking for a signal or when analyzing AEs/ADRs from a known signal, data can be obtained from multiple sources (e.g., FDA AERS database, Uppsala Monitoring Centre, teratology databases, poison control center databases, etc.) to obtain sufficient cases to create a case series or to do epidemiologic analyses. Another common use is in meta-analyses of data for safety and/or efficacy in which multiple, similar clinical trials are combined to obtain sufficiently large volumes of patients to draw clinical and statistical conclusions.

Authors' note: Data pooling is always risky and many biases (unintentional or intentional) can be introduced into the analysis. On the other hand, when little data are available and are scattered through multiple databases, data pooling may play a very useful role. Of course if all studies suffer from the same bias, the meta-analysis will not be helpful.

DATA PRIVACY

In the US in 1999 the US Health Insurance Portability and Accountability Act (HIPAA) became law. This act, amongst other things, was passed to ensure patient privacy in regard to healthcare information. Its provisions include:

- Patient education on privacy protections. Providers and health plans are required to give patients a clear written explanation of how they can use, keep, and disclose their health information.

- Ensuring patient access to their medical records. Patients must be able to see and get copies of their records and request changes and corrections. In addition, a history of most disclosures must be made accessible to patients.
- Getting patient consent to release information.
- Patient authorization to disclose information must be obtained before sharing their information for treatment, payment, and healthcare operations purposes. In addition, specific patient consent must be obtained for other uses, such as releasing information to financial institutions determining mortgages, selling mailing lists to interested parties such as life insurers, or disclosing information for marketing purposes by third parties (e.g., drug companies). Getting consent must not be coerced.
- Providing recourse if privacy protections are violated.
- Disclosures of information must be limited to the minimum necessary for the purpose of the disclosure.
- Entities covered by the act must adopt written privacy procedures, train employees, and designate a privacy officer.
- Establish grievance processes for patients to make inquiries regarding the privacy of their data.

In addition, the EU in 1995 passed a directive (Directive 95/46/EC on the protection of individuals with regard to the processing of personal data and on the free movement of such data) with similar provisions. Each member state has since passed local legislation implementing this and other requirements for privacy and data protection.

Data may not be "processed" (that is, collected, recorded, organized, stored, adapted, altered, retrieved, consulted, used, disclosed) except in the following circumstances:

- The person in question has given consent.
- The processing is necessary for the performance of a contract.
- The processing is necessary to meet a legal obligation.
- The processing is needed to protect the vital interests of the person in question.
- The processing is needed to carry out a task that is in the public interest or is done in exercise of official authority.
- The person in question has the right to be informed when his or her data are processed.
- The person has the right to see all the data processed about him or her as well as the right to changes and corrections for data that are not correct or are incomplete.

- The data must be accurate and relevant to the purpose they are collected for and should not contain more information than is necessary and should not be kept longer than necessary.
- Data may not be transferred to a third country where there is an inadequate level of data protection.

Authors' note: In the world of drug safety, the US HIPAA law is not fully applicable to drug safety and pharmacovigilance data, allowing companies and healthcare practitioners to submit personal safety information to the FDA though patient privacy is expected to be protected. In the EU, however, many modifications have been required to anonymize and protect personal information. The privacy rules protect both the patients and the reporters (nurses, pharmacists, physicians, etc.).

DATA PRIVACY DIRECTIVE

See Data Privacy.

DATA RETENTION AND STORAGE

In drug safety, the retention of all data related to the safety of all products. This includes source documents, handwritten notes, memos, emails, etc. In general these data should be retained as paper if they originated as paper and electronically if they originated in that manner. Storage (retention) times vary by country or region. They should be stored in a secure, fire- and waterproof area. Electronic storage should be backed up and kept on a medium that can be read by current technology and future technology (which may require periodic transfer of the data to new media).

Authors' note: In general, safety data is often kept indefinitely, though some companies and health authorities have defined finite timeframes. Some store the data as long as the drug is actively marketed anywhere in the world plus some additional time (e.g., three years) after sales stop, as the product often has an expiration date of several years and remains in stores and medicine cabinets for long lengths of time. In addition, litigation may also occur years after an AE has occurred.

DATA SHEET

The British term for drug labeling.

DATA SHEET COMPENDIUM

The British national collective listing of drug labeling. Produced by the Association of the British Pharmaceutical Industry (see this term).

DATA AND SOFTWARE VALIDATION AND VERIFICATION

See Validation and Verification of Data and Software.

DATA WAREHOUSE

A central repository for data collected from many sources or different parts of an organization. In drug safety, this could mean that safety data from postmarketing, clinical trials, literature, health agencies, and other sources is all kept in one central location (whether on one server or on many). This implies that the data from many sources can thus be retrieved and analyzed from this single repository.

DAVIES, THE

Davies DM, Ferner RE, & de Glanville H, Eds. *Davies's Textbook of Adverse Drug Reactions*, 5th ed. London, Lippincott-Raven, 1998.

Authors' note: A unique textbook of drug-induced diseases, a developing new field of human pathology that deserves to be recognized in its own right, that should be part of medical schools curriculum, and that should inspire many more textbook authors. An update, printed and electronic, would certainly benefit the world of drug safety and those in charge of initial and continuing medical education.

DEAR DOCTOR (HEALTHCARE PROFESSIONAL) LETTER

As defined by the FDA, a letter drafted by a licensed product manufacturer, or the Agency addressed to doctors, pharmacists, and health professionals regarding important new product issues, e.g., new warnings, other safety information, or other important changes to the prescribing information (labeling). See http://www.fda.gov/cber/regsopp/8108.htm.

Authors' note: Such letters are usually sent to many types of healthcare professionals in addition to physicians and thus the term "Dear Doctor Letter" is somewhat outdated but remains in use most probably because of euphony and alliteration. In Japan it is called a "Yellow Letter."

DEATH AND SERIOUSNESS

In the postmarketing domain, death is always "serious" (see this term) for regulatory reporting purposes (e.g., expedited reports).

DEATH, RELATED

This expression designates the consequences and outcome of an AE/ADR. It implies three notions:

1. An outcome (death).
2. A suspicion of causality between the ADR and the death.
3. A suspicion of causality between the product in question and the AE (i.e., Is it an ADR?).

There is a double causality judgment here and the degree and strength of the judgment of causality can differ in points 2 and 3. For example, a death would probably be unrelated if the person died of a ruptured cerebral aneurysm while reading the newspaper a week after receiving a flu vaccine, even if there was an ADR (e.g., fever) that was due to the vaccine immediately after receiving it.

The true level of death due to medication in the general population is not known for several reasons:

- The level of underreporting of drug-related fatalities is high and variable, sometimes attaining 100%. Oncologists, for example, often do not notify manufacturers or drug agencies about drug-related deaths, though it is clear that a significant number of their patients die from chemotherapy.
- The level of medication use in the general population is not known; it is only inferred from sales figures.
- It is also not clear how to calculate risk in a way that is meaningful to the clinician. A patient who takes a few doses a year of a drug (e.g., an antihistamine for seasonal allergic rhinitis) cannot be counted with the same weight as someone who takes it daily (e.g., for perennial rhinitis). To try to get around this, statisticians convert the data, where available, into episodes of "AEs per patient-days of exposure." This allows relative comparisons of drugs, but does not always aid the clinician in deciding a specific patient's risk.

DECHALLENGE

The removal or the stopping of use of a drug by a patient. This is a critical maneuver both in medical practice and in drug safety to help assess whether the drug has produced the adverse event (causality assessment).

The AE/ADR can have the following courses:

- worsening
- persisting
- abating (improving)
- disappearing (resolving).

The correct interpretation of the course upon dechallenge can prove to be difficult, because it requires a clinician familiar not only with the medical assessment of the patient but also with the disease or AE in question and with the safety profile of the suspect drug or drugs.

If the AE disappears after the drug is stopped this is known as a "positive dechallenge," and if it persists it is a "negative dechallenge." Finally, a dechallenge may be inconclusive if

- The patient improves, but the improvement is felt to be "spontaneous" (e.g., a drug-induced headache improves spontaneously a few hours after taking a suspect drug and without any treatment).
- The problem persists but is "pathophysiologically" irreversible (e.g., the ADR is an infarct or a stroke and the damage remains).
- The event disappears as a result of corrective treatment (e.g., a drug-induced rash starts disappearing after stopping the drug and applying a topical corticoid).
- The drug has a very long half-life; stopping it cannot lead to a quick positive dechallenge (e.g., amiodarone toxicity).

In general, if a patient has a particular AE and the suspect drug is stopped (the dechallenge), and the AE abates or disappears, this may be (weakly) suggestive of the AE being caused by the drug. A stronger piece of evidence would be the recurrence of the same AE upon rechallenge (see this term).

A positive dechallenge is usually considered a strong argument in favor of causality, but it still needs to be medically interpreted because some AEs are self-limited and disappear by themselves. Similarly, a negative dechallenge needs interpretation because some AEs may be permanent whether pathogenic or iatrogenic.

Authors' note: It is appropriate and feasible to do a dechallenge if there are alternatives to the drug in question. If, however, the drug is used in a critical situation and/or if there are no or few alternatives available, and if the AE/ADR in question is not life-threatening, it may be medically and ethically appropriate to continue the drug even if the AE seems to be due to the drug. This is yet another example of the need to analyze the benefit/risk situation in the individual patient.

An interesting aspect of dechallenge is when it is collective or occurs within a large population rather than just in a single patient's case. This can occur when there is a decrease in the incidence of an AE following a reduction in exposure to a suspect drug, either through negative publicity or following withdrawal from the market. See Dechallenge, Collective.

DECHALLENGE, COLLECTIVE (POPULATIONAL)

By analogy to the stopping of a drug in an individual patient, a collective dechallenge refers to either the withdrawal from the market of a product, forcing all patients taking the drug to stop using it, or from negative publicity that decreases the use of the drug. A positive collective dechallenge has occurred if the event in question disappears from the population after withdrawal as demonstrated by public health statistics, registry information, a case-control study, or a secular trend. A positive collective dechallenge argues in favor of a drug etiology for the event.

Two examples:

- The withdrawal of thalidomide from the market was followed by a return to the baseline very low incidence of phocomelia. Clear cell cancer of the vagina again became a very rare event following the withdrawal of use of DES in pregnant women.
- In 2002 and 2003 there was a drop in new breast cancers detected in the US following the publication in 2000 of the Women's Health Initiative randomized trial about hormone-replacement therapy and the occurrence of breast cancer. Prescription rates almost halved between 2001 and 2004. The rates of cancer started to fall by 8.6% per year mid-2002 for estrogen-receptor-positive tumors in women aged 50+ years. It is believed by the authors of a NEJM special report in 2007 that the most probable explanation is a direct effect of hormone-replacement therapy on preclinical disease. See http://content.nejm.org/cgi/reprint/356/16/1670.pdf.

See Dechallenge.

DECHALLENGE, NEGATIVE

In case causality assessment, this determination is a medical judgment made when a theoretically reversible adverse reaction persists in spite of having stopped the suspect drug. In making this decision one must take into account the natural course of the event and the pharmacokinetics of the suspect drug.

A negative dechallenge is said to occur if the event worsens or persists after stopping the suspect drug. A well-interpreted negative dechallenge may argue against drug causality for the AE.

See Dechallenge.

DECHALLENGE, POSITIVE

In drug causality assessment, a medical judgment made when a theoretically reversible adverse reaction regresses or disappears after the suspect drug is stopped. One should be careful in not ascribing too much weight to positive dechallenges because factors other than the suspect drug may be acting, such as:

- The event is naturally transient (e.g., a headache).
- The event may have been due to other medications that were stopped at the same time.
- Treatments may have been administered, causing the abatement of the event.
- The kinetics of the suspect drug are such that the quick abatement of the event is unlikely to be a true positive dechallenge.

A well-interpreted positive dechallenge is an argument in favor of a causality due to the suspect drug.

See Dechallenge.

DECLARATION OF HELSINKI

A document first established by the World Medical Organization in 1964 and amended five times since then with additional "notes of clarification." The most recent version is from 2004. The declaration deals with the standards for clinical research on humans. It covers the broad areas of what research is appropriate and what is not, the ethical constraints on and obligations of the researchers, the duties of physicians, ethics, oversight, and other critical points in clinical research. Some critical points—particularly regarding risks, benefit/risk analysis, and drug safety—are as follows:

"As a statement of principles, the Declaration of Helsinki is intended to establish high ethical standards that guide physicians and other participants in medical research involving human subjects."

It is the duty of the physician to promote and safeguard the health of the people.

The Declaration of Geneva of the World Medical Association binds the physician with the words, "The health of my patient will be my first consideration," and the International Code of Medical Ethics declares that, "A physician shall act only in the patient's interest when providing medical care which might have the effect of weakening the physical and mental condition of the patient."

In medical research on human subjects, considerations related to the well-being of the human subject should take precedence over the interests of science and society.

Medical research is subject to ethical standards that promote respect for all human beings and protect their health and rights. Some research populations are vulnerable and need special protection.

Research Investigators should be aware of the ethical, legal and regulatory requirements for research on human subjects in their own countries as well as applicable international requirements. No national ethical, legal, or regulatory requirement should be allowed to reduce or eliminate any of the protections for human subjects set forth in this Declaration.

It is the duty of the physician in medical research to protect the life, health, privacy, and dignity of the human subject.

Medical research involving human subjects must conform to generally accepted scientific principles, be based on a thorough knowledge of the scientific literature, other relevant sources of information, and on adequate laboratory and, where appropriate, animal experimentation.

The design and performance of each experimental procedure involving human subjects should be clearly formulated in an experimental protocol. This protocol should be submitted for consideration, comment, guidance, and, where appropriate, approval to a specially appointed ethical review committee, which must be independent of the investigator, the sponsor, or any other kind of undue influence. This independent committee should be in conformity with the laws and regulations of the country in which the research experiment is performed. The committee has the right to monitor ongoing trials. The researcher has the obligation to provide monitoring information to the committee, especially any serious adverse events. The researcher should also submit to the committee, for review, information regarding funding, sponsors, institutional affiliations, other potential conflicts of interest, and incentives for subjects.

Medical research involving human subjects should be conducted only by scientifically qualified persons and under the supervision of a clinically competent medical person. The responsibility for the human subject must always rest with a medically qualified person and never rest on the subject of the research, even though the subject has given consent.

Every medical research project involving human subjects should be preceded by careful assessment of predictable risks and burdens in comparison with foreseeable benefits to the subject or to others. This does not preclude the participation of healthy volunteers in medical research. The design of all studies should be publicly available.

Physicians should abstain from engaging in research projects involving human subjects unless they are confident that the risks involved have been adequately assessed and can be satisfactorily managed. Physicians should cease any investigation if the risks are found to outweigh the potential benefits or if there is conclusive proof of positive and beneficial results.

Medical research involving human subjects should only be conducted if the importance of the objective outweighs the inherent risks and burdens to the subject. This is especially important when the human subjects are healthy volunteers.

Medical research is only justified if there is a reasonable likelihood that the populations in which the research is carried out stand to benefit from the results of the research.

The subjects must be volunteers and informed participants in the research project.

The benefits, risks, burdens, and effectiveness of a new method should be tested against those of the best current prophylactic, diagnostic, and therapeutic methods. This does not exclude the use of placebo, or no treatment, in studies where no proven prophylactic, diagnostic, or therapeutic method exists."

Placebo use in clinical trials was addressed in the declaration and in an amendment in 2002: "The ethics of placebo use are a complex issue and were addressed by the World Medical Association in comments amended to the Declaration of Helsinki in 2002 stating the following: The WMA hereby reaffirms its position that extreme care must be taken in making use of a placebo-controlled trial and that in general this methodology should only be used in the absence of existing proven therapy. However, a placebo-controlled trial may be ethically acceptable, even if proven therapy is available, under the following circumstances:

- Where for compelling and scientifically sound methodological reasons its use is necessary to determine the efficacy or safety of a prophylactic, diagnostic, or therapeutic method; or
- Where a prophylactic, diagnostic, or therapeutic method is being investigated for a minor condition and the patients who receive placebo will not be subject to any additional risk of serious or irreversible harm.

All other provisions of the Declaration of Helsinki must be adhered to, especially the need for appropriate ethical and scientific review.

See http://www.wma.net/e/policy/b3.htm and http://www.wma.net/e/policy/pdf/17c.pdf.

DEFINED DAILY DOSE (DDD)

A concept developed by the WHO Collaborating Centre for Drug Statistics Methodology, "the assumed average maintenance dose per day for a drug used for its main indication in adults. . . . The DDD is nearly always a compromise based on a review of the available information including doses used in various countries when this information is available. The DDD is sometimes a dose that is rarely if ever prescribed, because it is an average of two or more commonly used dose sizes."

For combination products, "the DDDs assigned for combination products are based on the main principle of counting the combination as one daily dose, regardless of the number of active ingredients included in the combination."

See http://www.whocc.no/atcddd/atcsystem.html.

Authors' note: It should be emphasized that the defined daily dose is a unit of measurement and does not necessarily reflect the recommended or prescribed daily dose. Doses for individual patients and patient groups will often differ from the DDD and will necessarily have to be based on individual characteristics (e.g., age and weight) and pharmacokinetic considerations.

Drug consumption data presented in DDDs only give a rough estimate of consumption and not an exact picture of actual use. DDDs provide a fixed unit of measurement independent of price and formulation enabling the researcher to assess trends in drug consumption and to perform comparisons between population groups.

DDDs are not established for topical preparations, sera, vaccines, antineoplastic agents, allergen extracts, general and local anesthetics, and contrast media.

DENOMINATOR

In the fraction (X/Y), the denominator is Y and the numerator is X. In the world of drug safety, the issue revolves around incidence rates and reporting rates. In a simple case, the individual AE case reports received represent the numerator and the number of patients taking the product represent the denominator. In clinical trials, these numbers are easily obtained, the problem of underreporting of AEs does not apply, and the ratio is calculated reliably.

In spontaneous reporting of AEs, however, the numerator is always underestimated since not all—often very few—AEs are reported to companies or health authorities. Similarly, the denominator is unclear because the number of patients actually exposed to the drug is usually at best a rough estimate. As an esteemed drug safety expert has said, "the numerator is bad; the denominator is worse, and the ratio is meaningless."

DEPENDENCE (DRUG)

As defined in the consensus document of the American Academy of Pain Medicine, The American Pain Society, and the American Society of Addiction Medicine (www.cpmission.com/main/

addiction.html): "Physical dependence is a state of adaptation that often includes tolerance and is manifested by a drug class specific-withdrawal syndrome that can be produced by abrupt cessation, rapid dose reduction, decreasing blood level of the drug, and/or administration of an antagonist."

See also Addiction.

DERMATOVIGILANCE

The field of pharmacovigilance relating to adverse events involving the skin and mucous membranes. These reactions may be topical or systemic. The main systemic ones include acne, alopecia, eczema, erythema, exanthema, erythroderma, fixed-drug reactions, lupus, photosensitivity, hyperpigmentation, porphyria, isolated pruritis, purpura, vesico-bullus toxiderma (Stevens–Johnson and Toxic Epidermal Necrosis), urticaria, vasculitis, and others. The main local reactions are eczema, irritation, urticaria, and photo-stimulation. As always, allergic reactions are possible.

DES

See Diethylstilbesterol.

DES-ACTION

A movement created in the United States in 1977, in Canada in 1982, in France in 1987, and in the United Kingdom in 1989. Its mission is "to identify, educate, provide support to, and advocate for DES exposed people, and to educate health care professionals." *See* Diethylstilbesterol.

See their websites:

http://www.desaction.org/index.htm (US)
http://www.web.ca/~desact/ (Canada—in French and English)
http://www.desaction.org.au/ (Australia)
http://www.des-action.org.uk/index.html (UK)
http://www.des-france.org/accueil/default.asp   (France—in French)
http://www.descentrum.nl/ (Netherlands—in Dutch)
http://www.desaction.ie/ (Ireland)

DEVELOPMENT SAFETY UPDATE REPORT (DSUR)

A proposed document by the CIOMS VI Working Group (2005) for drugs in clinical development. This document would parallel the PSUR used for marketed drugs. It would replace periodic documents used in the US, EU, and elsewhere. The CIOMS VII Working Group is now attempting to define and clarify the document and its contents, which would include:

- All relevant, new, clinical, and non-clinical safety information.
- Cumulative and interval reviews of key safety findings.
- Patient exposure data and AEs.
- Marketing authorization information, if any.
- Summary of emerging and urgent safety issues.
- Comment on changes already made or possible new changes to the investigator brochure, the clinical trial protocol(s), and informed consent(s).

DEVICE

As defined by the FDA (http://www.fda.gov/cdrh/devadvice/312.html): "An instrument, apparatus, implement, machine, contrivance, implant, in vitro reagent, or other similar or related article, including a component part, or accessory which is:

Recognized in the official National Formulary, or the United States Pharmacopoeia, or any supplement to them, intended for use in the diagnosis of disease or other conditions, or in the cure, mitigation, treatment, or prevention of disease, in man or other animals, or intended to affect the structure or any function of the body of man or other animals, and which does not achieve any of its primary intended purposes through chemical action within or on the body of man or other animals and which is not dependent upon being metabolized for the achievement of any of its primary intended purposes."

"Medical devices range from simple tongue depressors and bedpans to complex programmable pacemakers with micro-chip technology and laser surgical devices. In addition, medical devices include in vitro diagnostic products, such as general purpose lab equipment, reagents, and test kits, which may include monoclonal antibody technology. Certain electronic radiation emitting products with medical application and claims meet the definition of medical device. Examples include diagnostic ultrasound products, x-ray machines and medical lasers."

As defined by the EMEA (93/42EEC): "Medical device" means any instrument, apparatus, appliance material or other article, whether used alone or in combination, including the software necessary for its proper application intended by the manufacturer to be used for human beings for the purpose of:

- Diagnosis, prevention, monitoring, treatment, or alleviation of disease.
- Diagnosis, monitoring, treatment, alleviation of, or compensation for an injury or handicap—investigation, replacement, or modification of the anatomy or of a physiological process—control of conception.

and which does not achieve its principle intended action in or on the human body by pharmacological, immunological, or metabolic means, but which may be assisted in its function by such means."

DEVICES, SAFE MEDICAL (FDA)

The Safe Medical Devices Act of 1990 required nursing homes, hospitals, and other facilities that use medical devices to report to the FDA incidents that suggest that a medical device probably caused or contributed to the death, serious illness, or serious injury of a patient. Manufacturers are required to conduct postmarket surveillance on permanently implanted devices whose failure might cause serious harm or death, and to establish methods for tracing and locating patients depending on such devices. The act authorizes the FDA to order device product recalls and other actions.

DIA

See Drug Information Association.

DIETARY SUPPLEMENT

In the US, a dietary supplement is a product taken by mouth that contains a "dietary ingredient" intended to supplement the diet. The "dietary ingredients" in these products may include vitamins, minerals, herbs or other botanicals, amino acids, and substances such as enzymes, organ tissues, glandulars, and metabolites. Dietary supplements can also be extracts or concentrates, and may be found in many forms such as tablets, capsules, softgels, gelcaps, liquids, or powders. They can also be in other forms, such as a bar, but if they are, information on their label must not represent the product as a conventional food or a sole item of a meal or diet. Whatever their form may be, DSHEA places dietary supplements in a special category under the general umbrella of "foods," not drugs, and requires that every supplement be labeled a dietary supplement.

Authors' note: So-called dietary supplements may carry a health risk, either through abuse, intrinsic toxicity (due to labeled components or to an unacknowledged active ingredient added fraudulently), or extrinsic toxicity (due to an excipient, a metabolite, or an involuntary contaminant). In addition, counterfeit products and poorly manufactured ones may also be more at risk, including those purchased from unknown or nebulous Internet suppliers.

DIETHYLSTILBESTROL (DES)

DES is an estrogen that was first synthesized in 1938. In 1941 DES was approved for human use by the FDA. In 1947 the agency approved the use during pregnancy for the treatment/prevention of spontaneous abortion (miscarriage) based largely on the work of two researchers that eventually proved to be wrong; the drug did not prevent miscarriages. The suspicion of a problem arose in 1970, when clinicians observed a rare vaginal cancer occurring in women aged 14 to 22 years. This cancer, clear cell adenocarcinoma (CCA), was classically and rarely seen only in women in their seventies. No explanation seemed apparent until the mother of one of the young cancer patients mentioned that she had taken DES to prevent a miscarriage. Questioning of the other mothers revealed that they, too, had taken DES, and others confirmed the association between DES and CCA in a case control study in 1971. This situation is an example of long latency of onset after the last dose and is among the longest ever seen even after exposure *in utero*. It has subsequently been noted that male offspring of DES mothers may also suffer from genital abnormalities. There may also be effects in the third generation offspring, although the question requires more follow-up.

In 1971, the FDA banned the use of DES in pregnant women. In the same year, a registry was established and in 1978 the DESAD Project was developed to study DES-exposed women with adenosis. In 1973 the US National Institutes of Health notified medical schools and gynecologic oncologists about increased cancer risk.

DIRECT (PRIMARY) EFFECT

An ADR produced directly by the suspect product. The opposite is a secondary or indirect effect that is triggered by the primary AE, producing a sort of cascade effect.

DIRECTIVES, EU

Legislation that binds European Union member states to the objectives of the legislation within a certain time period but allows each member state to create its own form of national law to so achieve it. That is, each member state may modify the wording and requirements of the directive as long as the objectives of the directive are met.

DISABILITY

The FDA has defined this term as "a substantial disruption of a person's ability to conduct normal life functions." [21 CFR 314.80(a) and 310.305(b)]

The EU has multiple definitions of disability from country to country and language to language. It has issued a 239-page guide to comparative definitions (http://ec.europa.eu/employment_social/publications/2004/cev502004_en.pdf).

DISABILITY, PERSISTENT

There is no formal definition of a "persistent disability" by the FDA or EMEA or E2A. A standard dictionary definition of "persistent" is "continuing or not-ending." An AE producing persistent disability is considered having a serious outcome.

Authors' note: In practice, this refers to a disability or incapacity that lasts longer than would normally be expected in the view of a medical professional, or that is really permanent. Some call it a sequelum.

DISCLAIMER

A term designating the denial or refusal of legal responsibility.

DISCONTINUATION

In regulatory matters, this is a more neutral term than the *suspension* or *withdrawal* of a product from the market. In pharmacotherapy matters, this term is equivalent to the cessation or interruption of the suspect product in a patient. It may be permanent or temporary.

DISCOVERY PROCESS (IN LITIGATION)

The formal procedures used to obtain compulsory disclosure of pertinent information and documents by one or both parties before trial in a civil lawsuit. This allows each party to find out ("discover") the opponent's version of the issues. A newer concept is "electronic discovery" (e-discovery or ediscovery), in which electronic data (email, memos, reports, spreadsheets, etc.) are similarly obtained.

In drug safety, this usually means a litigant requesting from a company all AE records and other documents relating to a particular drug for use in a lawsuit.

DISPROPORTIONALITY METHODS

Disproportionality methods (also called proportionality methods) rely on the proportion of a particular AE or series of AEs for a specific drug compared with the same AE or series of AEs for other drugs either in the same database or in a larger database. If there is a greater proportion of a particular AE for drug X compared to the rest of the drugs in the database, this "disproportion" is suggestive of a signal and may be worth further investigation. It is usually expressed as a whole number and fraction. For example, a dispro-portionality statistic of 1.33 for AE X with drug Y means that, com-pared to the rest of the database, the AE X is 33% more frequent with drug Y compared to the rest of the database. A figure below 1.0 (e.g. 0.97) means it is less frequently seen than compared to the rest of the database.

Authors' note: In safety databases, there is always background noise and there will always be some level of disproportionality with some AE–drug combinations appearing more or less frequently com-pared to the rest of the database due to random errors. In practice, the critical issue is determining what the threshold is to begin a sig-nal investigation. A low threshold will have higher sensitivity but lower specificity than a higher threshold. This will produce more real signals but more false positives. Thus users may set higher thresholds or avoid thresholds altogether and simply look at the top ten or twenty AE–drug combinations.

DMC (DATA MONITORING COMMITTEE)

See Data Monitoring Committees.

DOCUMENTED REACTION

This phrase, which implies a well-documented reaction, refers to a previously confirmed ADR with the suspect product in previously reported cases. It concerns an adverse reaction that is clearly ac-cepted to be associated with the suspect medication. It means the suspect drug is recognized to be capable of producing the AE in question, but it does not mean it did so in a new given case being assessed.

DOCUMENTED REPORT

This phrase, which implies a well-documented report, is synony-mous with a "valid report" in the broadest sense of the word and means a report whose validity includes factual correctness, plau-sibility, and relatedness to the drug (causality).

DOPING

The use of substances, often prescription medications, with the aim of improving sports performance (in humans or animals such as race horses). The objective is neither medical nor therapeutic because the subjects are in good health and are not "patients." The substance is either obtained illicitly or with the complicity of a medical professional who writes a prescription that is filled through normal channels. The prescriber should bear in mind his or her responsibilities concerning the prevention, detection, and correction of adverse reactions—some of which may be severe, have long latency periods, or even be fatal.

DOSE DEPENDENT ADR

An adverse drug reaction whose occurrence, frequency, or severity increases with the amount of the drug taken.

Authors' note: It may appear after the first dose or the first augmentation of dosing, and then disappear upon dose reduction or complete withdrawal. The mechanism is pharmacologic, predictable, and type A in safety jargon. It may be an exaggeration of the desired effect, or an effect on undesired targets/receptors (lateral, side effect). It may occur after a normal dose in susceptible individuals as a result of a concomitant drug interaction or a concomitant pathology (e.g., low body weight, low renal function).

DOSE, TIME, SUSCEPTIBILITY CLASSIFICATION (DoTS)

This recently proposed classification aims at facilitating the implementation of recent E2E guidelines about pharmacovigilance planning.

Dose

- Supratherapeutic doses (alias toxic effects; includes overdose, equivalent to type A, predictable, exaggerated action on desired targets).
- Standard therapeutic doses (collateral effects, alias side effects, equivalent to type A, predictable, action on undesired targets).
- Subtherapeutic doses in susceptible patients (equivalent to type B, unpredictable; allergic or idiosyncratic).

Time

- Time-dependent reactions: Rapid, first dose, early, intermediate, late, delayed.
- Time-independent reactions: May occur at any time during long-term treatment.

Susceptibility

- Risk factors include genetic variability, age, sex, physiological condition, exogenous factors (drug interactions, etc.), concomitant diseases.

DOSSIER

In medical practice, a file containing information on a patient, including his or her drug history and associated ADRs. In drug regulation, a submission made to a health agency requesting the permission to study a drug in humans (e.g., IND) or to market a drug (e.g., NDA).

Authors' note: The documents presented to the authorities to obtain the marketing authorization for a new product or formulation include the results of the phases I, II, and III studies. In the case of a product already on the market, new data must be submitted containing additional studies for a new indication or formulation. The dossier is usually confidential under the terms of "industrial secrets" or "proprietary information." This unfortunately prevents the medical and pharmacoepidemiology world from obtaining full knowledge of all the ADRs observed in the course of the clinical trials. (See Erice Declaration on Effective Communication in Pharmacovigilance).

DOUBLE OR DUPLICATE REPORTING

The sending, receiving, or having in a drug safety database the same case more than once. This is to be strenuously avoided as it gives a falsely elevated number of AEs reported to be associated with a drug. When two reports of the same case are found, all data should be combined into one case and the other case removed from the active database ("archived"). Initial and follow-up reports on the same case should be recognized as such and combined and not carried as two separate cases with two separate identification numbers.

Authors' note: This usually occurs because the same case is reported to the health authority or pharmaceutical company by the patient, the pharmacist, and/or the physician without each knowing the other was reporting it. Other situations occur when a case that was previously reported and entered into the safety database is found in a literature publication or a data collection from another source (e.g., another health agency or a poison control center). It is the duty of the database owner to ensure that all efforts are made to minimize duplicate reporting.

Duplicate reporting can present major problems in pharmacovigilance when the case in question is a very serious or critical reaction (e.g., aplastic anemia, Stevens–Johnson syndrome, torsades de pointes, fulminant liver failure, etc.) and it cannot be ascertained whether there are two reports or only one.

How duplicate reports come about is interesting. Sometimes it is malevolent, especially in regard to the published medical literature, with the same report initially published in slightly different contexts in different journals. More innocently it might be published alone and then later published as one of a series of similar events but with insufficient detail to be sure it is a true duplicate. In other cases an event might be reported to a national agency, which then reports it to the WHO Collaborating Centre, where it is not always clear that it is a duplicate report. Similarly, a spontaneously reported AE sent to the national agency may also be reported to the manufacturer and/or other national agencies (e.g., a report originating in Canada is reported by the company to Health Canada but also to the US FDA and the European national agencies). Transcription errors, recoding into different drug dictionaries, and incomplete data may also produce multiple duplicate reports.

A more subtle problem arises when there is a single AE in question but the information in the two reports is complementary. For example, a pharmacist reports a case that does not contain exactly the same demographic or medical details as the report of the prescribing physician. Another problem occurs when the telephone report to the manufacturer does not contain the same information as the written or electronic version sent to the authorities.

Finally, a new problem is arising with the tightening of privacy (data protection) laws around the world. In many cases the identity of the patient must be anonymized with the removal of any identifiers such as birthdate, age, initials, sex, or even country of origin. In these situations, it is often hard to know whether similar reports represent one or two different instances of the reaction.

DRUG, DRUG PRODUCT, MEDICATION

A chemical substance used to modify the functioning of a biologic organism for medical reasons and administered in the form of a pharmaceutical product. For the WHO, a drug is:

"Any substance administered to man for the prevention, diagnosis or treatment of a disease or for the modification of a physiologic function."

A medication is prepared as a commercial product whose galenic form includes the active ingredient (moiety) and excipients.

Whatever the purpose of its use, a molecule that affects human biology can present a serious safety problem.

- *Illicit drugs (i.e., street drugs):* Usage of the products here is not approved and is considered "recreational." The drugs may be commercial products produced by the pharmaceutical industry (either unchanged or adulterated on the street) or they may be products of questionable origin, content, and quality. The word "drugs" thus has two senses in English: drugs that are "good," i.e., drugs that are used for medical purposes to treat disease, and "bad," i.e., drugs that are used for recreational ends.

- *Sports drugs:* The use of illicit or commercial drugs with the aim of improving athletic performance. Drugs used include anabolic steroids, erythropoietin, amphetamines, and others. Their use is almost always outside of approved indications (for legal drugs) and is forbidden by the International Olympic Committee and most other professional and organized amateur sports. *See* Doping.
- *Food supplement:* This expression refers to substances that are used for nutritional reasons (vitamins, minerals, etc.). However, in some countries the definition is rather broad. In the United States, this includes such products as melatonin and St. John's Wart.
- *Iodine:* Iodine given to populations at risk for goiter is considered to be a nutritional supplement in some countries. It has also been used as a preventative when given to people living near nuclear reactors from which radioactive iodine accidentally escaped. The iodine serves as a competitor to the radioactive iodine that was accumulating in the thyroid, thus decreasing the risk of hypothyroidism.
- *Melatonin:* For the physiologists, melatonin is a hormone secreted by the pineal gland. For others, it is a natural product and a food supplement not governed by the drug laws of the country and easily available in health food stores and supermarkets. To researchers in the pharmaceutical industry, it is the starting point for the development of analogues (drugs) with fewer adverse drug reactions and better targeted efficacy for the treatment of jet lag or sleep problems. To be a drug or a food supplement is simply a question of point of view.
- *Diagnostic agent:* The clinician can administer a pharmaceutical product whose goal is purely diagnostic (radiocontrast agents, glucose for a glucose tolerance test, etc.).
- *Pharmacologic agent:* This term refers to the use of products for biologic testing (e.g., in receptor research).

The regulatory definition of a drug and a device can differ from country to country, with the same product being considered a device in one country and drug in another, producing peculiar and even paradoxical reporting situations. Note that in some pharmacovigilance regulatory situations, the term drug may also include biologics.

DRUG ALLERGY
See Allergy, Drug.

DRUG ANALYSIS PRINT

Complete listings of the suspected adverse drug reactions reported to the British MHRA through the Yellow Card Scheme (see this term) by healthcare professionals and patients are available online for the benefit of prescribers, scientists, and patients. Generic names are entered and ADRs are compiled by organ-system and MeDDRA preferred terms. This is an example to follow by other countries. See http://www.mhra.gov.uk.

DRUG CATEGORIES (IN AN INDIVIDUAL CASE SAFETY REPORT)

As proposed by ICH E2B, a drug or drugs may be categorized by the reporter, the manufacturer, or the health authority in one of three ways in a spontaneous report of an AE/ADR:

- *Suspect drug:* The drug is suspected of having contributed to the AE/ADR.
- *Concomitant drug:* The drug is not suspected of having contributed to the AE/ADR, but was taken by the patient.
- *Suspected of interaction:* Two drugs that are suspected of interacting together to produce the AE/ADR.

DRUG CODE

A number assigned to each drug/formulation in drug coding dictionaries for use in computerized systems to record and track drugs involved in AE cases. For example, WHO-ART uses a complex numbering system of up to 17 digits to identify a drug according to its name, market authorization holder, country, dosage form, and strength. See for further information http://www.umc-products.com/DynPage.aspx?id=2829.

Combination drugs pose additional problems as a product may have as many as five different active ingredients, each with a code as well as one for the overall product in some dictionaries.

Authors' note: Drug coding is a very tricky business and is often the source of error or confusion in AE reports. Care should be taken to be sure the proper formulation is found and correctly coded.

DRUG DICTIONARIES

There are several listings of drugs sold around the world. The Uppsala Monitoring Centre maintains the WHO-ART dictionary (http://www.umc-products.com/DynPage.aspx?id=2829), which is widely used either as is or modified by pharmaceutical companies. Another dictionary is the EudraVigilance Medicinal Product Dictionary from the EMEA (http://eudravigilance.emea.eu.int/human/evMpd01.asp).

Authors' note: Unlike AE coding dictionaries such as MedDRA (where there are few new diseases and codes now that the dictionary is fairly "mature"), drug dictionaries are very difficult to maintain as new drugs are introduced or withdrawn somewhere in the world every day. There are also issues of language and alphabet that can add to the confusion.

See Data Dictionary.

DRUG FACTS LABEL

The labeling on OTC products in the US that went into effect in 2002. It lists in a standardized format using large type:

- The product's active ingredients, including the amount in each dosage unit.
- The purpose of the medication.
- The uses (indications) for the drug.
- Specific warnings, including when the product should not be used under any circumstances, and when it is appropriate to consult with a doctor or pharmacist. The warnings section also describes side effects that could occur and substances or activities to avoid.
- Dosage instructions addressing when, how, and how often to take the medication.
- The product's inactive ingredients, which is important information for those with specific allergies.

It generally appears on the outside packaging of the product and on the bottle, tube, etc., itself. See http://www.fda.gov/fdac/features/2002/402_otc.html.

DRUG HOLIDAY

Withdrawing a single product at a time in a patient exposed to multiple pharmaceutical products (polypharmacy), which are suspected at various degrees of causing an adverse event. If the adverse event abates afterward, the dechallenge is termed positive and the product is stopped, replaced, or its dosage reduced.

This term is also used to refer to the time a patient chooses (often against medical advice) to stop taking his or her medications for a short while (e.g., over a holiday).

DRUG-INDUCED HEPATITIS

See Hepatitis.

DRUG INFORMATION ASSOCIATION (DIA)

The largest professional association for those in the pharmaceutical industry, health authorities, academia, and others with interest in the pharmaceutical world. Membership is inexpensive. Extensive educational offerings are available both online and in person. The annual US meeting is held in June, the EU meeting in March, and the Canadian meeting in the autumn. They have several publications and services, including a job bank. See http://www.diahome.org/DIAHome/Home.aspx.

DRUG INFORMATION CENTER

A phone service offered to prescribers, pharmacists, and sometimes the public, freely or upon a small fee, providing information on the safe use of drugs. Several are academically based and/or merged with a poison control center. They are mostly handled by pharmacists and often are associated with colleges/faculties of pharmacy and less frequently with medical schools. In Europe some are combined with a pharmacovigilance center. They often communicate with a manufacturer's safety unit and with their national drug agency.

DRUG INTERACTIONS

The modification of the action of a first drug in a patient by the consumption of a second product. The effects produced may or may not be desirable. The mechanism may be pharmacokinetic (the second product altering blood or tissue levels of the first drug with or without pharmacologic consequences) or pharmacodynamic (the second product producing an effect of its own on the body and interfering with the first drug).

There are several types of interactions:

- *Drug–drug interactions:* two or more drugs interact with each other to produce alterations in the kinetics and/or dynamics of one or more of the drugs in question.
- *Drug–food interactions:* Taking a drug with food in which absorption is altered, or which produces changes in kinetics (as is the case with grapefruit juice and several drugs) or dynamics of the drug (e.g., broccoli and cranberry juice reduce the action of the anticoagulant warfarin).
- *Drug–alcohol interactions:* Similar to drug–food interactions, but with reference to alcoholic beverages.
- *Drug–herb interactions:* Similar to drug–food interactions, but with reference to nutraceuticals.

See http://www.fda.gov/cder/consumerinfo/druginteractions.htm.

DRUG INTERACTION STUDIES

These clinical studies, which are usually done in phase II or phase III, look at the most common and predictable drug–drug, drug–food, and (sometimes) drug–alcohol interactions. For most drugs, this is done in normal volunteers.

For drug–drug studies, a typical drug from one or more of the main cytochrome P450 isoenzyme groups involved in drug metabolism by the liver (e.g., CYP1, CYP2, and CYP3) is chosen for study.

Authors' note: If not determined by studies, new drug–drug interactions are discovered by spontaneous reporting after the marketing of a new product. In this respect pharmacovigilance is irreplaceable.

DRUG LABELING

For drugs that are not yet on the market (i.e., not yet approved for sale) the labeling used for adverse event (AE) reporting is considered to be the official Investigator Brochure (see this term).

After a New Drug Application (NDA) in the US or request for Marketing Authorization in the EU or elsewhere is approved and the drug is marketed, the labeling that is used for regulatory reporting of AEs now changes to the document prepared by the sponsor and submitted to, negotiated with, and approved by the health authority, such as the US Package Insert, the EU Summary of Product Characteristics, or the Canadian Product Monograph.

In the US, the official definition of labeling for a marketed NDA product is noted in 21CFR1.3(a):

(a) Labeling includes all written, printed, or graphic matter accompanying an article at any time while such article is in interstate commerce or held for sale after shipment or delivery in interstate commerce.

(b) "Label" means any display of written, printed, or graphic matter on the immediate container of any article, or any such matter affixed to any consumer commodity or affixed to or appearing upon a package containing any consumer commodity.

Thus, drug labeling includes the FDA-approved written material describing a drug, such as the "package insert," and the packaging and box that a drug is shipped or sold in.

Labeling for an OTC product in the US is known as the "Drug Facts Label" (see this term) and is printed on the package and/or container.

Synonyms for labeling include "package insert," "professional labeling," "direction circular," and "package circular." Canadians often use the term "product monograph" and "official product monograph."

In the EU, the approved labeling is known as the Summary of Product Characteristics (SPC or SmPC). The EU situation is complex, with labeling being dependent on whether the drug was approved at the EMEA level or at the national level (or by "mutual recognition") and whether it was "harmonized" or not. Thus the labeling may be the same throughout the EU or may differ from country to country.

Note that the generic term "labeling" (sometimes called the "package insert") is used to refer to the official FDA-approved US product information. The word "labeling" is also used in the United States for the SPC when referring to European labeling. Some in the EU, conversely, use the term SPC (or SmPC) when they are referring to their own official European labeling or to the US labeling. Thus one might hear a reference to the US SPC—a concept that does not really exist in the United States. This refers, in practice, to the US official labeling.

DRUG MONITOR

Also known as the Local Safety Officer. This term refers to the person responsible for pharmacovigilance, either during clinical trials or after marketing, in the pharmaceutical industry.

The term may also refer to the medical personnel surveilling patients in a clinical trial at the study site.

DRUG MONITORING

1) In drug safety, this refers to the system or systems put in place to track or do surveillance on AEs and ADRs reported with drugs. In the clinical trial setting this refers to AEs reported by the investigator to the sponsor and noted in the case report form. For marketed drugs, this refers to the "spontaneous reporting systems" (see this term) set up in many countries around the world as well as to any additional surveillance systems set up as part of a risk management program such as registries, informed consent, and sentinel sites, comprising the duties of collection, processing, analysis, and signaling of adverse drug events. Equivalent to pharmacovigilance, drug surveillance, and safety surveillance.

2) In pharmacotherapy, it refers to the very tight and scrupulous surveillance of the patient under drug therapy with the goal of

maximizing the benefits (efficacy) and minimizing the adverse drug reactions (risk). Also referred to as therapeutic drug monitoring. Often includes the measurement of plasma drug level/activity, such as lithium levels in bipolar patients or INR (coagulation test) in patients on warfarin (antivitamin K).

DRUG NAMES

What a drug is called. A drug may have multiple names, which poses frequent problems in drug safety.

A drug may have a chemical name of the active moiety (e.g., cimetidine), a chemical name (N- cyano-N'-methyl-N"-((E)-2-([(5-methyl-1H-imidazol-4-yl)methyl]sulfanyl)ethyl)guanidine,1-cyano-2-methyl-3-(2-(((5-methyl-4-midazolyl)methyl)thio)ethyl)g uanidine,2-cyano-1-methyl-3-(2-(((5-ethylimidazol-4-yl)methyl)thio)ethyl)guanidine), a US Adopted Names Council (USAN) name (cimetidine), an International Nonproprietary Name (INN) (cimetidine), and one or more trade names (Tagamet®, Stomedine®, etc.).

Authors' note: Some drugs use the same trade name in different countries for different active moieties. This prompted the FDA to warn the public in 2006 that "for example, in the United States, 'Flomax' is a brand name for tamsulosin, a treatment for an enlarged prostate, while in Italy, the active ingredient in the product called 'Flomax' is morniflumate, an anti-inflammatory drug. In the United States, 'Norpramin' is the brand name for an antidepression drug containing desipramine but, in Spain, the same brand name, 'Norpramin,' is used for a drug that contains omeprazole, a treatment for stomach ulcers."

It is thus wise for people in drug safety to get as many names as possible as well as the formulation for drugs that are to be noted in AE reports.

Drug names may be found at health agency websites or in books such as Martindale—The Complete Drug Reference and the Merck Index.

DRUGS

A well-respected journal published 18 times a year by the ADIS group in New Zealand. It covers emerging and contentious issues in pharmacology, narrative reviews of drugs and drug classes, guides to drug treatment, drug evaluations, and product profiles reviewing innovations in patient management. It is not concerned primarily with drug safety, which is covered by its sister publication, *Drug Safety*. See the website http://drugs.adisonline.com.

DRUG SAFETY

1. The generic term referring to the surveillance of investigational and marketed drugs for their untoward effects. The term is often used, by extension, to include biologics, devices, nutritionals, etc. Equivalent to pharmacovigilance when marketed drugs are concerned.
2. The group or department in a pharmaceutical company charged with receiving, tracking, databasing, analyzing, and reporting AEs.
3. The group within a governmental health authority charged with organizing and monitoring postmarketing drug surveillance.

This expression has two additional meanings, according to context:

4. In medical practice: Describes the danger or lack of danger that a particular medication presents ("safety of a drug") as in "Drug safety in Mr. Jones is of primary importance since he is 96 years old, in moderate renal failure, and is also taking four different medications."
5. In regulatory affairs: Equivalent to pharmacovigilance ("drug safety surveillance"), as in "Every pharmaceutical company must, by law, have a department of Drug Safety."

DRUG SAFETY

A major journal published monthly by the ADIS group in New Zealand. It is the official journal of the International Society of Pharmacovigilance (ISoP). The journal publishes reviews on the epidemiology, clinical features, prevention, and management of adverse effects of individual drugs and drug classes, benefit-risk assessments, and original research on drug safety issues. See http://drugsafety.adisonline.com.

DRUG SAFETY BOARD, FDA

A panel formed in 2005 consisting of FDA staff and representatives from the National Institutes of Health and the Veterans Administration. The Board advises the Director, Center for Drug Evaluation and Research, FDA, on drug safety issues and works with the agency in communicating safety information to health professionals and patients.

DRUG SAFETY OVERSIGHT BOARD

See Data Management Committee.

DRUG SAFETY RESEARCH UNIT (DSRU)

An independent organization associated with the University of Southampton in the UK whose work is principally concerned with the detection of AEs and ADRs associated with selected newly marketed drugs. The specific technique used is known as Prescription-Event Monitoring (PEM), a form of cohort follow-up where 'recorded medical events' are compared during and after exposure to a new drug. This approach generates signals which, through pharmacoepidemiology, can be investigated in order to determine relevant concerns over drug safety. The Unit publishes its findings in international peer-reviewed journals. It has inspired a related approach in New Zealand, the Intensive Medicines Monitoring Programme (IMMP). See http://www.dsru.org/main.html.

DRUG WATCH WEBSITE (FDA)

In a guidance article published in May 2005, the FDA described a website entitled "Drug Watch" that they will create to disseminate important emerging drug safety information to healthcare professionals and patients concerning marketed drug products. The intent is to identify drugs for which the FDA is actively evaluating early safety signals. See http://www.fda.gov/cder/guidance/6657dft.pdf.

DRUG–DRUG INTERACTION

See Drug Interactions.

DRUG–EVENT RELATIONSHIP

The association of the taking of a drug product and the occurrence of an AE. The analysis of the relationship, with the aim of trying to determine whether the drug caused the event, is a fundamental function of drug safety and pharmacovigilance.

Authors' note: The analysis may be quite easy (e.g., cutaneous injection site reactions) or very difficult and complex. Data may be lacking or contradictory and one may never be able to come to a definitive conclusion about an individual case, especially if the background noise or prevalence rate of the AE is high. In the latter cases, it may be necessary to do clinical or epidemiologic trials to clarify the relationship. See Causality.

DRUGS AND THERAPEUTIC BULLETIN

A journal published by the British Medical Journal Publishing Group. DTB's main aims are:

- To provide informed and unbiased assessments of drugs and other treatments (concentrating on their efficacy, safety, convenience, and cost—in particular in relation to other available treatments).

- To comment on how those drugs or other treatments should be used.
- To assess a drug's place in overall patient management.
- To review evidence and give practical advice on the overall management of disease.
- DTB's related aims are to comment on how treatments are marketed and promoted, on the quality of the information available to prescribers and patients, and on the indication(s) for which the treatment has been licensed.

See www.dtb.bmj.com.

DRUGS OF CURRENT INTEREST (AUSTRALIA)

A section of the Australian health authority's (TGA) bimonthly bulletin on drug safety. (*See The Australian Adverse Drug Reactions Bulletin.*)

"The initial months and years of a drug's availability are crucial for gaining new information on safety in a large, diverse population. For this reason, ADRAC established its "Drugs of Current Interest" (DOCI) scheme in August 1990. This list generally includes all new drugs that are expected to be used widely in Australia, or those for which the Committee has identified an area of safety concern or uncertainty. Drugs normally remain on the list for 2 years, as this is the time period when the reporting of suspected adverse reactions is usually highest. It should be noted that removal of a drug from the DOCI list does not necessarily mean that all safety concerns have been answered. The DOCI scheme is a simple method to obtain safety information about marketed medicines."

The current list of such drugs appears on the front of every *Bulletin*. These drugs are reviewed regularly by the TGA for safety issues arising from spontaneous reports, the published literature, overseas regulatory agencies, or any other source. The agency asks that all suspected adverse reactions to these drugs be reported to them.

DRUGS UNDER SURVEILLANCE

In pharmacovigilance bulletins, this refers to a list of products that are the subject of intensified reporting of AEs (either a specific AE or all AEs seen with the product). This is done because the product is very new on the market or belongs to a family of drugs for which there is a specific risk, or because a signal regarding this drug has already been reported and a call for intensified scrutiny and reporting of AEs is required.

The placing of a drug on the intensified scrutiny list is done purely for scientific reasons to gain further information in order to be able to decide whether the signal is confirmed or rejected.

DSM-IV

The Diagnostic and Statistical Manual of Mental Disorders is a handbook published by the American Psychiatric Association and is used to diagnose and classify mental disorders. It is now in its fourth edition. It is "multi-axial," meaning it classifies the disorders in five areas or "axes":

Axis I: Major mental disorders, clinical disorders
Axis II: Underlying pervasive or personality conditions, developmental disorders, and learning disabilities, as well as mental retardation
Axis III: Medical conditions contributing to the disorder
Axis IV: Psychosocial and environmental factors contributing to the disorder
Axis V: Global Assessment of Functioning

In drug safety, mental disorders and AEs are generally coded in MedDRA rather than in DSM-IV.

DSUR

See Development Safety Update Report.

DUE DILIGENCE REVIEW

A review usually done by a pharmaceutical company before it purchases or licenses a new drug to investigate and/or sell. This includes the review of manufacturing data, animal toxicology and pharmacology data, clinical data, safety data, and regulatory correspondence with the FDA, European Medicines Evaluation Agency, and others.

The drug safety department may be called in during this "due diligence" review to examine the clinical safety data, including MedWatch and CIOMS forms, NDA periodic reports, IND annual reports, PSURs, rapporteur responses to PSURs, "raw" clinical trial and postmarketing safety data, regulatory correspondence, and animal toxicology data. Attention should be paid, in clinical trial data, to dropouts, deaths, lack of efficacy, and lost-to-follow-up cases and any other areas where safety data might be less than obvious.

DUPLICATE CASE

See Double Reporting.

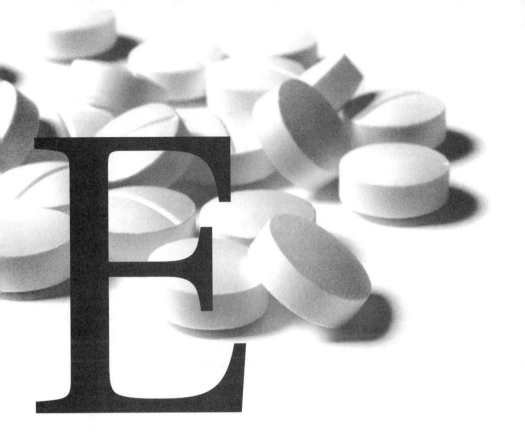

E2A DOCUMENT AND REPORTING RULES

A 1994 document from ICH officially entitled *Clinical Safety Data Management: Definitions and Standards for Expedited Reporting.* It is an early and key document in drug safety that set many of the standards now in use. Some key points:

The document described definitions and terminology for safety reporting as well as how to handle expedited (alert) reporting. The document was originally developed to cover clinical trial safety reporting, but its concepts have been extended to postmarketing (approved) drugs as well. It defined adverse events (AEs), adverse drug reactions (ADRs), and unexpected ADRs (serious and severe).

The document set the standard that all ADRs that are both serious and unexpected should be expedited. This means that, for clinical trial reports, all three categories (causality, seriousness, and unexpectedness) for AEs must be present to make a report expedited. They should be submitted in 7 calendar days if fatal or life-threatening followed 8 calendar days later with a 15-day report. Other serious unexpected ADRs should be submitted in 15 calendar days.

It defined the minimum criteria for a valid AE: an identifiable patient, a suspect medicinal product, an identifiable reporting source, an event or outcome that is serious and unexpected and, for clinical trial cases, a reasonable suspected causal relationship. Follow-up information should be sought and reported as soon as it becomes available. Reporting should be on the CIOMS I form.

The document also recommended that although advantageous to retain the blind for all patients before study analysis, when a serious adverse reaction is reportable on an expedited basis, the blind should be broken only for that specific patient by the sponsor even if the investigator has not broken the blind.

See http://www.ich.org.

E2B DOCUMENTS

The output of two working groups (1997–2000) set up by ICH to develop the means for the Electronic Transmission of Individual Case Safety Reports (ICSRs) among companies and health authorities. This would replace the use of paper-based MedWatch and CIOMS I forms. The data elements, fields, and contents of the electronic report were rigidly standardized. There are two series of documents in question, which are very technical.

The first are the E2B documents, which were prepared by the medical representatives and specified in detail the data elements to be included in the transmission. The second are the M2 documents, prepared by the informatics representatives and that provide technical informatics specifications for structured messaging; electronic data interchange; data definitions to incorporate structured data formats (SGML); security to ensure confidentiality, data integrity, authentication, and nonrepudiation; documents to handle heterogeneous data formats; and physical media for storage and transferability of data.

There are several documents that cover the various aspects of electronic transmission:

- E2B(M): Maintenance of the Clinical Safety Data Management, including Data Elements for Transmission of Individual Case Safety Reports.
- E2B(R): Revision of the E2B(M) ICH Guideline on Clinical Safety Data Management: Data Elements for Transmission of Individual Case Safety Reports.
- E2B(M): Maintenance of the Clinical Safety Data Management, including Questions and Answers.
- SGML DTD (Document Type Definition), Version 1.0 and related files for structured electronic data interchange data.

- DTD Version 2.0, ICSR Acknowledgment Message and related files.
- DTD Version 2.1, ICSR Acknowledgment Message and related files, which includes M2 Version 2.3 Specification Document.

See http://www.ich.org.

E2B TRANSMISSION

Data Elements For Transmission Of Individual Case Safety Reports between companies and/or health authorities.

The electronic equivalent of a MedWatch or CIOMS I report of a case. They are now obligatory for 15-day expedited reports in many EU countries and Japan and are optional (for now) in the US and other countries.

E2C DOCUMENTS

Clinical Safety Data Management: Periodic Safety Update Reports for Marketed Drugs.

Two documents (the original and addendum) from ICH describing the format and content of safety updates, which need to be provided at intervals to health authorities after products have been marketed.

The *original document* was published to ensure that the same worldwide safety information is provided to authorities at defined times after marketing. It defined the Periodic Safety Update Report (PSUR), which has been adopted by many countries.

Key points are:

- One report for one active substance. The PSUR should cover all dosage forms, formulations, and indications. The PSUR should be a "standalone" document.
- For combination products also marketed individually, safety information may be done as a separate PSUR or included in the PSURs prepared for one of the components with cross-referencing.
- The report should present data for the interval of the PSUR only except for regulatory status information, renewals, and serious unlisted ADRs, which should be cumulative.
- The report should focus on ADRs. All spontaneous reports should be assumed to be reactions (i.e., possibly related). Reports should be from healthcare professionals. For clinical trial and literature reports, only those cases believed by the reporter and sponsor to be unrelated to the drug should be excluded.

- Lack of efficacy reports (which are considered to be AEs) should not be included in the tables, but should be discussed in the "other information" section.
- Increased frequency reports for known reactions should be reported if appropriate.
- Each product should have an international birth date (IBD), usually the date of the first marketing authorization anywhere in the world. This date should be synchronized around the world for PSUR reporting such that all authorities receive reports every 6 months or multiples of 6 months based on the IBD.
- The report should be submitted within 60 days of the data lock-point.
- The reference document for expectedness should be the company core data sheet (CCDS), the safety section of which is known as the company core safety information (CSI).
- The verbatim reporter term as well as standardized coding term (i.e., MedDRA, which was approved after E2C was finished) should be used.
- ADR cases should be presented as line listings and summary tabulations. Individual CIOMS I or MedWatch forms are not included.

The sections of a PSUR are as follows:

- Introduction.
- Worldwide market authorization status.
- A table with dates of market authorization and renewals, indications, lack of approvals, withdrawals, dates of launch, and trade names.
- Update of regulatory authority or MAH actions taken for safety reasons.
- Changes to the Reference Product Information.
- Patient exposure.
- Presentation of individual case histories from all sources (except nonmedically confirmed consumer reports).
- Line listings.
- Studies.
- Other information (lack of efficacy cases, late-breaking information after database lock).
- Overall safety evaluation by system organ class with a discussion of:
  —changes in characteristics of listed reactions
  —serious unlisted reactions, placing into perspective the cumulative reports
  —nonserious unlisted reactions

—increased frequency of listed reactions
—new safety issues
—drug interactions
—overdose and its treatment
—drug misuse or abuse
—pregnancy and lactation
—experience in special patient groups
—effects of long-term treatment
—conclusion, as well as any action recommended or initiated.

The *addendum* (2003) provided clarification and guidance on the original document and addressed some new concepts:

International Birth Dates (IBDs)

PSURs should be based on IBDs. To transition to a harmonized IBD, the company may submit the already prepared IBD-based PSUR plus (1) line listings PSURs and/or tabular summaries for the additional period or (2) an Addendum Report (see below).

In attempting to harmonize IBDs, it is possible that a drug will be on a 5-year cycle in one country and a 6-month cycle in another. If harmonization is not possible, the company and regulators should try to find a common birth day and month so that reports can be submitted on the same month and day whether every 6 months, yearly, or every 5 years (or every 3 years).

Summary Bridging Reports

A summary bridging report integrates two or more PSURs to cover a specific time period for which a single report is requested. Thus two 6-month PSURs could be used to create a summary bridging report to cover the full year or ten 6-month reports to cover a 5-year PSUR. The bridging report does not contain new data but briefly summarizes the data in the shorter reports.

Addendum Reports

An addendum report is used when it is not possible to synchronize PSURs for all authorities requiring submissions. The addendum report is an update to the most recently completed PSUR. It should be used when more than 3 months for a 6-month PSUR and more than 6 months for a longer PSUR. It is not intended as an in-depth report (which will be done in the next regularly scheduled PSUR). It should contain an introduction, any changes to the CSI, significant regulatory actions on safety, line listings, and/or summary tabulations and a conclusion.

Restarting the Clock

For products in a long-term PSUR cycle (e.g., 5 years), the return to a 6-month reporting schedule may occur if a new indication is approved, a previously unapproved use in a special population is approved, or a new formulation or route of administration is approved. The restarting of the reporting clock should be discussed with the regulatory authorities.

Additional Time for Submissions
In rare circumstances, the company may request an additional 30 days to submit a PSUR. This might occur if there is a large number of case reports and there is no new safety issue, if issues are raised by the authorities in the previous PSUR for which additional time is needed for further analysis for the next PSUR, or if issues are identified by the company needing further analysis.

Reference Safety Information
The MAH should highlight differences between the CSI and the local product labeling in the cover letter accompanying the PSUR. For 6-month and 1-year PSURs, the CSI in effect at the beginning of the period should be used as the reference document.

For PSURs longer than 1 year, the CSI in effect at the end of the period should be used as the reference document for PSURs and Summary Bridging Reports.

Other Issues
An executive summary should be included.

Patient exposure data are often difficult to obtain and not always reliable. If the exposure data do not cover the full period of the PSUR, extrapolations may be made. A consistent method of exposure calculations should be used over time for a product.

The section containing individual case histories should describe the criteria used to describe the cases summarized. The section should contain selected cases, including fatalities, presenting new and relevant safety information and grouped by medically relevant headings or system organ class.

Consumer listings (AEs reported by non-medical professionals and not validated or verified by a healthcare professional), if required by regulators, should be done in the same way that other listings and summary tabulations are prepared.

The studies section should contain only those company-sponsored studies and published safety studies (including epidemiology studies) that produce findings with potential impact on safety. The company should not routinely catalogue or describe all studies.

Discussion and analysis for the "Overall Safety Evaluation" section should be organized by system organ class and not by listedness or seriousness. Risk management programs may be discussed.

When a more comprehensive safety or risk-benefit analysis has been done separately, a summary of the analysis should be included here.

See http://www.ich.org.

E2D DOCUMENTS

Post Approval Safety Data Management: Definitions and Standards for Expediting Reporting

These documents (2003) provide a standardized procedure for postapproval safety data management, including expedited reporting. It parallels and adds to the E2A document, which covered preapproval (clinical trial) safety data management. Key points:

Definitions

Adverse Event: The definition is nearly identical to the E2A version, leaving out the reference to clinical trials. "An AE is any untoward medical occurrence in a patient administered a medicinal product and which does not necessarily have to have a causal relationship with this treatment. An adverse event can therefore be any unfavorable and unintended sign (for example, an abnormal laboratory finding), symptom, or disease temporally associated with the use of a medicinal product, whether or not considered related to this medicinal product."

Adverse Drug Reaction: This definition is similar to the preapproval definition (E2A) but defines the causality component in the postmarketing setting ("at least a possibility" of a causal relationship). "All noxious and unintended responses to a medicinal product related to any dose should be considered adverse drug reactions. The phrase 'responses to a medicinal product' means that a causal relationship between a medicinal product and an adverse event is at least a possibility (refer to ICH E2A). A reaction, in contrast to an event, is characterized by the fact that a causal relationship between the drug and the occurrence is suspected. If an event is spontaneously reported, even if the relationship is unknown or unstated, it meets the definition of an adverse drug reaction."

Serious AE/ADR: This definition is the same as the one in E2A for preapproval issues. "Any untoward medical occurrence that at any dose that results in death, is life-threatening, requires inpatient hospitalization or results in prolongation of existing hospitalization, results in persistent or significant disability/incapacity, is a congenital anomaly/birth defect, is a medically important event or reaction. Medical and scientific judgment should be exercised in deciding whether other situations should be considered as serious such as important medical events that may not be immediately life-threatening or result in death or hospitalization but may jeopardize the patient or may require intervention to prevent one of the other outcomes listed in the definition above. These should also be considered serious."

Unexpected ADR: The definition of expeditedness is somewhat different from that in E2A for preapproval cases because the reference documents are different (investigator brochure for preapproval and the local labeling for marketed drugs). In addition, class labeling is discussed. This is summarized briefly: "An ADR whose nature, severity, specificity, or outcome is not consistent with the term or description used in the official product information should be considered unexpected. An ADR with a fatal outcome should be considered unexpected, unless the official product information specifies a fatal outcome for the ADR. In the absence of special circumstances, once the fatal outcome is itself expected, reports involving fatal outcomes should be handled as for any other serious expected ADR in accord with appropriate regulatory requirements." Note that the term "listedness" is not applicable for expedited reporting (refer to ICH E2C for definition in which listedness refers to whether the reaction is noted in CSI for PSURs). "Class ADRs" should not automatically be considered to be expected for the subject drug. "Class ADRs" should be considered to be expected only if described as specifically occurring with the product in the official product information.

Healthcare professional: "Any medically-qualified person such as a physician, dentist, pharmacist, nurse, coroner, or as otherwise specified by local regulations." The person does not have to be the prescriber of the suspected product.

Unsolicited Sources of AEs

Spontaneous reports: These are unsolicited communications by healthcare professionals or consumers to a company, regulatory authority, or other organization (e.g., World Health Organization, Regional Centers, Poison Control Center) that describe one or more ADRs in a patient who was given one or more medicinal products and that does not derive from a study or any organized data collection scheme.

Stimulated reporting: AE/ADR reports that are "provoked" by some external driver, such as a "call for reporting," the sending of *'Dear Healthcare Professional'* letters, a listing of suspected products among "drugs of special interest or drugs under surveillance" in a National Drug Bulletin, a publication in the press, or questioning of healthcare professionals by company representatives. Also known as prompted reporting, active pharmacovigilance. These reports should be considered spontaneous.

Consumer reports: These should be handled as spontaneous reports irrespective of any subsequent "medical confirmation," a process required by some authorities for reportability. Emphasis should be placed on the quality of the report and not on its source. Even if reports received from consumers do not qualify for regulatory reporting, the cases should be retained in the database.

Literature: The Marketing Authorization Holder (MAH) is expected to regularly screen the worldwide scientific literature (not just in English) by accessing widely used systematic literature reviews or reference databases according to local requirements or at least every 2 weeks. Cases of ADRs from the scientific and medical literature, including relevant published abstracts from meetings and draft manuscripts, might qualify for expedited reporting.

Clock Start: The regulatory reporting time clock starts once it is determined that the case meets minimum criteria for reportability. If the product source, brand, or trade name is not specified, the MAH should assume that it was its product, although reports should indicate that the specific brand was not identified.

Internet and E-mail: MAHs are not expected to screen external websites for ADR information. However, if an MAH becomes aware of an adverse reaction on a website that it does not manage, the MAH should review the case and determine whether it should be reported. Unsolicited cases from the internet should be handled as spontaneous reports. Regarding e-mail, identity of the reporter needs to be evaluated to see whether it refers to the existence of a real person. That is, it is necessary to verify that the patient and reporter exist.

Other Sources: Cases from nonmedical sources, such as the lay press, should be handled as spontaneous reports.

Solicited sources of AEs: This refers to cases from organized, structured data collection systems, which include clinical trials, postapproval named patient use programs, other patient support and disease management programs, surveys of patients or healthcare providers, or information gathering on efficacy or patient compliance. AE reports obtained from any of these should not be considered spontaneous. For the purposes of safety reporting, solicited reports should be handled as if they were study reports and therefore should have an appropriate causality assessment.

Contractual Agreements
If companies make contractual arrangements to market a product in the same or different countries or regions, explicit agreements

must be made to specify the processes for exchange of safety information, including timelines and regulatory reporting responsibilities, though the MAH is ultimately responsible. Duplicate reporting should be avoided.

Individual serious unexpected ADR reports originating from foreign regulatory authorities are always subject to expedited reporting. Resubmission of serious ADR cases without new information to the originating regulatory authority is not usually required, unless otherwise specified by local regulation.

Standards for Expedited Reporting

For reports from studies and other solicited sources, all cases judged by either the reporting healthcare professional or the MAH as having a possible causal relationship to the medicinal product qualify as ADRs. For the purposes of reporting, spontaneous reports associated with approved drugs imply a possible causality.

Other Observations

Any significant unanticipated safety findings, including in vitro, animal, epidemiologic, or clinical studies, that suggest a significant human risk and could change the benefit-risk evaluation should be communicated to the regulatory authorities as soon as possible.

Lack-of-efficacy observations should not be expedited but should be discussed in PSURs unless local requirements oblige their being expedited.

Overdoses with no associated adverse outcome should not be reported as adverse reactions. The MAH should collect any available information on overdose related to its products.

Minimum criteria for reporting include an identifiable reporter, an identifiable patient, an adverse reaction, and a suspect product. The MAH is expected to exercise due diligence to collect missing data elements.

Reporting time frames for expedited reports are normally 15 calendar days from initial receipt of the minimal information by any personnel of the MAH, which is day 0. Additional medically relevant information for a previously submitted report restarts the clock.

Good Case Management Practices

One or more of the following automatically qualifies a patient as identifiable: age (or age category; e.g., adolescent, adult, elderly), gender, initials, date of birth, name, or patient identification number. In the event of second-hand reports, every reasonable effort should be made to verify the existence of an identifiable patient and reporter. All parties supplying case information or approached for case information should be identifiable.

In the absence of qualifying descriptors, a report referring to a definite number of patients should not be regarded as a case until the minimum four criteria for case reporting are met.

The objective of the narrative is to summarize all relevant clinical and related information, including patient characteristics, therapy details, medical history, clinical course of the event(s), diagnosis, and ADR(s), including the outcome, laboratory evidence, and any other information that supports or refutes an ADR. The narrative should serve as a comprehensive standalone "medical story." The information should be presented in a logical time sequence; ideally, this should be presented in the chronology of the patient's experience rather than in the chronology in which the information was received. In follow-up reports, new information should be clearly identified.

Abbreviations and acronyms should be avoided, with the possible exception of laboratory parameters and units.

An ADR report should be reviewed by the recipient for the quality and completeness of the medical information. This should include, but is not limited to, the following: Is a diagnosis possible? Have the relevant diagnostic procedures been performed? Were alternative causes of the reaction(s) considered? What additional information is needed? The report should include the reporter's verbatim term (and, in the case of consumer reports, the consumer's description of the event). Staff receiving reports should provide an unbiased and unfiltered report of the information from the reporter. Clearly identified evaluations by the MAH are considered acceptable and, for some authorities, required.

Follow-up information: The information from ADR cases when first received is generally incomplete. Efforts should be made to seek additional information on selected reports. The first consideration should be prioritization of case reports by importance: cases that are (1) both serious and unexpected, (2) serious and expected, and (3) nonserious and unexpected. In addition to seriousness and expectedness as criteria, cases "of special interest" also deserve extra attention as a high priority (e.g., ADRs under active surveillance at the request of the regulators), as well as any cases that might lead to a labeling change decision. Follow-up should be obtained by a telephone call, site visit, and/or a written request. The MAH should provide specific questions it would like answered. The MAH should tailor the effort to optimize the chances of obtaining the new information. Written confirmation of details given verbally should be obtained whenever possible. Ideally, healthcare professionals with thorough pharmacovigilance training and therapeutic expertise should be involved in the collection and the direct follow-up of reported cases.

Pregnancy Exposure

MAHs are expected to follow up all reports, from healthcare professionals or consumers, of pregnancies where the embryo/fetus could have been exposed to one of its medicinal products. The CIOMS I form has been widely accepted. MedDRA should be used for coding. E2B should be implemented for electronic transmission of individual cases.

See http://www.ich.org.

E2E DOCUMENTS

Pharmacovigilance Planning

These documents (2004) cover planning pharmacovigilance activities and risk management, especially in preparation for the early postmarketing period of a new drug. It is recommended that company pharmacovigilance experts get involved early in product development. Planning and dialogue with regulators should also start long before license application. For products with important identified risks, important potential risks, or important missing information, the pharmacovigilance plan should include additional actions designed to address these concerns. For products for which no special concerns have arisen, routine pharmacovigilance should be sufficient for postapproval safety monitoring, without the need for additional actions (e.g., safety studies). During the course of implementing the various components of the plan, any important emerging benefit or risk information should be discussed and used to revise the plan.

A Pharmacovigilance Plan for a product has three sections: Safety Specification, Pharmacovigilance Plan, and an Annex (Pharmacovigilance Methods).

Safety Specification

The safety specification is a summary of the important identified risks of a drug, important potential risks, and important missing information. It should also address the populations potentially at risk (where the product is likely to be used) and outstanding safety questions that warrant further investigation to refine understanding of the benefit-risk profile during the postapproval period.

It should focus on the identified risks, important potential risks, and important missing information. It should refer to the three safety sections in the Common Technical Document. The following elements should be considered for inclusion.

Nonclinical. This section should present nonclinical safety findings that have not been adequately addressed by clinical data, for example, toxicity (including repeat-dose toxicity, reproductive/developmental toxicity, nephrotoxicity, hepatotoxicity, genotoxicity, carcinogenicity, etc.), general and safety pharmacology (cardiovascular, including QT/QTc interval prolongation, nervous system, etc.), drug interactions, and other toxicity-related information. If the product is intended for use in special populations, consideration should be given to whether specific nonclinical data need to exist.

Clinical. Limitations of the human safety database (e.g., related to the size of the study population, study inclusion/exclusion criteria) should be considered and discussed. Particular reference should be made to populations likely to be exposed during the intended or expected use of the product in medical practice. The worldwide experience should be discussed, including the extent of the worldwide exposure, any new or different safety issues identified, any regulatory actions related to safety, and populations not studied in the pre-approval phase (children, elderly, pregnant or lactating women, patients with relevant comorbidity such as hepatic or renal disorders, patients with disease severity different from that studied in clinical trials, subpopulations carrying known and relevant genetic polymorphism, patients of different racial and/or ethnic origins).

AEs/ADRs: This section should list the important identified and potential risks that require further characterization or evaluation. Discussion of risk factors and potential mechanisms should draw on information from the Common Technical Document and other relevant information, such as other drug labels, scientific literature, and postmarketing experience.

Identified risks that require further evaluation: More detailed information should be included on the most important identified AEs/ADRs, which would include those that are serious or frequent and that also might have an impact on the balance of benefits and risks of the product. This information should include evidence bearing on a causal relationship, severity, seriousness, frequency, reversibility, and at-risk groups, if available. Risk factors and potential mechanisms should be discussed. These AEs/ADRs should usually call for further evaluation as part of the pharmacovigilance plan (e.g., frequency in normal conditions of use, severity, outcome, at-risk groups).

Potential risks that require further evaluation: Important potential risks should be described and the evidence that led to the conclusion that there was a potential risk should be presented. It is anticipated that for any important potential risk, there should be further evaluation to characterize the association.

Identified and potential interactions, including food–drug and drug–drug interactions, should be discussed with consideration of the evidence, and the potential health risks posed for the different indications and in the different populations should be discussed.

Epidemiology. The epidemiology of the indication should be discussed, including incidence, prevalence, mortality, prognosis when untreated, and relevant comorbidity, and should take into account whenever possible stratification by age, sex, and racial and/or ethnic origin. Differences in the epidemiology in the different regions should be discussed (because the epidemiology of the indication(s) may vary across regions), if this information is available. For important AEs that may require further investigation, it is useful to review the incidence rates of these events among patients in whom the drug is indicated (i.e., the background incidence rates).

Pharmacologic class effects. The safety specification should identify risks believed to be common to the pharmacologic class.

Summary: This should include (a) the important identified risks, (b) potential risks, and (c) missing information on an issue-by-issue basis.

Pharmacovigilance Plan

The pharmacovigilance plan should be based on the safety specification and developed by the sponsor. It can be discussed with regulators during product development, before approval (i.e., when the marketing application is submitted) of a new product, or when a safety concern arises postmarketing. It can be a standalone document. For products for which no special concerns have arisen, routine pharmacovigilance should be sufficient for postapproval safety monitoring, without the need for additional actions (e.g., safety studies). However, for products with (a) important identified risks, (b) important potential risks, or (c) important missing information, additional actions designed to address these concerns should be considered. It should be updated as important information on safety becomes available and milestones are reached. The format and content should include the following:

- Summary of ongoing safety issues, including the important identified risks, potential risks, and missing information.
- Routine pharmacovigilance practice should be conducted for all medicinal products, regardless of whether or not additional actions are appropriate as part of a pharmacovigilance plan. This routine pharmacovigilance should include the following:
  - Systems and processes that ensure that information about all suspected adverse reactions that are reported to the per-

sonnel of the company are collected and collated in an accessible manner.

- o The preparation of reports for regulatory authorities including expedited ADR reports and PSURs.
- o Continuous monitoring of the safety profile, including signal detection, issue evaluation, updating of labeling, and liaison with regulatory authorities.
- o Other requirements, as defined by local regulations.
- o Action plan for safety issues. The plan for each important safety issue should be presented and justified according to the safety issue, objective of proposed action, action proposed, rationale for proposed action, monitoring by the sponsor for safety issue and proposed action, and milestones for evaluation and reporting. Any protocols for specific studies may also be provided.
- Summary of actions to be completed, including milestones:
  - o An overall pharmacovigilance plan for the product bringing together the actions for all individual safety issues should be presented and organized in terms of the actions to be undertaken and their milestones.
  - o It is recommended that milestones for completion of studies and for submission of safety results be included in the pharmacovigilance plan. The milestones should reflect when exposure to the product will have reached a level sufficient to allow potential identification/characterization of the AEs/ADRs of concern or resolution of a particular concern and when the results of ongoing or proposed safety studies are expected to be available.
  - o These milestones might be aligned with regulatory milestones (e.g., PSURs, annual reassessment, and license renewals) and used to revise the pharmacovigilance plan.
- Pharmacovigilance methods:
  - o The best method to address a specific situation can vary, depending on the product, the indication, the population being treated, and the issue to be addressed. When choosing a method to address a safety concern, sponsors should use the most appropriate design.
- Design and conduct of observational studies:
  - o Carefully designed and conducted pharmacoepidemiologic studies, specifically observational (noninterventional, nonexperimental) studies, are important tools in pharmacovigilance.
  - o A protocol should be finalized and experts from relevant disciplines (e.g., pharmacovigilance experts, pharmacoepidemiologists, and biostatisticians) should be consulted. It is

recommended that the protocol be discussed with the regulatory authorities before the study starts. A study report after completion, and interim reports if appropriate, should be submitted to the authorities according to the milestones within the pharmacovigilance plan.

- The sponsor should follow good epidemiologic practice for observational studies and also internationally accepted guidelines, such as the guidelines endorsed by the International Society for Pharmacoepidemiology.

Annex

- A detailed discussion of pharmacovigilance methods is appended to the document to which the reader is referred for further details.

See http://www.ich.org.

ECOPHARMACOLOGY AND ECOPHARMACOVIGILANCE

This new concept, introduced by Klaus Kümmerer at the 2005 meeting of the International Society of Pharmacovigilance, deals with the environmental aspects of medical products. Whereas the highest stability is needed for human use, environmental protection needs compounds quickly metabolized to harmless substances after release in water, air, and soil. Residues of drugs have been found in the London sewage system.

ELDERLY

There is actually no universally accepted definition. Some use the so-called mandatory retirement age (65) that some companies or governments use. Others use the age when a pension or governmental social security starts (e.g., 66 in the US for some people). Some geriatricians will say 80 years of age but most will make an individual evaluation of a patient independent of age.

In clinical research, studies in the "elderly" vary with regard to the minimum age of inclusion; 65 is commonly used but studies in the "very elderly" may use 80 years of age.

Authors' note: The term should be replaced by the ages in scientific publications because safety issues may differ markedly between 65- and 85-year-olds.

ELECTRONIC DATA CAPTURE (EDC)

Also known as "remote data entry" (RDE). In clinical trials, the system whereby the investigator enters case report data for the study directly into a computer located at the study site rather than writing the information down in a paper case report form (CRF). This includes the safety data (adverse events), which arrive at the sponsor's or CRO's site in real time (immediately). It saves the investigator from having to create a separate written safety report for a patient with an AE that is then faxed or scanned and emailed to the sponsor.

ELECTRONIC SIGNATURE (DIGITAL SIGNATURE)

This refers to the issue surrounding the verification of authenticity of an electronically transmitted file. It is the counterpart of the written signature on a paper document. AE reports are now sent electronically (see *ICH E2B*) to health authorities and the assurance that a signature given currently on paper documents will be required for the electronic transmissions. Two definitions of an electronic signature have been proposed:

"An electronic sound, symbol or process attached to or logically associated with a record and executed or adopted by a person with the intent to sign the record."

"Information in electronic form that a person has created or adopted in order to sign a document and that is in, attached to or associated with that document."

In the US Code of Federal Regulations (21 CFR11) , an FDA regulation describes the criteria under which the agency considers electronic records, electronic signatures, and handwritten signatures executed to electronic records to be trustworthy, reliable, and generally equivalent to paper records and handwritten signatures executed on paper. Databases and submissions to the FDA must be compliant with these requirements.

ELECTRONIC RECORD ARCHIVING

See Archiving.

ELECTRONIC TRANSMISSION

The sending of an individual case safety report from a company or sponsor to a health authority. The usual standard for such a transmission is the E2B/M2 standard. *See* E2B.

EMA (FORMERLY EMEA)

European Medicines Agency.

E-MAIL AE REPORTS

The receipt by a company or regulatory agency of spontaneous adverse events by email. Issues of privacy, secrecy, and follow-up have been raised. This issue has been addressed in the ICH E2D document (see this term). Email addresses that might receive AEs should be screened frequently to be sure such cases are not missed.

Some companies transmit AE reports either within the company or to other companies involved in comarketing or some other joint venture using e-mail. They may, for example, make a pdf version of a MedWatch or CIOMS I form, attach this to an e-mail, and send it to the other company. The same issues of privacy, secrecy, and so forth arise.

EMERGENCY USE PROGRAMS

See Compassionate Use Programs.

END POINT, SAFETY

In a clinical trial, a predefined event or series of events that will either end that patient's participation in the study or will end the study itself. The end point may be positive or negative.

For a positive example, in testing a new hypertension medication in a clinical trial in which the dose is escalated depending upon clinical response, the patient may stop having an increase in dose if his or her systolic pressure decreases to, say, 120 to 124 mmHg (the safety end point). This is both an efficacy end point (successful lowering of the blood pressure) but also a safety end point as anything lower might produce symptomatic hypotension.

For a negative example, in testing an angina pectoris medication, if the patient has more than a certain number of episodes of angina (e.g., 2 per day), the patient will stop participation in the study for safety reasons and resume standard therapy.

In clinical trials in which there is a drug and safety monitoring board or interim analyses, there may be certain safety criteria at which point the study will be stopped. For example, in testing a new lipid lowering agent in large groups of patients with hyperlipidemia, if the death rate in the treated group exceeds that of the control group (safety end point) the study may be stopped for safety reasons.

EOSINOPHILIA MYALGIA SYNDROME (EMS)

A severe syndrome characterized initially by myalgia, cramps, edema, fatigue, shortness of breath, skin rash, and other symptoms. After resolution of the acute symptoms neuropathy, myopathy, and skin changes persist. This may last years.

This was first seen in 1989 in the US and was traced to L-tryptophan (an essential amino acid found in foods) sold over the counter. The FDA initiated a nationwide recall in 1989 of all over-the-counter dietary supplements containing 100 milligrams or more of L-tryptophan due to a clear link between the consumption of L-tryptophan tablets and EMS. By 1990 the CDC noted over 1,500 cases of EMS, including 38 deaths. The FDA has prohibited the importation of L-tryptophan and has restricted domestic sales. It was never fully clarified whether the syndrome was due to the L-tryptophan, an excipient, or something else occurring with the product.

EUROPEAN MEDICINES AGENCY (EMA, EMEA)

The regulatory body covering the 27 countries in the European Union. The agency has many responsibilities, including drug safety and pharmacovigilance. Located in the Canary Wharf section of London, England. Formerly known as the European Medicines Evaluation Agency (EMEA).

From the EMEA website: Its main responsibility is the protection and promotion of public and animal health, through the evaluation and supervision of medicines for human and veterinary use.

The EMEA is responsible for the scientific evaluation of applications for European marketing authorization for medicinal products (centralized procedure). Under the centralized procedure, companies submit one single marketing authorization application to the EMEA.

All medicinal products for human and animal use derived from biotechnology and other high-technology processes must be approved via the centralized procedure. The same applies to all human medicines intended for the treatment of HIV/AIDS, cancer, diabetes, or neurodegenerative diseases and for all designated orphan medicines intended for the treatment of rare diseases. Similarly, all veterinary medicines intended for use as performance enhancers in order to promote the growth of treated animals or to increase yields from treated animals have to go through the centralized procedure.

The safety of medicines is monitored constantly by the Agency through a pharmacovigilance network. The EMEA takes appropriate actions if adverse drug reaction reports suggest changes to the benefit-risk balance of a medicinal product. For veterinary medicinal products the Agency has the responsibility to establish safe limits for medicinal residues in food of animal origin.

The Agency also has a role to stimulate innovation and research in the pharmaceutical sector. The EMEA gives scientific advice and protocol assistance to companies for the development of new medicinal products. It publishes guidelines on quality, safety, and efficacy testing requirements.

In 2001, the Committee for Orphan Medicinal Products (COMP) was established, charged with reviewing designation applications from persons or companies who intend to develop medicines for rare diseases (so-called 'orphan drugs'). The Committee on Herbal Medicinal Products (HMPC) was established in 2004 and provides scientific opinions on traditional herbal medicines.

The Agency brings together the scientific resources of over 40 national competent authorities in 30 EU and EEA-EFTA countries in a network of over 4,000 European experts. It contributes to the European Union's international activities through its work with the European Pharmacopoeia, the World Health Organization, and the ICH and VICH trilateral (EU, Japan, and US) conferences on harmonization, among other international organizations and initiatives.

The EMEA is headed by the Executive Director and has a secretariat of about 440 staff members.

http://www.emea.europa.eu/htms/aboutus/emeaoverview.htm

EPIDEMIOLOGY

The standard definition of classical epidemiology is, "the study of the distribution and determinants of health-related states or events in specified populations, and the application of this study to the control of health problems."

- Epidemiology involves studying the frequency, incidence, prevalence, distribution, and behavior of a disease within a population, as well as the effect of interventions on its course in a population.
- It also involves the studying of the who, where, when, what, and why people have a disease, to provide information and knowledge leading to decisions used in public health and community medicine for its control.

See also Pharmacoepidemiology and Clinical Epidemiology.

EPIDEMIOLOGY, CLINICAL

See Clinical Epidemiology.

ERICE DECLARATION ON EFFECTIVE COMMUNICATION IN PHARMACOVIGILANCE

Precepts set forth at a conference in Erice, Italy in 1997:

Preamble
Monitoring, evaluating and communicating drug safety is a public-health activity with profound implications that depend on the in-

tegrity and collective responsibility of all parties—consumers, health professionals, researchers, academia, media, pharmaceutical industry, drug regulators, governments and international organisations—working together. High scientific, ethical and professional standards and a moral code should govern this activity. The inherent uncertainty of the risks and benefits of drugs needs to be acknowledged and explained. Decisions and actions that are based on this uncertainty should be informed by scientific and clinical considerations and should take into account social realities and circumstances.

Declaration:
Flaws in drug safety communication at all levels of society can lead to mistrust, misinformation and misguided actions resulting in harm and the creation of a climate where drug safety data may be hidden, withheld, or ignored.

Fact should be distinguished from speculation and hypothesis, and actions taken should reflect the needs of those affected and the care they require. These actions call for systems and legislation, nationally and internationally, that ensure full and open exchange of information, and effective standards of evaluation. These standards will ensure that risks and benefits can be assessed, explained and acted upon openly and in a spirit that promotes general confidence and trust.

The following statements set forth the basic requirements for this to happen, and were agreed upon by all participants from 34 countries at Erice:

Drug safety information must serve the health of the public. Such information should be ethically and effectively communicated in terms of both content and method. Facts, hypotheses and conclusions should be distinguished, uncertainty acknowledged, and information provided in ways that meet both general and individual needs.

Education in the appropriate use of drugs, including interpretation of safety information, is essential for the public at large, as well as for patients and health-care providers. Such education requires special commitment and resources. Drug information directed to the public in whatever form should be balanced with respect to risks and benefits.

All the evidence needed to assess and understand risks and benefits must be openly available. Constraints on communication parties, which hinder their ability to meet this goal must be recognised and overcome.

Every country needs a system with independent expertise to ensure that safety information on all available drugs is adequately collected, impartially evaluated, and made accessible to all. Adequate nonpartisan financing must be available to support the system. Exchange of data and evaluations among countries must be encouraged and supported.

A strong basis for drug safety monitoring has been laid over a long period, although sometimes in response to disasters. Innovation in this field now needs to ensure that emergent problems are promptly recognised and efficiently dealt with, and that information and solutions are effectively communicated.

ERICE MANIFESTO FOR GLOBAL REFORM OF THE SAFETY OF MEDICINES IN PATIENT CARE

In 1997, 27 experts on drug safety met and issued the following manifesto (summarized):

The Erice Manifesto specifies the challenges that must be addressed to ensure the continuing development and usefulness of the science, in particular:

- The active involvement of patients and the public in the core debate about the risks and benefits of medicines, and in decisions about their own treatment and health
- The development of new ways of collecting, analyzing, and communicating information about the safety and effectiveness of medicines; open discussion about it and the decisions that arise from it
- The pursuit of learning from other disciplines about how pharmacovigilance methods can be improved, alongside wide-ranging professional, official, and public collaboration
- The creation of purposeful, coordinated, worldwide support amongst politicians, officials, scientists, clinicians, patients, and the general public, based on the demonstrable benefits of pharmacovigilance to public health and patient safety.

See http://www.who-umc.org/graphics/13286.pdf.

ESTRI

Electronic Standards for the Transfer of Regulatory Information. *See* E2B and M2 Documents.

ETHICS

A set of standards defined by the society or environment that defines or differentiates right from wrong.

In drug safety, the issue of ethics comes up in several areas:

Research Ethics Committee (Investigational Review Board): a group of individuals that determines whether a clinical trial may be performed based on scientific value, protection of volunteers (healthy or diseased), community/society legal and ethical standards.

Corporate ethics: Is the company acting not only in its own best interest (profit), but acting correctly ("ethically") in regard to patients, physicians, the public, pricing, and so forth?

Healthcare professional ethics: Is the person making a drug choice (to choose, start, or stop a drug) based on the patient's best interests or on some other grounds?

ETHICS COMMITTEE

Also known as "Institutional Review Board." A committee usually comprising medical scientists, medical professionals, and nonscientists (consumers, clergyman, lawyer, statistician, ethicist) who determine whether a proposed clinical trial is sufficiently safe, ethical, justifiable, and carried out in the appropriate manner. The committee may ask for modifications of the informed consent or the protocol, and may even turn down the study; it receives regular safety reports from the investigator (and sometimes the sponsor) and monitors the progress and completion of the study. The main goal is to protect the healthy volunteers (phase I) and patients (phase 2, 3, 4) involved in the study. In most countries the IRB does not do actual audits but instead reviews data supplied by the sponsor, clinical investigator, or others. Such committees are required by law in most countries for most studies. In the US the regulations are found at 21CFR56.

ETHNICITY

The sense or recognition of belonging to a particular group with a common heredity, environment, and/or culture. It may be based on such factors as country of birth, nationality, mother tongue, national or geographical origin, cultural difference, religion, and so forth.

In drug safety (as in medicine) this sometimes matters. For example, the cytochrome P450 system, which plays a major role in drug metabolism, is well known to exhibit enormous diversity (genetic polymorphism), producing major differences in metabolism of drugs from individual to individual or group to group.

EU DATA PRIVACY DIRECTIVE

See Data Privacy, Privacy.

EU PHARMACOVIGILANCE REGULATIONS, DIRECTIVES, AND GUIDANCES

There are a large number of regulations, directives, and guidances that the EMEA has published on pharmacovigilance. The key one is called "Volume 9A" and is entitled "Rules Governing Medicinal Products in the European Union—Guidelines on Pharmacovigilance for Medicinal Products for Human Use."

See http://eudravigilance.emea.eu.int/human/docs/vol9A_
2007-04.pdf for Volume 9A and http://eudravigilance.emea.eu.int/
human/euPoliciesAndDocs.asp for Volume 9A and the other EU
directives, guidances, and regulations.

EUDRANET

The European Telecommunication Network in Pharmaceuticals.
A platform for the exchange of information between health authorities and industry.

Objectives

The submission and evaluation of marketing authorization applications by pharmaceutical companies.

The pharmacovigilance of products on the market to ensure the
maintenance of high standards of quality as well as adhering to
European national and regional regulations.

The dissemination of relevant information to industry, scientific
experts, and regulators.

EUDRAVIGILANCE DATABASE

The European Union's database for the collection and storage of
adverse events.

EUROPEAN ECONOMIC AREA (EEA)

Austria, Belgium, Cyprus, Czech Republic, Denmark, Estonia,
Finland, France, Germany, Greece, Hungary, Ireland, Italy, Latvia,
Lithuania, Luxembourg, Malta, Netherlands, Poland, Portugal,
Slovak Republic, Slovenia, Spain, Sweden, United Kingdom,
Iceland, Liechtenstein, Norway.

EUROPEAN NETWORK OF TERATOLOGY (ENTIS)

A group of teratovigilance centers in some 15 countries whose aim
is to coordinate and collaborate the activities of the different
Teratology Information Services (TIS), and to collect and evaluate
data in order to contribute to the primary prevention of birth defects and developmental disorders. See also *Teratology Information
Services*. http://www.entis-org.com/section=home&lang=UK

EUROPEAN PUBLIC ASSESSMENT REPORT (EPAR)

The EMEA publishes information on the products assessed by the
Committee for Medicinal Products for Human Use (CHMP). Any
positive opinion given by the Committee is published in the first instance as a Summary of Opinion. More detailed information is published later, following the granting of a Marketing Authorisation by

the European Commission as a European Public Assessment Report (EPAR).

The European Public Assessment Report (EPAR) reflects the scientific conclusion reached by the Committee for Medicinal Products for Human Use (CHMP) at the end of the centralized evaluation process. It is made available by the EMEA for information to the public, after deletion of commercially confidential information.

The EPAR provides a summary of the grounds for the CHMP opinion in favor of granting a marketing authorization for a specific medicinal product. It results from the Committee's review of the documentation submitted by the applicant, and from subsequent discussions held during CHMP meetings. The EPAR is updated throughout the authorization period as changes to the original terms and conditions of the authorization (i.e., variations, pharmacovigilance issues, specific obligations) are made. EPARs also contain a summary written in a manner that is understandable to the public.

They are available by drug name at http://www.emea.europa.eu/htms/human/epar/a.htm.

EUROPEAN SOCIETY OF PHARMACOVIGILANCE (ESOP)

The original name of what is now the International Society of Pharmacovigilance (ISoP). See this term.

EUROPEAN TELECOMMUNICATION NETWORK IN PHARMACEUTICALS

See EUDRANET.

EUROPEAN UNION

A federation of 27 European countries (member states): Austria, Belgium, Bulgaria, Cyprus (Greek part), Czech Republic, Denmark, Estonia, Finland, France, Germany, Greece, Hungary, Ireland, Italy, Latvia, Lithuania, Luxembourg, Malta, Netherlands, Poland, Portugal, Romania, Slovakia, Slovenia, Spain, Sweden, United Kingdom of Great Britain and Northern Ireland.

The EMEA was created by the EU to handle drug safety and pharmacovigilance both centrally in London at the EMEA and in cooperation with the member states' national health authorities

EXCHANGE AGREEMENTS

See Data Exchange Agreements.

EXCIPIENT

An ingredient of a drug that is (in theory) inactive and is added to a drug as a vehicle, diluent, or space filler. They are usually added to solid dosage forms to allow sufficient volume to be formed into a tablet (that is stable and does not disintegrate before ingestion) or to fill a capsule.

Excipients should be inactive but occasionally they cause:

- Mild adverse reactions: lactose powder in tablets may produce diarrhea in lactose intolerant patients.
- Severe adverse reactions: in the early 20th century an elixir of sulfanilamide killed 50 adults and a similar number of children. It was discovered that the cause was the excipient diethylene glycol.
- Allergic reactions.

Most countries have lists of approved and excluded excipients.

Products, branded or generic, will contain the same active ingredients but may contain different excipients. This means that both the brand name and generic name of a suspected product should be listed and excipients considered as possible causes of unexplained ADRs.

EXCLUSION CRITERIA

In clinical study protocols, patient characteristics, diseases, and conditions that if present disqualify the patient from participating in the trial. They vary from protocol to protocol. For example, in a study of an outpatient antibiotic for urinary tract infections, exclusion criteria might include age <18, allergy to this drug or class of drugs, difficulty swallowing tablets, or other infections requiring antibiotics.

Authors' note: It is clear that many excluded categories of patients are more susceptible to ADRs than the included categories, and that the frequency/severity of ADRs in the population exposed after marketing may be greater than that observed during clinical trials.

EXPANDED ACCESS PROGRAMS

See Compassionate Use Programs.

EXPECTED, EXPECTEDNESS

An AE/ADR that is consistent with the labeling. *See* Unexpected.

EXPEDITED REPORT

Communication of a suspected adverse reaction to a medicinal product either in clinical trials or in the postmarketing situation to the competent health authorities within 15 calendar days after the marketing authorization holder becomes aware of it. Note that for clinical trial reports, a death or life-threatening ADR that is unexpected and possibly related also requires a 7-day report in certain countries.

Expedited reports are usually sent on standardized paper forms such as the MedWatch in the US and the CIOMS I in much of the rest of the world. With the trend to electronic transmission, the E2B mechanism will be widely used.

EXPERT OPINION ON DRUG SAFETY

A drug safety journal published by Informa Healthcare in the UK. http://www.expertopin.com/loi/eds

EXPORT OF DATA

See Electronic Transmission, E2B/M2.

EXTRINSIC AE/ADR

This expression is used to designate adverse drug reactions that are not due to the active ingredient but rather to such diverse causes as a reaction to an excipient; an accidental contamination; defective material; manufacturing, packaging, labeling, or storage problems; or inadequate preparation. Since patented and generic products may vary in their formulations, the brand name of suspected products must be known for identifying extrinsic ADRs.

Authors' note: An example: In 1981, the FDA was notified of the death of newborns exposed to a preservative in saline which was used to rinse central vein catheters in premature babies. In one hospital, 10 cases occurred in 6 months while in another hospital 6 cases were seen in 12 months. After the FDA recommended that the usage of this excipient be stopped, this "epidemic" ended. This can be considered as a positive "collective" dechallenge. This episode clearly illustrates the fact that deaths can occur due to ADRs that are related to excipients as well as to the active ingredient of a drug or product, as pointed out in the 1980s by Dr Edward Napke, founding director of the pharmacovigilance program at Health Canada.

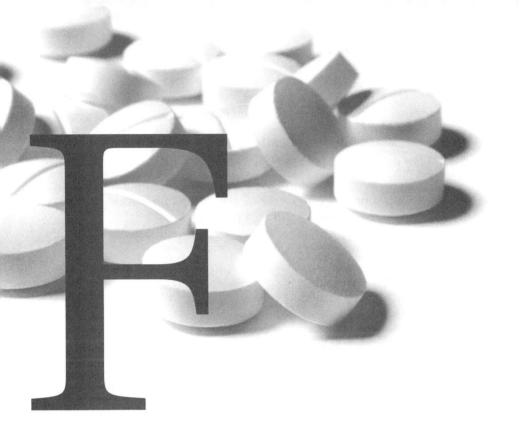

FACULTY OF PHARMACEUTICAL MEDICINE

Based in the UK, it is not a medical school but rather a professional membership organization with approximately 1,400 members who are practicing or retired pharmaceutical physicians or those with a professional interest in the specialty. The mission is to advance the science and practice of pharmaceutical medicine by working to develop and maintain competence, ethics, and integrity and the highest professional standards in the specialty for the benefit of the public.

http://www.fpm.org.uk/

See also Pharmaceutical Medicine.

FDA

See Food and Drug Administration.

FDLI

See Food and Drug Law Institute.

FDA REVITALIZATION ACT

See Food and Drug Administration Revitalization Act

FEDERAL FOOD, DRUG AND COSMETIC (FDC) ACT

A law passed in 1938 in the US, it contained new provisions:

- Extending FDA control to cosmetics and therapeutic devices.
- Requiring new drugs to be shown safe before marketing, starting a new system of drug regulation.
- Eliminating the requirement to prove intent to defraud in drug misbranding cases.
- Providing that safe tolerances be set for unavoidable poisonous substances.
- Authorizing standards of identity, quality, and fill-of-container for foods.
- Authorizing factory inspections.
- Adding the remedy of court injunctions to the previous penalties of seizures and prosecutions.

Authors' note: It is said that this act began the modern era of drug safety, requiring safety to be considered in drug development, manufacture, and marketing.

FEDERAL REGISTER

A publication of the US Government that contains public notices of government agencies including the FDA. It is published daily and includes proposed new rules, called a Notice of Proposed Rulemaking. There is usually a public comment period with written comments sent to the federal agency in question for review and possibly a public meeting. If the agency chooses, they will then issue a final rule or never put the proposed rule into effect. It is prepared by the Office of the Federal Register and printed by the Government Printing Office. Available at: www.gpoaccess.gov/fr/index.html.

FEDERAL REGULATIONS

In the US, regulatory law that is made by a federal agency after being "enabled" by a law passed by the US Congress and signed by the President. A regulation goes through the rulemaking process (see *Federal Register*) in order to be put into effect. The FDA makes such regulations. Some of these concern safety.

FEEDER GROUPS

Also called "line units." In a company, departments other than the drug safety department that may directly receive AEs, such as the legal, regulatory, and marketing/sales departments as well as telephone operators and the mail room. There must be SOPs in place instructing them on how to handle such AEs in order for the company to remain in full regulatory compliance.

FETAL ABNORMALITIES

A nonnormal occurrence in a fetus, usually first recognized at birth. Any congenital abnormality is considered a serious AE.

FETAL DEATH

If a drug is suspected of having contributed to fetal death or to a spontaneous abortion, the recommendation of ICH E2B is to routinely file a report on the mother. The report is known as a parent–fetus report or parent–child report.

FIALURIDINE (FIAU)

Fialuridine was a drug used to treat hepatitis B virus (HBV) in the early 1990s. Its use in one clinical trial in particular produced seven cases of severe hepatic toxicity in 15 patients (including five deaths). Several investigations were made to determine if there was any fault involved.

The lessons learned include:

- Serious and nonserious AEs due to drugs may occur that mimic the disease being treated. They may be called paradoxical ADRs.
- Clinical trial safety oversight by the company (sponsor) and the investigator must be "meticulous." All the regulatory requirements (protocol design, investigator qualification, AE collection, reporting and review, consent forms, investigational review board oversight, safety data review committees, etc.) must be followed strictly and completely.
- A data safety plan must be drawn up and in place before the study starts.
- Prestudy signals (from animal data or other clinical trials or class drugs) must be followed carefully.
- Investigator (and sponsor, monitor) training must be done before the study starts and during the study if new personnel become involved.
- A sponsor physician must be designated as clearly in charge of the ongoing safety review. A safety monitoring committee may also need to be in place.
- The use of qualified investigational review boards with high-quality experienced personnel who have sufficient time to

review safety data must occur. Sponsors and investigators must supply the investigational review boards with easily reviewable data sent at frequent periods.

- Companies and institutions doing clinical trials must have a crisis management plan in place to be able to do a preliminary investigation and to take appropriate actions on critical safety issues within a few hours.

FIDUCIARY RESPONSIBILITY

Originally, the obligation (sometimes legal, sometimes moral, sometimes both) to handle the finances of someone else in a trustworthy manner putting that person's interest above one's own. By extension, the comparable concept in medicine, per the Hippocratic Oath, is to put the patient's best interest ahead of the treating physician's interest.

Authors' note: In the pharmaceutical industry, outsourcing drug safety to clinical research organizations does not exempt the sponsor from its obligations and responsibilities.

FILE ROOM

See Archiving.

FILLER

See Excipient.

FIRST DOSE PHENOMENON

An ADR of type A that is seen almost exclusively after the first dose of the drug in most of the patients who experience this reaction. It can be due to an exaggerated pharmacologic effect (easily avoided if the drug is given in smaller and/or divided doses) or a paradoxic effect. Two examples:

- *Terfenadine.* Neuropsychiatric reactions have been reported following the first dose of this nonsedating H1 antihistamine, which was subsequently removed from the market because of cardiotoxicity.
- *Nifedipine.* A formulation of this calcium-blocker drug has been associated with angina following the first dose in some patients, possibly due to an exaggerated reflex tachycardia or coronary steal.

FIXED DRUG ERUPTION (REACTION)

A skin ADR that characteristically recurs in the same site or sites each time a particular drug is taken; with each exposure, however, the number of involved sites may increase. In dermatovigilance, this is the only cutaneous ADR whose etiology is clearly associated with a drug or xenobiotic taken systemically. It is usually of allergic origin.

The time to appearance varies from 30 minutes to 8 hours or more, though it is rare after 16 hours. Rechallenge by the same route of administration at a lower dose under medical supervision and with the consent of the patient is a very sensitive method to verify the causality of the suspect product.

FOI OR FOIA

See Freedom of Information Act.

FOLLOW-UP

The requirement that a pharmaceutical company must make due diligent efforts to obtain complete information on individual case safety reports of AEs. The FDA's 2005 guidance on good pharmacovigilance practices noted that the greatest efforts should be made to obtain follow-up information for serious cases, particularly ones that are not already known to occur with the drug in question. For consumer reports, an attempt should be made to obtain corroborative details from the consumer's healthcare practitioner and to obtain medical records. Follow-up reports should be properly identified in order to avoid duplicate case reports.

Authors' note: In general companies are expected to do follow-up on all serious cases—especially if they represent an important signal—unless the information at hand is known to be complete or there is no possibility of further information being obtained (e.g., certain reports from health authorities). At least two attempts to obtain information are usually made for serious cases. Follow-up is sometimes not done for nonserious cases that are labeled/listed and where the four reportability criteria are present. Follow-up should also be sought from healthcare professionals if the initial report is from a consumer or patient.

FOOD AND DRUG ADMINISTRATION (FDA)

The US regulatory agency handling drug safety amongst other functions. It is a part of the US Department of Health and Human Services. The two largest areas touching drug safety are the Center for Drug Evaluation and Research (CDER) and MedWatch. The FDA's website is extensive and very useful: www.fda.gov.

See CDER, CBER, MedWatch Program.

Note also that at least one other country (Thailand) uses this name for its health agency.

FOOD AND DRUG LAW INSTITUTE (FDLI)

A nonprofit organization located in Washington, DC, and committed to providing high quality education and a neutral forum for the generation of ideas and discussion of law and public policy for its legal, policy, and regulatory communities. FDLI does not engage in advocacy activities. There are more than 570 members comprising manufacturers and suppliers of medicines (pharmaceuticals, biologics, and biotechnologies), medical devices, food, and cosmetics subject to FDA regulation; law and consulting firms; associations; and individuals.

FDLI pursues two major priorities: (1) to present conferences and publications for comprehensive discussion of major policy, legislative, regulatory, and enforcement actions and judicial decisions; and (2) to provide education and training in the practice of food and drug law and regulation. FDLI's mission relates to the regulatory programs of the Food and Drug Administration (FDA) and other government agencies. http://www.fdli.org/about/

FOOD AND DRUG ADMINISTRATION (FDA REVITALIZATION ACT)

In late 2007 this act went into effect replacing and extending the Prescription Drug User Fee Act. Many new provisions were included. User fees were expanded for both drugs and devices. A new tracking system down to the lot and serial number for devices was introduced. FDA's authority over pediatric studies, labeling and vigilance was increased. The issues and restrictions on conflicts of interest for members of FDA Advisory Committees were clarified. A registry of essentially all controlled phase II, III and IV studies is to be created and made easily available to the public. By June 2009, the FDA must determine what safety is to be posted covering:

- Serious AEs—A table of anticipated and unanticipated serious adverse events grouped by organ system, with number and frequency of such event in each arm of the clinical trial.
- Frequent AEs—A table of anticipated and unanticipated adverse events that are not included in the table described above that exceed a frequency of 5 percent within any arm of the clinical trial, grouped by organ system, with number and frequency of such event in each arm of the clinical trial.

The FDA may require a sponsor to conduct a post-approval studies of a drug to assess a known serious risk related to the use of the drug, to assess signals and to identify an unexpected serious risk when available data indicates the potential for this.

If the FDA becomes aware of new safety information that it believes should be added to the labeling of the drug, it will tell this to the sponsor who will have 30 days to submit proposed label changes including changes to boxed warnings, contraindications, warnings, precautions, or adverse reactions or submit a state explaining why the change is not warranted. The FDA will promptly review this and may initiate discussions with the sponsor which will last no more than 30 days. The FDA may then within 15 days issue an order forcing the label change. The sponsor may appeal. The FDA has the right to accelerate the timelines if it wishes.

The FDA can force the sponsor to submit a risk management/minimization plan as part of an NDA submission or within 120 days for a drug already on the market. Such a plan must be reviewed at 1.5, 3 and 7 years.

The FDA may require special access conditions for drugs that have significant safety risks. FDA may require health care providers, pharmacists or other institutions who prescribe the drug or where the drug is prescribed to have particular training or experience or are specially certified to prescribe it. In other circumstances the drug may be dispensed only in certain health care settings, such as hospitals. The FDA may also require that particular evidence of safe use conditions, such as laboratory test results, before prescribing. FDA may also require that each patient using the drug be subject to certain monitoring or be enrolled in a registry.

The FDA will develop risk identification and analysis methods based on electronic health data for the reporting (in a standardized form) of data on all serious adverse drug and those adverse events submitted by patients, providers, and drug sponsors and to provide or active adverse event surveillance using the following data sources: Federal health-related electronic data (such as data from Medicare and the Department of Veterans Affairs); private sector health related electronic data (such as pharmaceutical purchase data and health insurance claims data); and other data to create a robust system to identify adverse events and potential drug safety signals; to identify certain trends and patterns with respect to data accessed by the system; to provide regular reports concerning adverse event trends, adverse event patterns, incidence and prevalence of adverse events which may include data on comparative national adverse event trends. A database of 100,000,000 patients is to be developed by 2012.

The FDA may contract with private (non-governmental) groups to classify, analyze, or aggregate data for prompt investigation of priority drug safety questions, including—unresolved safety questions for drugs or classes of drugs; and for a newly-approved drugs, safety signals from clinical trials used to approve the drug and other preapproval trials; rare, serious drug side effects; and the safety of use in domestic populations not included, or underrepresented, in the trials used to approve the drug (such as older people, people with co-morbidities, pregnant women, or children); perform advanced research and analysis on identified drug safety risks; focus post-approval studies and clinical trials more effectively on cases for which reports and other safety signal detection is not sufficient to resolve whether there is an elevated risk of a serious adverse event associated with the use of a drug.

FDA may require pre-approval of TV advertising (direct to consumer ads). Penalties for non-compliance can be up to $250,000 for individual violations and up to $10 million for repeated violations.

FDA was given the power to order a manufacturer to conduct post-marketing surveillance for class II or III devices. Surveillance of more than 3 years for pediatric devices may also be required.

The FDA is given several years to put all of the new requirements into place. The user fees may now be spent in the drug safety field in addition to being used for review of new drug applications. It is likely that this new act will have far reaching consequences.

FOOD SUPPLEMENT

A product or food that, when absorbed into the body, supplements a real or supposed lack of a nutrient. *See* Dietary Supplement.

FORMULARY

A preferred list of drug products that typically limits the number of drugs available within a therapeutic class for purposes of drug purchasing, dispensing, and/or reimbursement. A government body, third-party insurer or health plan, or an institution may compile a formulary. Some institutions, hospitals, or health plans develop closed (i.e., restricted) formularies where only those drug products listed can be dispensed in that institution or reimbursed by the health plan. From the US Health and Human Services Administration http://www.hrsa.gov/opa/glossary.htm.

Authors' note: The WHO has developed a list (formulary) of essential medicines, especially useful in developing countries, to improve patients' safety and limit unnecessary spending.

FRACTIONAL REPORTING RATES

Also known as Proportional Reporting Rates.

A type of data mining in pharmacovigilance databases (see this term). For a particular AE, the calculation of the proportion of that

AE as a fraction of all AEs reported for that drug compared with the proportion of that AE for all other drugs in a safety database. If the value for the AE/drug combination is greater than the value seen for the AE/total database, this may be considered as a possible signal.

Authors' note: One must adjust the specificity and sensitivity of this methodology in order to reasonably search for signals. Due to chance there will always be some AE/drug combinations above and below the AE/whole database proportion. Thus, it is usually necessary to set a threshold above which one will consider something to be a signal and below which one will consider something to be "noise."

See Disproportionality Methods.

FREEDOM OF INFORMATION ACT (FOI OR FOIA)

In the US, a law enacted in 1966 that established the legal right of public access to information in the federal government. Certain data are exempted (e.g., secret or proprietary information).

In terms of the FDA and drug safety, very large amounts of information, including the data in the AERS database, is available to the public. Other countries around the world are slowly adopting similar legislation. See http://www.fda.gov/foi/.

Authors' note: For the time being, consulting the FDA's AE database requires significant expertise. Database access could and should be made more user-friendly.

FREQUENCY OF AEs/ADRs

The number of occurrences of an event (e.g., AE/ADR) over a particular period of time. In drug safety, for example, a clinical trial may show an ADR to occur in x% of the drug-treated patients compared to y% in the placebo patients in a 4-week study.

Authors' note: In the postmarketing situation, it is impossible to determine the true frequency of an AE/ADR as the number of patients taking the drug is never clearly known. It is possible to track surrogates of drug use, such as the number of tablets sold or prescriptions filled, but it is not really possible to know who actually took the drug or for how long. Similarly, it is not possible to know the true number of a particular AEs/ADRs as many (if not most) never get reported. Hence creating a ratio based on such imperfect numbers is usually meaningless.

In certain controlled situations (e.g., in-hospital patients) it may be possible to measure AE/ADR frequency by controling exposure and recording adverse events.

The CIOMS III Working Group proposed the following definitions for defining frequency of AEs/ADRs.

Very frequent or common	> 10%	> 1 in 10
Frequent or common	1% to 10%	Between 1 in 10 and 1 in 100
Infrequent or uncommon	0.1% to 1%	Between 1 in 100 and 1 in 1,000
Rare	0.01% to 0.1%	Between 1 in 1,000 and 1 in 10,000
Very rare	0.001% to 0.01%	Between 1 in 10,000 and 1 in 100,000
Exceedingly rare	< 0.001%	< 1 in a million (1,000,000)

FREQUENT (AE/ADR FREQUENCY)

Under the CIOMS III definition, frequent (synonym "common") refers to an AE/ADR that occurs between 1% and 10% of patients who are exposed to the suspect drug.

FULL DATA SET

As defined by the FDA in its 2003 proposed new rules, a full data set for an individual case safety report (ICSR) is "completion of all the applicable elements" on the FDA form 3500A (or a CIOMS I form for foreign SADRs) and includes a narrative ("an accurate summary of the relevant data and information pertaining to an SADR or medication error."

FULMINANT HEPATITIS

See Hepatitis.

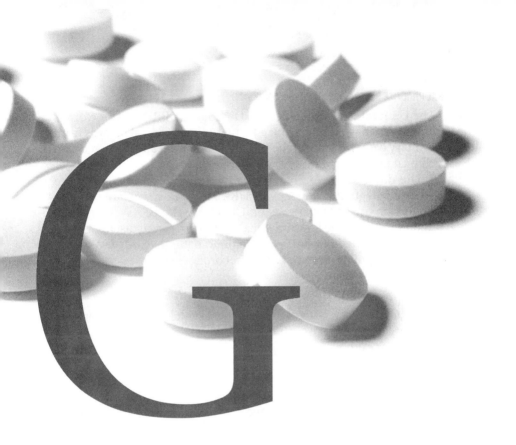

GALENICS

Pertaining to the branch of pharmacy handling the formulation of therapeutic agents into clinically useful and useable forms.

GENDER AND MEDICATION RESPONSES, FDA GUIDELINES

Revising a policy from 1977 that excluded women of childbearing potential from early drug studies, the FDA issued new guidelines in 1993 calling for improved assessments of medication responses as a function of gender. Companies are encouraged to include patients of both sexes in their investigations of drugs and to analyze any gender-specific phenomena and tolerance.

GENE THERAPY

A medical treatment in which genetic material is introduced into the cells of a person to replace a defective gene in that person. It is hoped by many that this type of treatment may be able in the future to prevent some adverse drug reactions by being more selective.

GENERAL PRACTICE RESEARCH DATABASE (GPRD)

The General Practice Research Database (GPRD) is the world's largest database of anonymized longitudinal medical records from primary care with comprehensive observational data from real-life clinical practice.

The database is managed by the Medicines and Healthcare Products Regulatory Agency (MHRA). Its data is available to customers online or as datasets on CD-ROM. The GPRD is regularly updated so that the latest medical, prescribing, and disease trends can be identified. It contains 46 million patient years of validated data on 3.4 million active patient records.

Data include:

Demographics, including age and sex
Medical symptoms, signs, and diagnoses, including comments
Therapy (medicines, vaccines, devices)
Treatment outcomes
AEs and events leading to withdrawal of a drug or treatment
Referrals to hospitals or specialists
Laboratory tests, pathology results
Lifestyle factors (height, weight, BMI, smoking, and alcohol consumption)
Patient registration, practice, and consultation details

It is able to link diagnoses to prescribing data, which allows the study of conditions common in general practice and their treatment. Adverse events may be studied in regard to drug prescribing and usage. See www.gprd.com.

GENERIC DRUG

A product containing the same active ingredient as a brand name (innovator) product that is now off patent (i.e., the patent or monopoly of sale has expired). For example, Zantac® has gone off patent and any other company may now manufacture and/or sell its active ingredient (randitidine) in their products.

Authors' note: Presuming that the manufacture of the product is the same, the branded product and the generic version(s) should have the same safety and AE profile. In practice this may not always be the case depending upon excipients and manufacturing processes.

By the time a drug is generic, most of the safety issues have been addressed and AE reporting and pharmacovigilance tend to be a "maintenance function" with few new data or signals appearing, except for interaction with recently marketed drugs. In addition, because it is often hard to identify the manufacturer of a generic prod-

uct, the AEs tend to get reported to the innovator regardless of whether the patient took the branded or generic product. The primary function of generic company safety departments is often limited to reviewing the published medical literature and including these AEs in their expedited and periodic safety reports.

GENERIC PHARMACEUTICAL COMPANY

A company that manufactures products that are off patent. They may be independent companies or subsidiaries of large multinational pharmaceutical companies. Sometimes a company will manufacture and sell both a branded and generic version of the same product. Generic companies may do little or no drug discovery or clinical research. They may do small studies to show bioequivalence.

GOOD CASE MANAGEMENT PRACTICES

A term used to mean the proper, careful, and complete collection and handling of safety data. It is discussed in detail in the ICH document Postapproval Safety Data Management: Definitions and Standards for Expedited Reporting (E2D). See http://www.ich.org/cache/compo/475-272-1.html.

GOOD CLINICAL PRACTICE (GCP)

A broad term referring to the methodology used in doing clinical research and drug safety. It covers the design, conduct, performance, monitoring, auditing, recording, analysis, and reporting of clinical trials. Such requirements have been existent for many years but not always referred to under this term. "Good Clinical Practice" now largely refers to the documents created primarily by ICH and CIOMS that have been adopted in whole or in part, changed or unchanged by most health authorities around the world. Thus "GCP" is now obligatory for most or all trials done in most countries.

GOOD LABORATORY PRACTICE (GLP)

Detailed regulations, laws, and guidelines that set standards and require specific operating procedures for basic research, data acquisition, and reporting of laboratory tests and research. This includes laboratories doing animal testing and laboratories doing tests on human blood, urine, tissue, and so forth.

GOOD MANUFACTURING PRACTICE (GMP)

Also known as Current Good Manufacturing Practice (cGMP). Detailed regulations, laws, and guidelines that set standards and require specific operating procedures for the production of pharmaceuticals, biological products, and medical devices. Standards apply that products have the correct ingredients, strength, quality, and purity characteristics and have not been changed during manufacture, packaging, or handling from creation to the finished product.

Authors' note: These requirements have been defined by the FDA and other health authorities. In addition, the International Organization for Standards (ISO) has defined certain manufacturing standards, particularly for device manufacture. See http://www.iso.org/iso/en/aboutiso/introduction/index.html.

GOOD PHARMACOVIGILANCE PRACTICE (GPVP)

A set of guidelines or recommendations intended to ensure:

- The authenticity and quality of the data collected in pharmacovigilance in order to allow the risks attributable to a drug to be evaluated at any time.
- The confidentiality of the information related to the identity of the persons submitting or reporting adverse reactions.
- The use of uniform criteria in the evaluation of reports and the generation of alert signals.

In addition, in March 2005 the US FDA issued three guidances summarizing the agency's views on risk management and good pharmacovigilance practices. In particular the document entitled "Good Pharmacovigilance Practices and Pharmacoepidemiologic Assessment Guidance" codified these practices. See http://www.fda.gov/cder/guidance/6359OCC.htm.

See also the document on Good Pharmacoepidemiologic Practices issued by the International Society of Pharmacoepidemiology (ISPE): http://www.pharmacoepi.org/resources/guidelines_08027.cfm.

GRADUATED PLAN (STUFENPLAN)

A risk management system set up by the German Health Authority (BfArM) whereby there is a "graduated" or "stepwise" plan to monitor and control drug risk. It requires the assigned person in the drug company (known as the Stufenplanbeauftragter in German) to put in place actions of increasing rigor to limit or prevent safety issues with products on the market. It is similar in some respects to the EU concept of Qualified Person. (See this term.)

GENERALLY RECOGNIZED AS SAFE (GRAS)

An ingredient that the FDA allows to be added to products without prior approval if it is considered to be safe by experts in the field.

See   http://www.cfsan.fda.gov/~dms/grasguid.html   and http://www.fda.gov/Fdac/features/2004/204_gras.html.

GUIDELINE

Also known as a Guidance. A suggested policy or method of handling certain safety issues issued by a health authority. They are not obligatory and do not carry the force of law. However, most companies will tend to comply with health authority guidelines where possible.

GXP

See Predicate Rules.

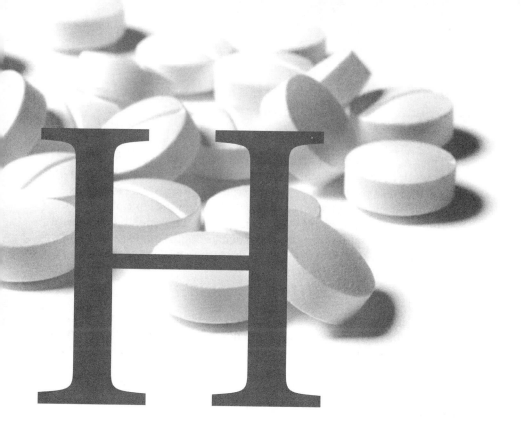

HARMONIZATION

The largely successful attempt to have the pharmaceutical world (sometimes narrowly defined as the US, EU, and Japan) agree on common procedures and requirements in drug development and surveillance.

This took the form of a series of international meetings and working groups, starting in 1990 and continuing to date, called the "International Conference on Harmonization" or ICH. (See this entry.)

In the pharmacovigilance world similar harmonization has been done by CIOMS (Council for International Organizations of Medical Sciences). *See* CIOMS.

The international harmonization of coding terms (MedDRA), of the definitions (ICH E2A) and forms (CIOMS 1 form), of procedures for periodic reporting of adverse events and reactions (ICH E2C), and of good pharmacovigilance practices are part of the objectives and results of several groups, most particularly CIOMS and the International Conference on Harmonization.

HAs (HEALTH AGENCIES OR AUTHORITIES)

See Health Agencies or Authorities.

HAZARD RATE

The hazard rate is the risk of an event (such as death) at a given point in time in a clinical trial and can be computed for the experimental and control groups in the trial. The hazard rate for the experimental group divided by the hazard rate for the controls defines the "hazard ratio." If this fraction is greater than one, the chances of succumbing to the health risk (such as death) increase with the treatment; if the ratio is less than one, the chances of the health risk decrease with treatment.

HEADER, E2B ELECTRONIC TRANSMISSIONS

The initial section of an E2B transmission that contains the technical information about the report needed for uploading. It is separate from the rest of the transmission which contains the data elements.

See E2B.

HEALTH ACTION INTERNATIONAL (HAI)

An independent, global network working to increase access to essential medicines and improve their rational use. The members are concerned with pricing, access, innovation, adverse reactions and their reporting by patients, promotion, education, and rational use. Member organizations include the British Consumers Association and the Swiss Agency for Therapeutic Products. The secretariat of this consumer advocacy organization is based in The Netherlands. See its website: www.haiweb.org.

HEALTH AGENCIES OR AUTHORITIES (HAs)

Governmental bodies responsible for some or all of the regulation of drugs, devices, food supplements, biologics, neutraceuticals, and herbal medicines. In the US it is the Food and Drug Administration, in the EU it is the European Medicinals Agency, in Canada it is Health Canada, in Germany it is BfArM, and in France it is AFSSAPS. In some countries there may be more than one HA.

HEALTH CANADA (SANTÉ CANADA)

The federal government agency in Canada that deals with the health and well-being of the people. "Build awareness and encourage reporting of adverse reactions by health professionals and consumers through initiatives such as MedEffect, which provides access to adverse reaction reporting forms, new product safety information advisories, warnings and recalls, an e-sign up for automatic notification about new product information, and a complete archive of the CARN (Canadian Adverse Reaction Newsletter).

Provide channels for reporting of adverse reactions to veterinary drugs." See http://www.hc-sc.gc.ca/dhp-mps/advers_react_neg/index_e.html.

HEALTHCARE PROFESSIONAL (HCP)

A professional, usually licensed by an official body or a licensing board, who is involved with medical treatment of people. In the context of drug safety, they report AEs to health authorities and companies. They receive information and promotional material ("detailing") from pharmaceutical companies and prescribe medications for their patients. They may receive urgent letters from the companies warning of new safety issues with drugs ("Dear Doctor Letter" or "Dear Health Professional Letter"). They play the key role in the voluntary AE reporting systems in place in the US, Canada, the EU, and elsewhere when communicating such reports to the health authorities or companies. In some countries, an HCP must "validate" a consumer report of an AE. In addition, healthcare professionals work in the health authorities and the companies handling AEs and safety issues.

HEMOVIGILANCE

Surveillance of the adverse events associated with blood products and blood derivatives. Not to be confused with hematovigilance, which is concerned with adverse reactions noxious to the blood cells and the blood-forming organs.

Authors' note: Scandals concerning blood contaminated with hepatitis virus and HIV have occurred in Canada, Japan, and France. For example, in Canada the Krever Report published in Ottawa in November 1997 reported on 1,148 people contaminated with HIV and 28,600 infected with hepatitis C. In France a physician had to serve a prison term because of his involvement in a scandal.

HEPATITIS

A general term for inflammation of the liver that may be produced by multiple etiologies including viruses, parasites, metabolic diseases, drugs, alcohol, toxins and other causes.

The liver is a common site for drug toxicity and injury and there is an enormous literature on drug-induced hepatitis or liver disease. When hepatic failure becomes permanent and severe, liver transplantation may be the only solution.

The clinical presentations vary:

- Acute hepatic injury may be seen with nausea, loss of appetite, malaise, fatigue, weakness, jaundice, abdominal discomfort, and hepatomegaly.
- Fulminant hepatitis is occasionally seen with rapid deterioration, leading to liver failure in a few days to a couple of weeks.
- Chronic hepatitis may present with minimal or no symptoms or signs until very late in the course. Early diagnosis requires laboratory examinations.

There are several types of drug-induced liver injury:

- *Metabolic:* This occurs when the liver metabolizes a drug into a toxic metabolite. The classic example of this is the activation of acetaminophen (paracetamol) into a toxic intermediate metabolite if the primary metabolic pathway is unable to handle a high dose (usually over 1 gm). This may produce fulminant and often fatal hepatitis. Other metabolic hepatitis may be produced only in certain people who metabolize drugs in a particular way.
- *Direct toxicity:* This occurs when a drug produces hepatic injury in all or almost all patients exposed. It is usually dose related. Alcohol (though not really a drug) is the classic example of this, producing various types of liver injury often depending upon the dose.
- *Idiosyncratic toxicity:* Usually immunologic and unpredictable. With an immunologic idiosyncrasy the patient's body recognizes the metabolized drug by-products as foreign. This leads to the destruction of liver cells containing the by-product via the immune system resulting in hepatitis. An immunologic idiosyncrasy is seen in less than one person per 10,000 (0.01%) people and is more than twice as common in women.

Authors' note: Not all drug-induced liver toxicity leads to hepatitis (inflammation). Some drugs may produce a benign "fatty liver," whereas others may produce "steatohepatitis" with a serious or even fatal outcome. The diagnosis may be tricky and a high level of suspicion must be kept. The possibility of drug–drug interactions producing unsuspected toxic levels of one or more drugs should be kept in mind as should the possibility of OTC drug and other less usual causes. Usually withdrawal or lowering of the dose of the offending drug will end the problem. A gastroenterologist, hepatologist, and/or pharmacologist may need to be consulted.

HERBAL MEDICINAL, HERBS

Products made from botanicals that are claimed to maintain or improve health.

HEALTH MAINTENANCE ORGANIZATIONS (HMOS)

A type of group health insurance provider in the US. Many physicians, nurses, physical therapists, and pharmacists offer care and services at a flat rate through this kind of organization. The patient usually pays a small deductible or coinsurance fee for each visit though some HMOs do not charge any fee per visit. However, only visits to caregivers affiliated with the HMO are covered. Visits to nonaffiliated healthcare professionals are not covered or are only partially covered (with the remainder paid for out of pocket by the patient) unless agreed to in advance by the HMO management. Each patient usually has a primary physician ("gatekeeper") who provides routine treatment and handles referrals. Some HMOs now allow the patient to get specialist treatment without referral from the primary care physician.

The healthcare professionals are usually paid a flat salary (rather than a "fee for service") and the administration, paperwork, and office management are provided by the HMO.

Many HMOs maintain their own pharmacies with controlled formularies. Their claims databases represent an important source of information for conducting data mining and pharmacoepidemiologic investigations.

There are now many variants of HMOs in the US.

HEMATOVIGILANCE

Surveillance of AEs affecting the blood (red and white cells, platelets) and blood-forming organs.

HEPATOTOXICITY

The term is used in two ways:

1. The capacity of a drug or other substance to damage the liver ("the hepatotoxicity of drug X").
2. Damage to the liver from whatever cause. ("The patient has marked hepatotoxicity and we suspect that drug X caused it.")

Drugs, chemicals, viruses, fungi, natural products, and other substances may be hepatotoxic.

HERBAL MEDICINES

Also known as herbalism, herbology, phytotherapy, or traditional medicines. The use of plant and plant extracts for treating or preventing disease. This use dates back to ancient times and has been found on all continents. In general, testing for safety and efficacy, as is done for regulated drug products, is seldom performed. The manufacture and importation of such products into countries is often unregulated or minimally regulated.

Authors' note: There is now much discussion and controversy regarding whether health authorities should regulate herbal medicines and other food and nutritional supplements. See http://ntp.niehs.nih.gov/ntp/htdocs/liason/factsheets/HerbMedFacts. pdf. The US FDA will track serious adverse events associated with food supplements starting in late 2007.

The EMEA has issued several documents regarding food supplements and herbals (http://www.emea.europa.eu/pdfs/human/ hmpc/18232005en.pdf). It is likely that regulation of these products will increase over the next several years.

HIGH LEVEL GROUP TERM (HLGT)

In MedDRA, the second highest level of codes (terms) that is just below the System Organ Class terms (SOCs) and above the High Level Terms (HLTs). There are approximately 330 HLGTs. These terms are more "granular" (specific) than SOCs but less granular than HLTs. *See* MedDRA.

HIGH LEVEL TERM (HLT)

In MedDRA, the third highest level of codes (terms) that is just below the High Level Group Terms (HLGTs) and above the Preferred Terms (PTs). There are approximately 1600 HLTs. These terms are more "granular" (specific) than the HLGTs but less granular than the PTs. *See* MedDRA.

HIPAA (HEALTH INSURANCE PORTABILITY AND ACCOUNTABILITY ACT)

See Data Privacy.

HIPPOCRATIC OATH

An ancient oath attributed to Hippocrates that binds physicians to treat the sick to the best of their ability, to preserve the privacy of the patient, and to teach medicine to future physicians. It should be held sacred by the medical community and represents the correct and appropriate ethical conduct expected of physicians. Most medical students swear to an updated version of the oath upon graduation from medical school. In regard to drugs, it states that "I will neither give a deadly drug to anybody who asked for it, nor will I make a suggestion to this effect."

Authors' note: Things are not so simple anymore now that it is known that all drugs may produce adverse drug reactions and that many drugs, particularly oncology drugs, can be "deadly."

HOSPITALIZATION

The act of admitting a patient to a hospital. This generally refers to being admitted to an in-patient unit and not simply being held or observed in an emergency room. "Hospitalization" is a criterion for "seriousness." *See* Serious Adverse Event (SAE).

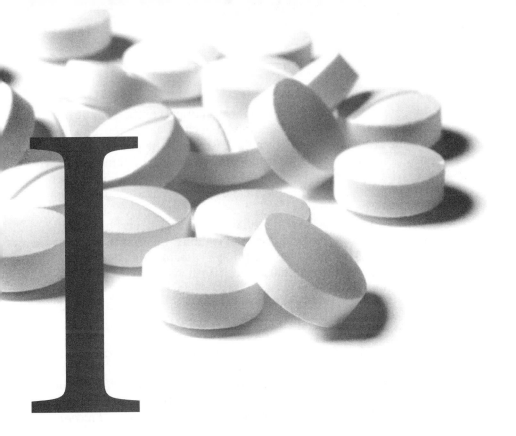

IATROGENIC ILLNESS (OR DISEASE)
A medical problem induced by the use of medicines or medical treatments or by the actions of physicians or other healthcare professionals.

IBD
See International Birth Date.

ICH
See International Conference on Harmonization.

ICSR
See Individual Case Safety Report.

IIS
See Investigator-Initiated Study/Trial.

IIT
See Investigator-Initiated Study/Trial.

IDENTIFIABILITY (OF REPORTER AND PATIENT)

This refers to the ability of the pharmaceutical company or health authority, upon receipt of an individual case safety report, to determine if it is a valid (reportable) case. Both the patient and reporter must have at least one documented piece of demographic data. The reporter and patient are two of the four minimum criteria (along with an identifiable AE and an identifiable suspect drug) needed for a valid report.

A patient is considered identifiable if there is at least one documented piece of demographic data establishing that the patient really exists. This includes: age (or age category, e.g., adolescent, adult, elderly), gender, initials, date of birth, name, or patient identification number.

A reporter is considered identifiable if there is a name, initials, address, relationship to the patient (e.g. patient's mother), profession.

Authors' note: There is some controversy over the criteria for patient identifiability. Some authorities feel that a report of "two patients with headaches" is considered sufficient for identifiability for two individual case safety reports but that "a few patients with headaches" is not. There is no clear agreement in spite of recommendations from CIOMS.

IDIOSYNCRATIC ADR

A type B reaction (see this term). An unpredictable ADR that is unrelated to the known pharmacologic actions of the drug.

IFPMA

See International Federation of Pharmaceutical Manufacturers and Associations.

IMPORTANT MEDICAL EVENTS

Also called significant medical events. In the definition of a serious adverse event, an event that a trained and experienced medical reviewer in the pharmaceutical company or health authority feels is serious even though it does not meet the specific criteria for a serious AE (such as death or hospitalization).

As noted by ICH E2A and captured in many HAs' regulations around the world: "Medical and scientific judgment should be exercised in deciding whether expedited reporting is appropriate in other situations, such as important medical events that may not be immediately life-threatening or result in death or hospitalization but may jeopardize the patient or may require intervention to prevent one of the other outcomes listed in the definition above. These should also usually be considered serious.

"Examples of such events are intensive treatment in an emergency room or at home for allergic bronchospasm; blood dyscrasias or convulsions that do not result in hospitalization; or development of drug dependency or drug abuse." *See* E2A.

The WHO Uppsala Monitoring Center has issued a list of so-called critical terms that corresponds more or less to the same concept. *See* Critical Term.

IMPORTING AND EXPORTING SAFETY DATA

There are many instances when safety data (either individual case safety reports or aggregated data) must be sent to or received from somewhere else. This occurs, for example, when a company sends an expedited report to a health authority or when two companies agree to comarket a drug and they agree to send AEs to each other.

The most efficient way to do this for individual cases is to use the standardized and official method of transmitting individual case safety reports: E2B (see this term). When this is not feasible the informatics and safety departments of the sender and receiver must develop a tested and validated mechanism to transmit the data.

Authors' note: In general, the transfer of data should be simple, but in practice the devil is in the details. Companies may use different drug dictionaries, different ways of storing laboratory data (e.g., tables vs. free text), MedDRA versions, etc. This produces complexity and difficulties in data exchange that must be resolved before data can be exchanged.

IMPUTABILITY

The result of a causality assessment. It reflects the confidence of the analyst in the causality relationship between the administration of a drug and the occurrence of an AE/ADR, leading to assignment of a causality category. The categories of imputability range from excluded, not assessable, and unlikely to possible, probable, or definite.

An imputability determination may vary between healthcare professionals interpreting the same case report as well as between algorithms, questionnaires, and decision tables. It may vary over time in the same case when a follow-up report becomes available and also when new information is provided by the literature and by safety databases.

This term is used mainly in France ("imputabilité").

IMPUTATION

An individual, case-by-case analysis of the causal relationship between administration of a drug and occurrence of an adverse reaction. It is an individual analysis for a given report that is not intended to categorize the overall potential hazard of the drug or the significance of the risk caused by the drug in the population. The result of the case-by-case analysis is called the imputability or causality assessment result for that particular case.

See Appendix I for a proposed Imputation Guide.

IN SITU, ADR

In situ ADRs include administration site reactions (e.g., cutaneous, subcutaneous, venous, mucosae), transit site reactions (e.g., esophagus, bowel), concentration site reactions (e.g., thyroid, kidneys, brain), and excretion site reactions (e.g., biliary lithiasis, renal calculi). The causality assessment of these reactions is usually clear and thus felt to be "definite" because the concentration site is often evident and obvious.

INTENSIVE MONITORING BY LAREB

The Netherlands Pharmacovigilance Centre Lareb has implemented a program of observational cohort studies of new drugs.

This method is an addition to the regular system of spontaneous reporting. Patients' experiences with drugs are the main focus of this system. Patients starting with the drug included in the Lareb monitoring system are selected in the pharmacy. After registration on www.larebmonitor.nl patients are sent questionnaires via e-mail with questions about adverse events occurring during treatment with the drug. The combination of using patient as reporters of adverse events and using e-mail to distribute the questionnaires makes it possible to obtain a lot of information about a drug in a short period of time.

Lareb Intensive Monitoring makes it possible to detect adverse reactions from new drugs at an early stage. The system will be an addition to our current system and is not intended to replace spontaneous reporting from doctors and pharmacists.

Other national systems for following cohorts of patients exposed to new products include the Prescription Event Monitoring (PEM) based in Southampton, UK, and the New Zealand Intensive Medicines Monitoring Program (IMMP).

INCAPACITY, PERSISTENT

Not well defined in regulations or guidances. The FDA gives an example in its 2001 draft guidance: "Persons incarcerated because of actions allegedly caused by a drug (e.g., psychotropic drugs and rage reactions) have sustained a substantial disruption in their ability to conduct normal life functions. Thus, these adverse experiences would qualify for the significant or persistent disability/incapacity outcome." The incapacity may be a direct or an indirect (cascade) effect of the drug.

INCIDENCE RATE

The number of new occurrences of an AE (or a disease) in a population over a period of time. For example, 17 new myocardial infarcts for each one hundred thousand patients taking drug X each year. It is usually very difficult if not impossible to get a true incidence rate in postmarketing situations due to incomplete knowledge of the number of AEs occurring and the number of patients using the drug.

See also Prevalence Rate.

INCIDENCE RATES VS. REPORTING RATES

Incidence rates represent the "true" number of AEs in the population over a period of time—that is, if all cases were known. The reporting rates represent the actual number of AEs in the population reported to the company, health authorities, etc., over a period of time.

In the postmarketing setting, the reporting rate is always less than the incidence rate. A reporting rate of only about 10% compared to the true incidence rate is often loosely quoted—meaning that we are missing 90% of the actual number of AEs that occur but are not reported. For most ADRs the reporting rate may be much different from 10% due to many reasons:

- The drug is late in its life cycle and the AE is felt by the patient or reporter not to be worth reporting.
- The degree of suspicion is low as the AE is felt not to be drug related.
- The AE is hard to pick up: for example, skin AEs are usually very visible and easy to discern whereas a blood cell abnormality requires a laboratory test.
- The severity is minimal and the reporter feels it is not worth taking the time to report.
- The AE is expected and well known.
- The influence of media, the reporting culture of health professionals in a region at a given time, a request from a health authority to report specific AEs, and so forth.

In a clinical trial, however, where full data capture is expected, the reporting rate should equal the incidence rate.

INCIDENTAL AE

As noted in CIOMS V (2001), this is an event that occurs in reasonable clinical temporal association with the use of the drug product but is not the intended subject of the spontaneous report (it did not prompt the contact with the company or regulator). There is also no implicit or explicit expression of possible drug causality by the reporter or the company's safety review staff. They should be included as part of the medical history and not be the subject of expedited reporting. Incidental events should be captured in the company database.

INCLUDED TERM

AE terms in the WHO-ART dictionary that are synonymous with "lower-level terms" in MedDRA. They are a hierarchical step below "preferred terms" and are more specific than preferred terms.

INCLUSION CRITERIA

In clinical trials, requirements that the patients must meet in order to participate.

INCORRECT ROUTE OF ADMINISTRATION

This type of medication error can be committed by the dispenser (e.g., anesthesiologist, nurse, pharmacists) or patient. The reaction may occur locally if the mistake involves the site of administration.

A case series from the coroner of Birmingham, England (Ferner 1994) illustrates the diversity of possible errors. A total of 3,277 inquests were opened during the period 1986–1991. Ten of the deaths were identified as due to errors of prescribing or giving drugs. During the same period, 36 deaths were caused by adverse drug reactions.

- A premature newborn received 2.5 mg/kg/day rather than 2.5 mmol/kg/day of potassium chloride.
- A manic-depressive patient off lithium for 6 months believed her daily dose had been 1.2 gm/day. This dose in fact had been a dose given only in an emergency. Her usual daily dose was 600 mg/day; that is 2 times her normal dose.
- A woman with severe lumbar pain on propoxyphene received during the course of one day: delayed release dihydrocodeine, meperidine (pethidine) IM in the early evening, and 4 hours later morphine. She did not wake up.
- A patient with bronchitis received 4.5 l/min of oxygen by nasal cannula rather than 1 ml/min. She died from respiratory depression.

- An Englishman who required emergency anticoagulation while abroad was given one warfarin 2.5 mg tablet per day. Upon returning to his own physician in Britain he was given one warfarin 3.0 mg tablet per day (the formulation available in the UK). This increase in warfarin of 20% may have led to his fatal hemorrhage.
- A man in atrial fibrillation took the NSAID azapropazone and the anticoagulant warfarin together. This is contraindicated. A fatal cerebral hemorrhage occurred.
- A psychotic patient overdosed on propoxyphene, diclofenac, and dihydrocodeine and required peritoneal dialysis. Bouts of agitation required repeated doses of chlorpromazine both orally and intramuscularly, which produced fatal respiratory arrest.
- A schizophrenic was well controlled for 10 years on 5 mg of haloperidol three times a day. A computerized prescription by his general practitioner for a markedly lower dose led to fatal catatonia and pneumonia.

INCREASED FREQUENCY OF AEs

The calculation of a greater reporting rate of AEs in one period of time compared to the reporting rate in a previous period. This was a requirement by the FDA in periodic reports but later dropped. It is a requirement in PSURs.

It generally applies to serious and nonserious labeled/listed AEs/ADRs. This is used to see if conditions have changed (e.g., new population using the drug, product quality issues, etc.) producing more known AEs/ADRs where the general level of surveillance might be lower than for unexpected serious and nonserious AEs.

The periods used may be month to month, quarter to quarter, or year to year. Various statistical methods have been proposed including the use of the Poisson distribution analysis.

Authors' note: This concept appears at first glance to be very useful in pharmacovigilance but in practice it has been found to be very insensitive. The FDA had this requirement in place for many years only to drop it in July 1997 when it was found to be of limited use. The FDA has proposed to restart it in the Tome (see this term) but has not put this into effect. It is sometimes included in PSURs.

IND

See Investigational New Drug Application.

IND ANNUAL REPORT

A summary of the status of a drug under investigation required by the US FDA (21CFR312.33). The sponsor must submit within 60 days of the anniversary of the date that the IND went into effect a report of the progress of the investigation.

It includes information on the study, including:

- A summary of the status of the study during the previous year: study title, purpose, the patient population, whether the study is completed.
- Total number of subjects planned, number entered to date tabulated by age, gender, and race; number of subjects who completed the study; number of subjects who dropped out.
- A description of any available study results.
- Safety data: A summary of the most frequent and most serious AEs by body system. A summary of all IND expedited reports submitted during the past year. A list of all deaths with the cause of death. A list of drop-outs because of AEs.
- A description of information that was learned regarding the drug.
- A list of preclinical studies completed or in progress during the past year and a summary of the findings.
- A summary of any significant manufacturing or microbiological changes made during the past year.
- The general investigational plan for the coming year.
- A copy of the investigator brochure.
- A description of any significant protocol modifications made during the previous year and not previously reported to the IND in a protocol amendment.

IND REPORTS

A 7- or 15-day expedited report of a serious, unlabeled/unlisted, possibly related (associated) AE or death (7-day report) filed to a US IND.

INDEX CASE

In drug safety, the first reported case of a particular AE/ADR.

INDEX OF SUSPICION

The need to consider a drug as the cause when a new medical problem remains unexplained. Healthcare professionals, patients, consumers, and family members must always consider that medications taken by a patient may be the cause of his or her new problem.

Authors' note: Published data suggest that medicinals do indeed produce significant numbers of unrecognized medical problems.

The teaching of iatrogenic diseases by medical faculties might be a step in the right direction.

INDIVIDUAL CASE SAFETY REPORT (ICSR)

A clinical observation regarding a patient who received a drug and experienced one or more AEs/ADRs. The most common written formats for presentation of a case report are the MedWatch form and the CIOMS I form. The standard electronic format is the E2B transmission. Some are also published as short reports in medical journals.

INFORMATICS OR INFORMATION TECHNOLOGY (IT)

The general term used in drug safety encompassing the use of computers and other means of data collection, storage, manipulation, analysis, retrieval, reporting, and mining to handle drug safety data.

Authors' note: Given the massive amounts of data (millions of AE cases in the databases of companies, the FDA, EMEA, Uppsala Monitoring Center, etc.), it is impossible to store and use this data without sophisticated and high maintenance computers, computer programs, and the people who keep them running.

INFORMED CONSENT

In clinical trials, the document signed by the patient (or guardian) and witness that describes the clinical trial, benefits, risks, options to leave the trial at any point without compromising health care, whom to call, etc. It signifies that the patient has freely chosen to enter the trial and understands the consequences, both good and bad.

Occasionally used in drug safety to allow records (hospital, laboratory, physician, insurance, etc.) of a possible AE to be released to the pharmaceutical company, HA, etc. It may also be used if the data is to be used for marketing purposes.

Informed consents are also used occasionally in the general practice of medicine when certain drugs are prescribed that are known to be toxic in certain situations. For example, in the US, female patients of child-bearing potential must sign an informed consent before being given Accutane® (isotretinoin) against severe acne refractory to less dangerous treatments because of the teratogenic risks.

INJECTION SITE REACTION

A cutaneous ADR that occurs at the place on the skin where a parenteral drug has been given. What is most interesting about these reactions is that the causality is in almost all cases clearly due to the drug in question and thus can be classified as "very probable" or even "certain." There are very few other adverse events that have such clear causality.

This type of reaction can be of type A or type B. It can be due to the active product, an excipient, or the mode of administration (needle, catheter, etc.). It may also be due to an error of administration which may or may not be evident such as intravenous injections which are, in fact, given subcutaneously or intra-arterially.

INNOVATOR DRUG

A product marketed by the company that first created it. The "original brand" of the product.

INSPECTIONS

See Audit.

INSTITUTE OF MEDICINE (IOM)

An organization within the US National Academy of Sciences. They are a nonprofit, nongovernmental research group that provides evaluation and counsel on healthcare issues.

The IOM recently performed an analysis of the US drug safety system (www.iom.edu/CMS/3793/26341/37329.aspx) and noted that:

There is a perception of crisis that has compromised the credibility of the FDA and of the pharmaceutical industry. Most stakeholders—the agency, the industry, consumer organizations, Congress, professional societies, healthcare entities—appear to agree on the need for certain improvements in the system.

The drug safety system is impaired by the following factors: serious resource constraints that weaken the quality and quantity of the science that is brought to bear on drug safety; an organizational culture in CDER that is not optimally functional; and unclear and insufficient regulatory authorities particularly with respect to enforcement.

The FDA and the pharmaceutical industry do not consistently demonstrate accountability and transparency to the public by communicating safety concerns in a timely and effective fashion.

Recommendations include:

- Labeling requirements and advertising limits for new medications.
- Clarified authority and additional enforcement tools for the FDA.
- Clarification of the FDA's role in gathering and communicating additional information on marketed products' risks and benefits.

- Mandatory registration of clinical trial results to facilitate public access to drug safety information.
- An increased role for the FDA's drug safety staff.
- A large boost in funding and staffing for the FDA.

The FDA and the US Congress have acted on many of these recommendations. *See* the FDA Revitalization Act.

INSTITUTIONAL REVIEW BOARD (IRB)

See Ethics Committee.

INSURANCE COMPANIES (ROLE IN PHARMACOVIGILANCE)

Many insurance companies or governmental agencies that "insure" or cover patients' health (e.g., the US Department of Veterans Affairs, Canadian provinces, etc.) maintain large databases of information in that database or with such medical information available in other "linked" databases. These databases may then be used for epidemiologic studies of adverse events and drug toxicity.

Insurance companies may also choose which newly marketed drugs they will allow on their formulary and provide reimbursement to the patient when purchased. Their selection is determined by the price and the benefit:risk balance, compared with older products. Drugs that are excluded from the formulary must be paid for out of pocket by the patient.

INTENSIFIED MONITORING

This term represents a call for reporting by healthcare practitioners of one or more AEs/ADRs with the aim of acquiring more data. This is done either in the case of a pharmacovigilance investigation because the product is new on the market and is a member of a pharmacologic family of drugs that may produce significant risk ("reporting focused on a product to see if there is a true signal") or in follow-up to a known signal ("reporting focused on an AE/ADR"). Other terms have been used, including: enhanced, requested, facilitated, reinforced, encouraged, incited, active, or stimulated reporting. It must be emphasized that this is a scientific measure taken to (a) confirm, (b) clarify, or (c) refute a hypothesis raised by a signal.

- *Focused on a product.* The specific product is added to the table of medications under formal surveillance in the national bulletin of pharmacovigilance. In Australia the list is called "Drugs of Current Interest." In Great Britain, being under such surveillance can last 2 years or more and a list of products under intensive monitoring is published in the national bulletin. Such a medication is identified in the labeling by a black triangle.

- *Aimed at an ADR.* It is possible in the course of a pharmacovigilance investigation produced as the result of a signal to ask for intensified monitoring of a particular ADR felt to be possibly due to the drug. An example of this might be a specific ADR such as torsades de pointes or a suspected new drug interaction that has only become suspect since the marketing of the product. The first step consists of placing the drug on the list of "products under surveillance" in the national bulletin of pharmacovigilance. However, if the situation is very serious, additional measures such as a request for cases can be addressed to healthcare professionals by use of a "Dear Healthcare Professional" letter using all the modern means of communication (traditional mail, e-mail, the Internet, announcements in professional journals) as well as a call to the public using mass media (e.g., television and radio) as appropriate from either the health authority or the manufacturer or both.
- *Global or universal surveillance.* Intensified reporting of all suspected ADRs for all products. This can be directed, usually by a health agency, at the clinicians in an entire country, region, hospital, etc. To be effective it is necessary to ensure that sufficient budget, logistics, and competent and motivated personnel are available and the reasons are adequately explained to the reporting clinicians. This may occur when a country introduces pharmacovigilance at the national level for the first time or revamps its older drug surveillance system.

INTERACTION STUDY

See Drug Interaction Studies and Drug Interactions.

INTERIM PERIODIC SAFETY REPORTS (IPSRs)

A report defined in the 2003 FDA proposed regulations ("The Tome"). This is an abbreviated report to be submitted to the FDA at 7.5 and 12.5 years after US approval. The FDA did not accept the 5-year interval between a PSUR at years 5, 10 and 15.

This report is similar to a PSUR but excludes summary tabulations, new information after the data lock point, summary tabulations of spontaneous consumer SADRs, summary tabulations for SADRs with unknown outcomes, summary tabulations for reports from class action lawsuits, and summary tabulations for US MEs.

As of late 2007 it has not been put into effect.

INTERNATIONAL BIRTH DATE (IBD)

The date that the first regulatory authority anywhere in the world approved a drug for marketing.

Authors' note: This date is used for establishing the periodicity and timing of PSURs and should be synchronized around the world such that all authorities receive the PSUR every 6 months, 1 year, 3 years, etc., based on the IBD. If harmonization is not possible, the MAH and regulators try to find a common birth month and day so that reports can be submitted on the same month and day whether every 6 months, yearly, etc.

INTERNATIONAL CLASSIFICATION OF DISEASE (ICD-10)

A standardized classification put out by the World Health Organization (WHO) of diseases for use in epidemiology, healthcare institutions, insurance companies, the pharmaceutical industry, etc.

See the website http://www.who.intclassifications/icd/en/.

INTERNATIONAL CONFERENCE ON HARMONIZATION (ICH)

The International Conference on Harmonization (spelled with an "s" instead of a "z" on their website) of Technical Requirements for Registration of Pharmaceuticals for Human Use (ICH) is a unique project that brings together the regulatory authorities of Europe, Japan, and the United States and experts from the pharmaceutical industry in the three regions and elsewhere to discuss scientific and technical aspects of product registration.

The purpose is to make recommendations on ways to achieve greater harmonization in the interpretation and application of technical guidelines and requirements for product registration in order to reduce or obviate the need to duplicate the testing carried out during the research and development of new medicines.

The objective of such harmonization is a more economical use of human, animal and material resources, and the elimination of unnecessary delay in the global development and availability of new medicines whilst maintaining safeguards on quality, safety, and efficacy, and regulatory obligations to protect public health.

Multiple plenary and working group meetings have been held since 1989 with the result that many guidances have been written and adopted by health authorities around the world. This has served to standardize many aspects of pharmaceutical development, clinical trials, reporting, etc. In terms of drug safety, many of the recommendations from ICH (and CIOMS, see this term) have been adopted as regulations producing much uniformity in AE data collection, storage, analysis, expedited and PSUR reporting, E2B use, etc.

See their website: www.ich.org. *See also* E2A, E2B, E2C, E2D, E2E.

INTERNATIONAL FEDERATION OF PHARMACEUTICAL MANUFACTURERS AND ASSOCIATIONS (IFPMA)

From their website: A non-profit, non-governmental organization of national industry associations and companies from both developed and developing countries. Member companies are research-based pharmaceutical, biotech and vaccine companies.

The main objectives of IFPMA are:

- To encourage a global policy environment that is conducive to innovation in medicine, both therapeutic and preventative, for the benefit of patients around the world.
- To contribute industry expertise and foster collaborative relationships and partnerships with international organizations, national institutions, governments and non-governmental organizations that are dedicated to the improvement of public health, especially in developing and emerging countries.
- To assure regular contact and experience-sharing and coordinate the efforts of its members towards the realization of the above objectives.

See their website: http://www.ifpma.org/index.aspx.

THE INTERNATIONAL JOURNAL OF RISK & SAFETY IN MEDICINE

A journal published by IOS Press in Amsterdam covering patient safety, pharmacovigilance, and liability. From their website: "The Journal is concerned with rendering the practice of medicine as safe as it can be; that involves promoting the highest possible quality of care, but also examining how those risks which are inevitable can be contained and managed. This is not exclusively a drugs journal. Our journal wants to publish high quality interdisciplinary papers related to patient safety, not the ones for domain specialists."

The founding editor is Dr M.N. Graham Dukes. See http://www.iospress.nl/loadtop/load.php?isbn=09246479.

INTERNATIONAL NONPROPRIETARY NAME (INN)

The International Nonproprietary Name Program of the World Health Organization (WHO) assigns international "generic" names to drugs. Each INN is a unique name that is globally recognized and is public property. See their website: http://www.who.int/medicines/services/inn/en/index.html.

Authors' note: The name of a drug is usually the same from country to country, but there are instances in which the names differ. For example, acetaminophen is the designation in the United States (the United States Adopted Name—USAN), whereas paracetamol is the designation in France. Another example is cephalexin, which is the designation in the US (USAN), Great Britain (British Approved Name—BAN), and in Canada, whereas the French designation (Dénomination commune française—DCF) is cefalexinum and INN is cefalexine.

INTERNATIONAL NORMALIZED PROTHROMBIN TIME RATIO (INR)

In pharmacotherapy: A laboratory test that is used to monitor the pharmacologic action of oral anticoagulants. The results are used to adjust the dosage to stay within the narrow therapeutic window.

In drug safety: This test is used to discover new drug interactions between an oral anticoagulant and recently marketed drugs. That is, if a patient has a stable INR and a new drug is added to the regimen taken by the patient with a subsequent change in the INR, the patient should be worked up for a drug interaction (e.g., dechallenge and, if safe and ethical, a rechallenge with the new drug) and a readjustment of the anticoagulant accordingly if the new drug is medically required.

INTERNATIONAL SOCIETY FOR PHARMACOEPIDEMIOLOGY (ISPE)

An organization dedicated to advancing the health of the public by providing a forum for the open exchange of scientific information and for the development of policy; education; and advocacy for the field of pharmacoepidemiology, including pharmacovigilance, drug utilization research, and therapeutic risk management.

It is a nonprofit international professional membership organization dedicated to promoting pharmacoepidemiology, the science that applies epidemiologic approaches to studying the use, effectiveness, value, and safety of pharmaceuticals. ISPE is firmly committed to providing an unbiased scientific forum to the views of all parties with interests in drug development, drug delivery, drug use, drug costs, and drug effects.

ISPE members represent the various scientific disciplines involved in studying drugs. Members are employed by the pharmaceutical industry, academic institutions, government agencies, nonprofit and for-profit private organizations. Members have degrees in a number of fields, including epidemiology, biostatistics, medicine, nursing, pharmacology, pharmacy, law, health economics, and journalism. With members in 53 countries and national chapters in Argentina, Belgium, Denmark, and the Netherlands, ISPE provides an international forum for sharing knowledge and scientific approaches to foster the science of pharmacoepidemiology.

ISPE sponsors conferences and seminars, a quarterly newsletter, and an official journal called *Pharmacoepidemiology and Drug Safety* that is published by Wiley. See their website: www. pharmacoepi.org/.

INTERNATIONAL SOCIETY OF PHARMACOVIGILANCE (ISoP)

An international nonprofit scientific organization for promoting education, publication, and research in pharmacovigilance. Formerly the European Society of Pharmacovigilance founded by Pr René Royer in France, the membership comes from academia, regulatory agencies, industry, and health professionals. It maintains affiliations with the International Union of Pharmacology (IUPHAR) and the European Association for Clinical Pharmacology and Therapeutics (EACPT), maintains ties with the WHO Uppsala Monitoring Center (UMC) and the International Society of Pharmacoepidemiology (ISPE), and organizes a yearly scientific meeting and courses on pharmacovigilance. The official journal is *Drug Safety* published by Adis. The website is www.isoponline.org.

INTERVENTIONAL STUDY

Equivalent to Experimental Study or Clinical Trial. A type of study in which the treatment of participating patients is selected by a clinical investigator rather than by their treating physician and is administered to patients according to a written protocol. A drug treatment may be used either within the approved labeling or according to indication, dosage, and formulation as specified in a protocol. The number of control measures may vary, from the single arm open label trial typical of phase I to the sophisticated randomized double-blind comparative multicenter trial typical of phase III.

By comparison, during an observational (i.e., noninterventional) study the treatment of patients is selected by their physicians in the course of normal medical practice. Any drug treatment is used according to the labeled indication, dosage, and formulation. Such a study may also have a written protocol.

Authors' note: All studies should be done according to the laws, regulations, and good clinical practices in effect in that country no matter what the type of study.

INVESTIGATIONAL NEW DRUG APPLICATION (IND)

A dossier that a drug sponsor must submit to the US FDA before beginning tests of a new drug, formulation, patient population, indication, or dosage in humans. The IND contains the plan (protocol) for the study and is expected to provide a complete picture of the drug, including its structural formula, animal test results, and manufacturing information. The trial may not start until the IND is approved by the FDA.

INVESTIGATOR BROCHURE

For drugs that are not yet on the market (i.e., are not yet approved for sale), the labeling used for adverse event (AE) reporting is considered to be the official "investigator brochure" as prepared by the sponsor that contains a summary of the known information about the drug, including its chemistry, pharmacology, toxicology, clinical studies, and AEs. It is usually updated yearly or more frequently if new information is developed. It is this document that is used in the preparation of 7- and 15-day expedited (alert) reports to health authorities (FDA, EMEA, etc.) and for investigational new drug annual reports.

INVESTIGATOR, CLINICAL

A physician but also sometimes a nurse, pharmacist, dentist, or other medical professional (under the supervision of a physician) who is responsible for the conduct, supervision, and safety of the patients in a clinical trial at his or her site during a company designed and sponsored multicenter trial. The investigator is responsible for the reporting of AEs to the sponsor company and/or the FDA or other health authority.

When an academic physician initiates a trial, he is also responsible for the design of the trial. *See* Investigator-Initiated Study/Trial. In both situations he or she is also responsible for keeping the investigational review board up to date on the progress of the study.

INVESTIGATOR-INITIATED STUDY/TRIAL (IIS/IIT)

A clinical research study or trial in which new ideas (usually thought up by researchers in the academic world and proposed to pharmaceutical companies) are examined. This can be instrumental in the scientific development of a drug. The advantages of such studies are that new ideas are found and explored, costs are usually fairly small, and the studies can be done fairly quickly. The disadvantage is that many details that should be determined before doing trials are unanswered (e.g., effective dose, safety in this population, etc.).

Funding is usually from the pharmaceutical company in the form of a grant-in-aid, drug supply, protocol, or case report form support. A contract or agreement is usually signed by both parties. The legal sponsor of the study is not the pharmaceutical company but rather the investigator. It is he or she who opens the IND with the FDA (or equivalent with another HA), often with the help of the pharmaceutical company, if one is required. The usual safety provisions are followed: good clinical practices, investigational review boards, and SAE reporting to the FDA by the investigator. The SAEs should be reported to the company in addition to the health authority by the investigator so that a full safety database is maintained for all uses of a product by the company.

Authors' note: In earlier years, there were disputes over ownership of the data and the publication (or rather lack of publication) of negative results. These are resolving, in general, with the "ownership" of the data by both parties and with the right to publish retained by the investigator no matter what the results.

INVESTIGATOR NOTIFICATION

The regulatory obligation of the sponsor (usually a pharmaceutical company) to notify all "participating investigators" (21CFR32C(1)) as well as the FDA of a 15-day expedited report to the IND. The notification is often in the form of an "investigator letter" that either contains the case information as text or includes the MedWatch form sent to the FDA. In addition, 21CFR32(B)(ii) requires that "the sponsor shall identify all safety reports, previously filed with the IND concerning a similar adverse experience, and shall analyze the significance of the adverse experience in light of the previous, similar reports." Similar requirements exist in the EU and many other jurisdictions.

IPSR

See Interim Periodic Safety Reports.

IRB

See Ethics Committee.

ISPE

See International Society for Pharmacoepidemiology.

IT

See Informatics or Information Technology.

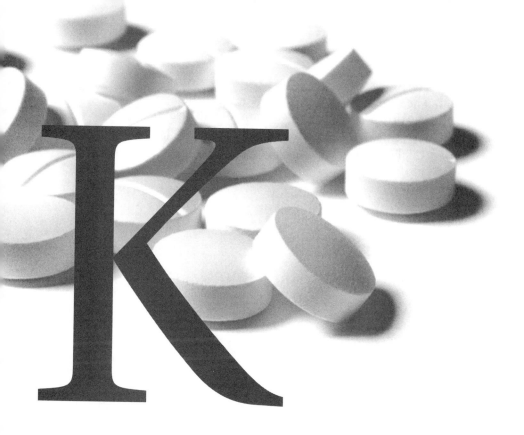

KOCH'S POSTULATES

A concept developed by Robert Koch in the 19th century to prove that a particular microorganism causes a particular disease:

1. The microbe must be found in all animals with the specific disease in question and it must be absent in healthy animals.
2. The microbe must be isolated from the diseased animal (e.g., from blood, skin lesion, etc.).
3. If the organism grown in culture from the first animal is introduced into an unaffected animal, this animal develops the disease.
4. The microbe is then isolated from the newly infected animal.

This concept has loosely been applied to drug safety to refer to the challenge/dechallenge/rechallenge situation. When the following scenario occurs some will say that this "meets Koch's postulates":

a. A patient receives a drug and experiences an AE.
b. The drug is withdrawn (dechallenge).

   c. The AE disappears.

   d. The drug is reintroduced and the AE recurs.

   e. The drug is withdrawn again and the AE disappears.

     This is highly suggestive that the drug in question caused the AE. *See* Challenge, Dechallenge, Rechallenge.

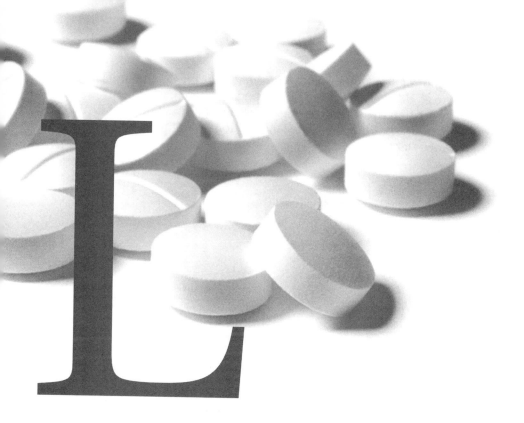

L-TRYPTOPHAN

See Tryptophan and the FDA.

LABELED

An AE/ADR that appears in the official (national) reference documentation of a drug. That is, if an AE/ADR appears in the AE section of the labeling (US package insert, EU SmPC, Drug Facts for OTC products, the investigator brochure for clinical study products, etc.), then the AE/ADR is considered to be labeled for purposes of expedited and aggregate reporting to health authorities. Conversely, if it does not appear in the reference document it is considered unlabeled.

The definition became more confusing and complex with the creation of the Core Safety Information and the Core Data Sheet in 1992 (CIOMS II). The core safety information is prepared by the manufacturer and contains all relevant safety information. This information should appear in all product labels worldwide. When an AE/ADR is found in the core information it is, under this newer definition, considered "listed." In addition to the core safety information, there is safety information printed in national labels (e.g., US package insert, European SmPC, etc.), which may differ, for various reasons, from the Core Safety Information. An AE/ADR that is now found in the local or national labeling is now considered "labeled."

Listed	*Labeled*	*Explanation*
In Core Safety Information (CSI) and used for PSUR expectedness	**In national labeling and used for expedited reporting expectedness**	
Yes	Yes	AE/ADR is in core and local labels. Used for PSUR and expedited expectedness.
Yes	No	In core but not local label. This should not occur as local labeling should contain all core AEs/ADRs.
No	Yes	In local label but not core. This may occur if a particular health authority wants something in the local label above and beyond the core safety information.
No	No	An AE/ADR or signal that has not attained a sufficient level of proof or concern to be included in the safety information.

Thus, in theory, all AEs/ADRs that are in the core should be in the national labels (listed and labeled). Some AEs in the national labels (that a particular country chooses to add to its local labels for whatever reason) might not appear in the core label.

LABELING

"Labeling" is a general term referring to the document or electronic file that summarizes all key information for the safe and effective usage of a drug. Labeling is usually prepared by the manufacturer and approved by the FDA or other health authorities.

The requirements for labeling in the US are summarized in 21CFR1. The official definition of labeling for a marketed product is 21CFR1.3(a): (a) Labeling includes all written, printed, or graphic matter accompanying an article at any time while such article is in interstate commerce or held for sale after shipment or delivery in interstate commerce. (b) Label means any display of written, printed, or graphic matter on the immediate container of any article, or any such matter affixed to any consumer commodity or affixed to or appearing upon a package containing any consumer commodity. Thus, it includes the FDA-approved written material describing a drug such as the "package insert" and the packaging and box that a drug is shipped or sold in.

Synonyms for labeling include "package insert," "professional labeling," "direction circular," and "package circular." It also includes the FDA-approved patient labeling where this exists: boxed warning (if applicable), indications and usage, dosage and administration, how supplied, contraindications, warnings, general precautions, drug interactions, drug and laboratory test interactions, laboratory tests, information for patients, teratogenic effects, nonteratogenic effects, labor and delivery, nursing mothers, pediatric use, geriatric use, carcinogenesis, mutagenesis, impairment of fertility, adverse reactions, controlled substance (if applicable), abuse, dependence, overdosage, description, clinical pharmacology, animal pharmacology/toxicology, clinical studies, and references.

In 2006, the FDA introduced new requirements for labeling, including structured product labeling (SPL) in which all labeling has three basic parts: (1) The header with general information about the label and product, (2) the sections with blocks of text (e.g., indications, contraindications, warnings, etc.), and (3) the data elements with product-specific information (e.g., active ingredient, dosage form, how supplied, etc.).

Most other countries have similar requirements for labeling but differences in style, content, philosophic approach to what should be in a label, language, and other factors contribute to labeling differing to some degree from country to country.

In the EU the approved labeling is known as the Summary of Product Characteristics (SPC or SmPC). The EU situation is complex with labeling being the same or similar for some products (often newer products) if the product was approved centrally or if the label was harmonized at the EU level. Many other products, however, have labels that differ from country to country within Europe.

In the United States, the generic term "labeling" (sometimes called the "package insert") is used to refer to the official FDA-approved US product information. The word "labeling" is also used in the United States for the SPC when referring to European labeling. Some in the EU, conversely, use the term SPC (or SmPC) when they are referring to their own official labeling or to the US labeling. Thus one might hear a reference to the US SPC—a concept that does not really exist in the United States. This refers, in practice, to the US official labeling.

In terms of pharmacovigilance the sections of labeling that are of most interest include the AEs, warnings, drug interactions, precautions, and pregnancy information. The labeling is used to determine whether a particular AE that is reported for that product is "labeled" or "listed" (see these terms).

LACK OF EFFICACY (LOE)

Lack of efficacy, or the failure of the drug to do what it is supposed to do, is considered by the regulations in the US, EU, and elsewhere as a reportable adverse event and thus this data should be collected and tracked. An increase in LOE may be a risk management clue to problems with a specific lot, a new group of patients now taking the drug, an alteration in the disease (e.g., new resistance to an antibiotic developing in various bacteria), etc.

In practice, LOE concerns the direct pharmacological efficacy, an effect that is expected in all cases and can be observed readily. For example, a bottle of beta-blocker tablets that do not lower the pulse rate when taken at therapeutic dosage would raise suspicion of a defective lot; but taking the same beta-blocker for 10 years and dying from a heart attack at the end of that period would not be considered a case of LOE.

Authors' note: LOE refers to approved indications. Failure of the drug to work in nonapproved indications may not be surprising at all and does not need to be collected as an LOE but may be collected as either "misuse" or "abuse" depending upon the circumstances. LOE poses something of a problem in certain situations, such as OTC products where patients often use the drug "loosely" for indications other than those approved.

LACTATION

Production of breast milk. In drug safety, the possibility that a drug taken by the mother may produce AEs in a breastfeeding child must be kept in mind because transmammary transmission of certain drugs may be harmful to the child. Not all drugs or their metabolites are found in milk. Information on whether a drug is found in breast milk is usually noted in the drug labeling.

LANDMARK ARTICLES ON DRUG SAFETY

David Coulter has chosen his top five papers in pharmacovigilance (Uppsala Reports #36, 2007)

- Finney DJ. "The design and logic of a monitor of drug use." *J Chron Dis* 1965, 18:77–98.

- Karch FE, Lasagna L. "Adverse Reactions. A critical review." *JAMA* 1975, 234:1236–1241.
- Skegg DCG, Doll R. "Frequency of eye complaints and rashes among patients receiving practolol and propranolol." *Lancet* 1977, ii:475–478.
- Venning GR. "Identification of adverse reactions to new drugs." *BMJ* 1983, 286 pages:199–202, 289–292, 365–368, 458–460, 544–547.
- Lazarou J, Pomeranz BH, Corey PN. "Incidence of adverse drug reactions in hospitalized patients. A meta-analysis of prospective studies." *JAMA* 1998, 279:1200–1205.

LAREB

A Dutch organization founded in 1991 and whose name was abbreviated LAREB which stood for, in Dutch, "The National Registration and Evaluation of Adverse Drug Reactions." The name is now the Netherlands Pharmacovigilance Centre Lareb but it is still known as Lareb.

Lareb collects and analyses reports of suspected adverse drug reactions that have been passed on by caregivers, patients and manufacturers.

The focus lies mainly on identifying as yet unknown negative adverse drug reactions. Lareb receives almost 4500 reports yearly. See http://www.lareb.nl/index.asp.

LARGE SIMPLE SAFETY STUDY (LSSS)

A type of study done in risk management programs. Originally derived from large efficacy trials, in drug safety, an LSSS is classically a randomized clinical trial with a control group looking at large numbers of patients for safety endpoints. These safety issues usually arose in previous clinical trials and warrant further study. These studies may be done before or after marketing (the latter as phase IV commitments). They are usually quite powerful statistically as the number of patients is large. They try to reflect real clinical use in patient populations at risk and they are randomized and controlled to minimize biases.

LATENCY PERIOD

1) The interval or duration between the last dose of a suspect product and the first manifestation of an ADR. Some drugs may have a very long latency period measured in weeks to months to years.

Often the latency period is short, such as seen in withdrawal or rebound syndromes. However, long and variable latency periods may render the diagnosis difficult:

- In teratovigilance, there is usually a delay between the administration of a drug in the first trimester and the diagnosis of a malformation either during the later stages of the pregnancy or after birth.
- In the case of retroperitoneal fibrosis due to the beta-blocker practolol, the physician would not recognize the lesion until the "cascade" or indirect effect of intestinal or ureteral occlusion occurred.
- In the case of clear cell adenocarcinoma of the vagina due to in utero exposure to diethylstilbesterol (DES), the latency period was about 20 years.
- A final disconcerting example occurs when the time to onset is expected to be short but in fact turns out to be long. As an example, the onset of severe cutaneous necrosis can occur rapidly in the surrounding tissues due to extravasation of an antineoplastic agent from the vein; but if it takes a week to develop after the end of the infusion, then we have a long latency period.

2) Some authors still use this term to designate a late occurring AE. (See that term.)

LATE OCCURRING AEs

Adverse events with very long times to onset or very long latency periods. Diethylstilbesterol produced vaginal cancers in the offspring of women taking this drug early in their pregnancy, some 20 years after the last exposure in utero. This latency period was thus measured in years and prevented the earlier detection of this catastrophic ADR.

LAW

An obligation on people or companies that is created by a legislature, executive, courts, etc., depending on the country. In drug safety, laws should be distinguished from regulations, guidelines, and directives. (See these terms.) In general, laws take effect in and of themselves, whereas other instruments might require another body (e.g., the FDA) to put out regulations or guidances.

Authors' note: As an example, the US Congress passed a law in late 2006 which was subsequently signed by the President requiring the FDA to set up regulations to ensure the collection of serious and nonserious AEs on over-the-counter products in the US. The law required the FDA to put the law into effect by the end of 2007.

LAWSUIT

An action or a proceeding brought to a court in order to recover a right or money or to obtain a remedy for a grievance. These actions are usually civil rather than criminal. They are usually between companies and individuals but occasionally the government (e.g., the FDA) may take civil or criminal action against companies or individuals. These phenomena are the most common in the US but are increasingly being seen elsewhere.

Authors' note: Pharmaceutical companies are exposed to numerous and costly civil and class action lawsuits, usually as a result of adverse events alleged as insufficiently labeled ADRs. Some of these lawsuits are settled without going to court; others are settled in court and can be decided in favor of either the plaintiff or the company. The lawsuits for widely used drugs may number in the thousands. Timely and transparent labeling of ADRs is an important step for avoiding lawsuits.

LEGACY DATABASE

In the context of installing a new database (e.g., an electronic system to collect adverse events), the data and the programming (software) in the old database that is being replaced are referred to as the legacy database.

Authors' note: Moving data from one database to another is full of pitfalls, as the two databases are never alike and certain changes, assumptions, alterations, and coding revisions must be made in the information being transferred from the old database to make the data transferable and acceptable to the new database. For example, the old database may refer to patient ages as baby, child, adolescent, adult, and elderly whereas the new database may have different categories (child, adult) or may use numerical ages or ranges. Moving this data set may prove to be a nightmare.

LEGAL REQUIREMENTS

In drug safety this generally refers to the governmental laws, regulations, directives, etc., that oblige (or, in some cases, request) companies, healthcare professionals, the health authority, and others to collect, process, analyze, and report adverse events to the health authority or elsewhere (e.g., investigators) within certain periods of time. Failure to do this may result in civil or criminal penalties.

Authors' note: Very often the situation arises where senior management in a company (mistakenly) chooses not to put certain procedures into effect that are recommended either by the safety department or by health authority guidances, arguing that the company does not have a legal obligation to do so. This is correct but usually unwise. Once, however, something becomes a legal obligation the safety department may (usually) argue that the company must take this action to be in full legal compliance. Thus legal requirements are usually the safety department's best friend.

LEGAL DEPARTMENT

In drug companies, the group of attorneys, paralegals, and others who deal with lawsuits, claims, patents, intellectual property, data privacy, etc. that involve the company. The legal group may be the first to receive notification of an AE (an alleged ADR) in the form of a lawsuit. The legal group also assists in analysis of safety regulations and laws as well as drawing up secrecy (confidentiality) agreements, contracts, and safety exchange agreements, obtaining follow-up information when attorneys are involved, etc. They also prepare contracts and confidentiality agreements with clinical investigators and with the medical institutions where the trial is carried out.

LICENSING AGREEMENT

A contract between two companies in which one company allows the other company to sell its drug in exchange for fees, royalties, etc. In such situations, there are safety obligations on both companies in regard to collecting, exchanging, storing, reporting, analyzing, etc., adverse events, medical errors, quality issues, and so forth, that must be spelled out in a written safety exchange agreement.

LIFE CYCLE MANAGEMENT

As used now in the pharmaceutical industry, the concept that a drug product has a natural life cycle from premarketing development until withdrawal from the market (which may be due to newer and better products making the drug outmoded due to safety related issues).

Thus the product needs to be looked after and interventions made in order for it to be profitable with the best possible benefit:risk evaluation throughout its existence. This implies review and analysis of its indications, uses, marketing and sales, areas of research, areas of concern or problems (e.g., safety), competitors, pricing, etc., from its earliest preclinical study until its withdrawal from the market.

In terms of drug safety and pharmacovigilance, this means that someone (usually from the drug safety department) in the company needs to follow the safety profile (and benefit:risk analysis) of the drug from its first animal pharmacology and toxicology trials through marketing. In particular, while on the market risk assessment, mitigation and management must be done, as well as looking at the safety aspects of possible new patient populations, formulations, and indications.

Authors' note: This concept is now very much in vogue, along with risk management. Anything that allows medical professionals to continuously examine the safety of drugs is a good thing.

LIFE THREATENING

A life-threatening adverse drug experience is any adverse drug experience that places the patient, in the view of the initial reporter, at immediate risk of death from the adverse drug experience as it occurred; i.e., it does not include an adverse drug experience that, had it occurred in a more severe form, might have caused death. [21 CFR 314.80(a) and 310.305(b)]

It does not matter whether the AE was treated immediately or not.

LINE LISTING

In pharmacovigilance, a computerized tabulation of data associated with a particular product. The columns contain the specific information on the product, the patient, and the AE/ADR while each row corresponds to individual cases.

In a Periodic Safety Update Report (PSUR) as prepared by the manufacturer to be submitted to health authorities, this table summarizes the AEs/ADRs associated with a product. The format has been standardized by ICH (following the original CIOMS II format very closely) and has been accepted by the EU, Japan, and the US. The columns of the line listing are as follows:

- Country
- Source (clinical trial, healthcare professional, literature)
- Age
- Sex
- Dose
- Time to appearance
- Description of the reaction reported
- Outcome (fatal, recovered, etc.)
- Comments
- Reference number of the manufacturer.

LINKAGE STUDY

This term is often used to refer to genetic studies. It is also used in the world of computers and information technology.

In clinical medicine and drug safety, it usually refers to record linkage. This is the exercise of identifying data records referring to the same person from different sources and creating a link between them so that the data from both sources can be used together for analysis. For example, data on patients may be linked from an insurance company's claims database to a hospital database and then to the pharmacy database of drug use to study the safety profile of drugs in hospitalized patients.

It may also mean the comparison of diseases (e.g., hypertension, arthritis), treatments given (drugs, surgery), and patient outcomes (hospitalization, death) in a given health database and linking them to individual patients through their medical record.

LISTED

An AE/ADR that is found in the Core Safety Labeling is considered "listed." It may or may not be "labeled" in the Summary of Product Characteristics, US Package Insert, or other local drug labeling. *See* Labeled.

LITERATURE REVIEW

The obligation of the pharmaceutical company to periodically (sometimes as frequently as every week or two) review the published literature worldwide looking for serious and nonserious adverse events/adverse drug reactions reported with that company's products. This is also known as literature surveillance. If, in the published report, the manufacturer is not specified (i.e., the product might be from another manufacturer or generic), it is still the company's obligation to review these publications. If the report meets the four minimum criteria for reportability, the company is obligated to database and report the case as required. This may lead to multiple notifications of the same case to the health authority if many companies manufacture generic versions of the product.

CIOMS V notes the following:

- Cases may appear in letters to the editor.
- There may be a long lag time between the first detection of a signal by a researcher and his or her publication of it.
- Publications may be a source of false information and signals.
- Companies should search at least two internationally recognized literature databases using the International Normalized Nomenclature (INN) name at least monthly.
- Broadcast and lay media should not ordinarily be monitored. If such information is made available to the company, it should be followed up.

- Judgment should be used in regard to follow-up with the strongest efforts made for serious unexpected ADRs.
- If the product source or brand is not specified, a company should assume it was its product. The company should indicate in any report made that the specific brand was not identified if this is the case.
- If there is a contractual agreement between two or more companies (e.g., for comarketing), the contract should specify the responsibility for literature searches and reporting.
- English should be the standard language for literature report translations.
- Regulators should accept translation of an abstract or of pertinent sections of a publication.
- References cited in a publication on apparently unexpected/unlisted and serious reactions should be checked against the company's existing database of literature reports. Articles not previously reported should be retrieved and reviewed as usual. Routine tracking down of all such sources is unrealistic unless faced with a major safety issue or crisis.
- The clock starts when a case is recognized to be a valid case (reporter, patient, drug, event).

LITIGATION

See Lawsuit.

LIVER FUNCTION TESTS (LFTs)

Laboratory tests of blood to determine the state and functioning of the liver. Drugs often cause abnormalities in liver tests. The tests are not necessarily specific to the liver as many of these tests will be elevated with diseases of other organs. The major tests used in clinical medicine include:

Alanine transaminase (ALT) or alanine aminotransferase (ALAT), also called serum glutamic pyruvate transaminase (SGPT), is an enzyme found in liver cells. Blood levels may rise when there is damage to the liver cells or when a drug or other chemical induces its synthesis. It is elevated in liver disease as well as other diseases including myocardial infarctions.

Aspartate transaminase (AST) or aspartate aminotransferase (ASAT), also called serum glutamic oxaloacetic transaminase (SGOT), is also an enzyme found in liver cells. When both ALT and AST are elevated, if the increase in ALT is greater than that of AST, drug-induced or viral hepatitis or fatty liver is more likely to be suspected. If the reverse is true with AST being higher than ALT, alcohol is more likely to be the cause of the liver enzyme elevations.

Alkaline phosphatase ("alk phos", or ALP) is an enzyme that is actually found in the biliary cells found in the liver rather than in the liver cells (hepatocytes), and tends to be elevated with diseases of the biliary tree as well as certain liver diseases.

Total bilirubin ("bili," or TBIL) is a breakdown product of the hemoglobin found in red blood cells that the liver pulls from the circulating blood, metabolizes, and secretes into the bile. Diseases of the bile ducts or the liver cells may cause elevations of bilirubin in the blood (also producing jaundice of the skin). Bilirubin is not specific to liver disease and may be elevated with blood disease, bile duct obstruction, and other diseases.

Other liver function tests include total protein, albumin, gamma glutamyl transpeptidase (GGT), 5' nucleotidase (5'NTD), prothrombin time, and the International Normalized Ratio (INR)—the latter may be elevated if the liver is unable to synthesize the proteins needed to coagulate blood, and the patient may be susceptible to bleeding.

Alanine aminotransferase/alkaline phosphatase ratio

It is sometimes useful to make the determination as to whether the liver problem is cytolytic or cholestatic, as some drugs are more prone to produce one or the other. As a rough rule of thumb, when the ratio of ALT/AP (or ALT/AlkPhos) is greater than 5, the hepatic lesion can be considered to be hepatocellular (cytolytic). When the ratio is under 2, the hepatic lesion is considered to be cholestatic. If the ratio is between 2 and 5 the picture is considered to be mixed. If ALT is not available, the AST may be used in the calculation.

LOCAL AUTHORIZATION

Also called national authorization and refers to one of the three methods to gain marketing approval for a drug in the European Union. The other methods are central authorization or mutual recognition. It involves the submission of the dossier to an individual country in the EU. Approval, if granted, is in general for that country only. It may be done for as many countries as desired. Some drugs may only be authorized centrally, however.

LOCKING CASES OR DATABASES

A date beyond which no further data will be entered into any AE case in a database. This then allows the case or database to be "cleaned" and prepared for analysis. Any additional data must be handled as an addendum or in an updated or new version of the report. For an individual case safety report that is due at the health authority by calendar day 15 after receipt, it is common to lock the case on day 10 or 11 in terms of data entry. The case is then medically reviewed, quality checked and printed out for mailing to the health authority or released into the "outbox" for E2B submission. Any data received after day 10 or 11 is entered into the next version of the case for submission as a follow-up report 5 days later.

LOE

See Lack of Efficacy.

LONG TIME TO ONSET

See Latency and Late Occurring AEs.

LONGITUDINAL STUDY

A prospective observational cohort or clinical trial conducted over some time period, in which multiple examinations or observations are done at fixed intervals. The study may include some control measures and control groups. Clinical trials are the most reliable designs to assess causality when studying medical interventions; the next best are cohort studies.

LONG-TERM AEs

See Latency and Late Occurring AEs.

LOW-LEVEL TERM (LLT)

In MedDRA, the most granular and specific of the five hierarchical levels of terms. There are over 60,000 such terms.

LUMPERS AND SPLITTERS (AE CODING)

The ongoing debate in AE coding (MedDRA). "Lumpers" prefer to use simple syndrome names to convey a constellation of signs and symptoms. "Splitters" prefer to list the individual symptoms and signs. Flu-like syndrome vs. fever, malaise, headache, muscle aches, etc.

Authors' note: Most coding conventions tend to make compromises between the two extremes. Most would accept "myocardial infarction" to include chest pain, sweating, arm pain, and ECG and laboratory changes consistent with this diagnosis. However, most would also want the specifics of the Hermansky Pudlak Syndrome spelled out (albinism, visual problems, platelet defects with bleeding, lung disease, and often kidney and gastrointestinal disease).

LYELL'S SYNDROME

See Toxic Epidermal Necrolysis (TEN).

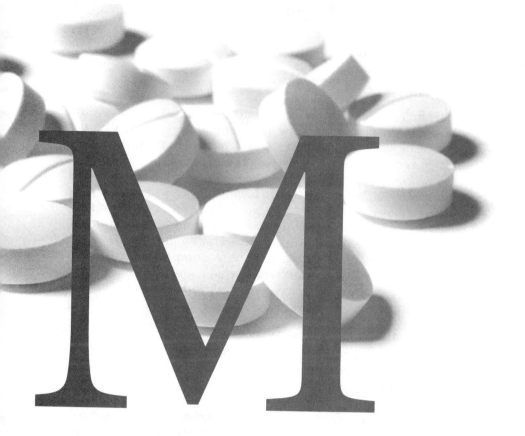

M1 DOCUMENTS (ICH)

The ICH Working Group formed in 1994 that established the concept and original ideas for MedDRA. Primarily of historical interest now. *See* MedDRA.

M2 DOCUMENTS (ICH)

Two working groups were set up in the ICH in 1994 to develop the means for the electronic transmission of individual case safety reports. One working group dealt with the contents of the transmission (E2B) and the other (M2) dealt with the informatics (information technology) issues of the transmission. They defined the Electronic Standards for the Transfer of Regulatory Information (ESTRI) in a series of technical documents available at the ICH website: http://estri.ich.org/. *See* E2B.

MA

Marketing authorization. *See* Marketed Drug.

MACULOPAPULAR RASH (ERYTHEMA)

A simple, benign skin eruption whose mechanism is not always clear. It constitutes one of the most commonly reported ADRs because of its frequency and visibility. They are not always drug related as there are other causes (e.g., viral).

Authors' note: The reporting frequency of this AE/ADR is even greater when the reporter is not a healthcare professional. The issue is even worse if the diagnosis is not reliable (i.e., made by an observer—even a health professional—who cannot distinguish among an exanthema, urticaria, dermatitis, febrile eruption, etc).

There is most probably a relative overreporting of cutaneous ADRs compared to more important renal, hepatic, and hematologic ones, which occur unnoticed when they are subclinical or picked up only by laboratory examinations.

MAINTENANCE AND SUPPORT SERVICES ORGANIZATION (MSSO)

The private organization that supports MedDRA. From their website: "Maintenance and Support Services Organization—serves as the repository, maintainer, and distributor of MedDRA as well as the source for the most up-to-date information regarding MedDRA and its application within the biopharmaceutical industry and regulators. MedDRA subscribers submit proposed changes to the terminology. The MSSO includes a group of internationally based physicians who review all proposed subscriber changes and provide a timely response directly to the requesting subscriber." The MSSO currently is a part of the Northrup Grumman Corporation. See http://www.meddramsso.com/MSSOWeb/index.htm.

MAJOR FINDING (AUDITS AND INSPECTIONS)

Qualifier used by the British MHRA, the EMEA, and others in regard to audits. A major finding is a deficiency in pharmacovigilance systems, practices, or processes that could potentially adversely affect the rights, safety, or well-being of patients, or that could potentially pose a risk to public health or that represents a violation of applicable legislation and guidelines.

Another definition in use is a finding that is a violation of a requirement, which individually would not directly impact data usability or validity or patient safety and regulatory compliance.

See Critical Finding, Minor Finding.

MALE PARTNERS OF PREGNANT WOMEN AEs

AEs/ADRs produced in the mother, fetus, or child due to exposure to a drug product in the semen of the male partner. This field is largely unexplored.

Theoretically a drug or its metabolite could be excreted in the semen or sperm and could produce untoward effects in the fetus or induce birth defects.

In addition, there is the possibility of transmission of the drug (or metabolite) in semen that reaches the partner through sexual contact. Some drugs that appear in the semen or which might alter sperm physiology and morphology include HIV drugs, chloroquine, and caffeine, while the effects of mesalazine (5-aminosalicylic acid), sulfasalazine, salicylate, propranolol, diltiazem, flunarizine, verapamil, caffeine, and nicotine.

There are rare reports of female allergic reactions to the semen or drugs contained in semen.

Ethics committees and sponsors are increasingly concerned about these risks, albeit very rare, and are increasingly asking for an informed consent of the pregnant or potentially pregnant partner of a male participating in a clinical trial of a new product.

MALPRACTICE, AS SOURCE OF AE/ADR INFORMATION

AEs/ADRs frequently are first reported to pharmaceutical companies as lawsuits against the company or against treating physicians for malpractice. These are usually serious AEs as nonserious ones are less likely to lead to lawsuits. Attorneys in companies must be aware of this possibility and report the AEs to the safety department within the required timeframes for reporting to health authorities. Follow-up requests from the company may have to be done through the attorneys and not directly to the patient or physician-reporter.

MANDATORY AE REPORTING FOR MANUFACTURERS AND LICENSE HOLDERS

Most countries now have obligatory reporting requirements for certain AEs/ADRs that pharmaceutical companies, distributors, licensors, etc., learn about. These are primarily for serious and nonserious cases in clinical trials, marketed drugs, and published literature. In some countries only unexpected (unlabeled, unlisted) AEs are obligatory, whereas other countries require all AEs to be reported. Many countries require reporting of global AEs, whereas other countries only require AEs from domestic sources.

Mandatory reporting is also required in some jurisdictions for hospitals and other healthcare institutions, though rarely for individual nurses, pharmacists, and physicians.

MANUFACTURER

This term is used loosely and interchangeably with other terms (sponsor, company, pharmaceutical company, wholesaler, distributor, licensor, licensee, authorization license holder, etc.) to designate one or more of the entities that have responsibility at some level for AE/ADR reporting. Companies at any stage of the drug process may in some countries have AE reporting responsibilities.

For example, if the package labeling of a product lists the company selling the drug and the manufacturer, then both companies may receive AEs/ADRs from consumers or healthcare professionals and need to have in place systems to ensure the proper handling of the cases.

MANUFACTURER CONTROL NUMBER

A number given to an AE/ADR case by the manufacturer. Of note is the fact that each governmental health agency receiving the case will give this report a number of its own. Thus the same case may have scores of identification numbers.

Authors' note: The situation is complex and it is always a challenge to avoid reporting duplicate cases because a single report may have multiple numbers: the manufacturer's subsidiary may assign a local control number; the manufacturer's home office safety group may assign a corporate control number; each health authority receiving the report will assign a (different) number, and if the case is transmitted by a health authority to the WHO Monitoring Centre in Uppsala, it will be assigned another number there. All of this presents a challenge in keeping track of cases and avoiding duplicate counting and reporting. The E2B/M2 Working Groups have attempted to address the issue of a unique control number for use in electronic data transmission.

MANUFACTURER AND USER FACILITY DEVICE EXPERIENCE DATABASE (MAUDE)

The database for device AEs maintained by the Center for Device and Radiological Health of the FDA. It contains data dating back to 1991 and is available at the FDA website: http://www.fda.gov/cdrh/maude.html.

MANUFACTURER RECEIVED DATE

On the MedWatch 3500A form, field G4: Date received by manufacturer. "This means the date when the applicant, manufacturer, corporate affiliate, etc., receives information that an adverse event or medical device malfunction has occurred. This would apply to a report received anywhere in the world. (mm/dd/yyyy format)." From the FDA's instructions on how to fill out the form. http://www.fda.gov/medwatch/report/instruc_10-13-06.htm#G4

Authors' note: This field is controversial. In many countries this field must be the initial received date—the date of the first receipt by anyone in the company and not the date received by the safety de-

partment or headquarters. Other countries do not always follow this rule and begin the clock when the AE is received by the safety department in that country (even if the case originated in another country and is processed centrally in the headquarter's safety department).

MARKET WITHDRAWAL

The extreme situation in the life cycle of a drug product when it is taken off the market. Although drugs may have a "natural lifespan" in which their use diminishes as newer, safer, and more efficacious products arrive, some drugs are withdrawn for safety reasons. This may be done voluntarily by the manufacturer or it may be forced by the health authorities. Drug withdrawal may engender multiple lawsuits (e.g., Vioxx®, Baycol®, and others), especially in the US. A withdrawal is usually permanent but occasional drugs do return either for different indications (thalidomide) or in limited markets (e.g., Bendectin® reintroduced in Canada as Diclectin®).

As conditions for the withdrawal, the health authority may require a patient registry or follow-up until all patient exposure comes to an end and all patients are accounted for.

A withdrawal should be distinguished from a recall. A recall may refer to a particular lot and may be for reasons other than an intrinsic ADR (e.g., manufacturing problem, mislabeling, contamination, tampering, etc.). A recall usually comes under the umbrella of product or quality problem. *See* Recall.

A withdrawal or recall may be done at various levels. If urgent, all means of media (TV, radio, Internet, emails to known users, etc.) may be used to instruct patients and healthcare professionals to stop using and prescribing or dispensing the drug. Letters ("Dear Doctor" or "Dear Healthcare Professional") will go out to wholesalers, retailers, and even patients instructing them to stop using the product and how to return the product for reimbursement or replacement. At other levels, communications may only go out to the wholesale or retail level to return unused stock and contact patients. Levels may vary from country to country.

MARKETED DRUG

A drug that has government approval for sale to the public either as a prescription product or over-the-counter, behind the counter etc. In the US it generally means an approved New Drug Application (NDA) or Abbreviated New Drug Application (ANDA) or Biologic License Application (BLA). In Europe it means a Marketing Authorization (MA). An over-the-counter drug in the US, if it conforms to the CFR monograph, may be marketed without obtaining a specific NDA. *See* Monograph Product.

Adverse events for marketed drugs must be reported to most health authorities around the world under conditions that are now quite well harmonized. Serious, unexpected adverse events must be reported in 15 calendar days in most countries. Serious expected and certain nonserious AEs must be reported in periodic aggregate reports (e.g., US NDA periodic reports or PSURs in most other countries).

MARKETING AND SALES

In terms of drug safety, the marketing and sales departments of companies must be instructed to report AEs to the drug safety department that are reported to sales representatives, marketers, advertising agencies, company-sponsored websites, market research studies, and partners (distributors, licensees, etc.). A written procedure is usually prepared with specific instructions on how to do this. It usually must be stressed that this is obligatory under the law and that reporting the case does not imply that the marketer admits its drug caused the AE.

MARKETING AUTHORIZATION (MA)

See Marketed Drug.

MARKETING AUTHORIZATION HOLDER (MAH)

Also called the license holder. Any physical or legal person (i.e., company) who has received the mandatory health authorization for marketing of a proprietary medicinal product. This holder (MAH), whether the manufacturer or not, is responsible for the safety, efficacy, quality, adequate identification, and appropriate and updated information on a medicinal product. The term is used primarily in reference to approved drugs in the EU. In the US the term is usually the NDA holder.

MARTINDALE'S, *THE COMPLETE DRUG REFERENCE*

Now in its 35th edition. It contains over 6,300 drug monographs covering 149,000 preparations from 14,700 manufacturers and 40,700 references. It is particularly useful for identifying drugs when only their trade name and country are known. It includes herbals, diagnostic agents, radiopharmaceuticals, pharmaceutical excipients, toxins, and poisons, as well as drugs and medicines. One of the standard references in the field and probably the most authoritative.

MedDRA

Medical Dictionary for Regulatory Activities. MedDRA is a terminology developed for drugs and devices used for standardized coding of medical terms, including AEs and medical history. It is hierarchical, which means that it has multiple levels (five) ranging from the most general to very specific. It is available in English with some or all of it also available in Dutch, French, German, Italian, Portuguese, Spanish, and Japanese. It has been "mandated" by the FDA, Japan, Canada, the EU, and others for use in AE reporting. It has largely replaced COSTART, WHO-ART, HARTS, JART, ICD-9, and other older drug coding systems, although WHO-ART is still used by the UMC in Uppsala.

MedDRA is updated twice yearly (April and October) and, in general, users update their own computer systems within 60 days of receipt of the upgrade. Users may request the addition of new codes to future versions of MedDRA by applying to the MSSO, which then reviews each request. Codes also may be moved, deleted, changed, demoted, and promoted by the MSSO in the updates.

MedDRA terms cover diseases, diagnoses, signs and symptoms, therapeutic indications, medical and surgical procedures, and medical, social, and family histories. MedDRA does not cover drug and device names, study design, patient demographic terms, device failure, population qualifiers (e.g., rare, frequent), and descriptions of severity or numbers. It does not give definitions of AEs. Originally, MedDRA was developed for postmarketing AEs, but it is now used widely for clinical trial AEs as well.

MedDRA presently (2007) has over 81,000 terms arranged into five hierarchical categories:

1. System organ classes (SOCs): 226
2. Higher-level group terms (HLGTs): 332
3. Higher-level terms (HLTs): 1,683
4. Preferred terms (PTs): 16,976
5. Lowest-level terms (LLTs): 62,950

Because there are so many terms, it is necessary to search for a needed term by computer rather than reading through a written version of the terminology. For this, the MSSO and other companies have developed browsing software to allow a user to find the terms he or she needs. *See* Browser.

MEDICAL DEVICE AMENDMENTS, FDA

Passed in 1976 to ensure safety and effectiveness of medical devices, including diagnostic products. The amendments require manufacturers to register with the FDA and follow quality control procedures. Some products must have premarket approval by the FDA. Others must meet performance standards before marketing.

MEDICAL DICTIONARY FOR REGULATORY ACTIVITIES

See MedDRA.

MEDICAL LETTER ON DRUGS AND THERAPEUTICS

A highly respected resource on drug therapy published in five languages with a circulation of about 200,000. From their website: "An independent, peer-reviewed, nonprofit publication that offers unbiased critical evaluations of drugs, with special emphasis on new drugs, to physicians and other members of the health professions. It evaluates virtually all new drugs and reviews older drugs when important new information becomes available on their usefulness or adverse effects. Published every other week in a four-page newsletter format, it carries no advertising and is supported entirely by subscription fees. A typical issue appraises two or three new drugs in terms of their effectiveness, toxicity, cost and possible alternatives. Occasionally, The Medical Letter publishes an article on a new non-drug treatment or a new diagnostic aid." http://www.medletter.com/html/who.htm

MEDICATION ERROR

From the US National Coordinating Council for Medication Error Reporting and Prevention: "Any preventable event that may cause or lead to inappropriate medication use or patient harm while the medication is in the control of the health care professional, patient, or consumer. Such events may be related to professional practice, health care products, procedures, and systems, including prescribing; order communication; product labeling, packaging, and nomenclature; compounding; dispensing; distribution; administration; education; monitoring; and use."

Authors' note: This is an area brought into focus in the last several years. Medication errors may produce significant numbers of serious and nonserious adverse events. These are, in theory, entirely preventable and represent "low-hanging fruit" (something that should be easily corrected) in the area of public health. It is now a major focus in the FDA and in healthcare facilities around the US.

A nonprofit US organization that is devoted to the safe use of medications is the Institute for Safe Medication Practices. They have a very interesting website: www.ismp.org. They publish a newsletter.

MEDICINES AND HEALTHCARE PRODUCTS REGULATORY AGENCY (MHRA)

The regulatory agency in the United Kingdom. From their website: "The MHRA is the government agency which is responsible for ensuring that medicines and medical devices work, and are acceptably safe. No product is risk-free. Underpinning all our work lie robust and fact-based judgments to ensure that the benefits to patients and the public justify the risks. We keep watch over medicines and devices, and we take any necessary action to protect the public promptly if there is a problem. We aim to make as much information as possible publicly available. We enable greater access to products, and the timely introduction of innovative treatments and technologies that benefit patients and the public." They are very active in the field of drug safety. http://www.mhra.gov.uk/home/idcplg?IdcService=SS_GET_PAGE&nodeId=5

It is also possible to register for periodic email alerts on drug safety and other topics from the MHRA at http://www.mhra.gov.uk/home/idcplg?IdcService=SS_GET_PAGE&nodeId=340

MEDLINE PLUS

A free service online from the US National Library of Medicine for consumers and healthcare professionals. It contains information from the National Institutes of Health and other sources on over 700 diseases and conditions. There are also lists of hospitals and physicians, a medical encyclopedia and a medical dictionary, health information in Spanish, extensive information on prescription and nonprescription drugs, health information from the media, and links to thousands of clinical trials. MedlinePlus is updated daily. Its URL is www.medlineplus.gov. There is no advertising on this site, nor does MedlinePlus endorse any company or product.

The section entitled Daily Med has the FDA-approved prescribing information on over 2200 drugs. The Drugs and Supplements section has patient-oriented information on drugs and supplements listed by generic and brand name.

A very useful site.

MEDSCAPE

A website from WebMD® with much medical information, including extensive information on drugs covering prescribing information, news, cost, pictures of the product, and other data. There is a tool to look up drug interactions in which one types in the names of the two (or more) drugs in question and known interactions are listed. There is also a search engine that covers MedScape, Medline, and the drug reference. There is a section on information from the pharmaceutical industry. www.medscape.com

An interesting and useful website.

MEDWATCH FORM (3500 AND 3500A FORMS)

The form used to submit individual case safety reports to the FDA for marketed or clinical trial cases (Appendix 4). *See* MedWatch Program.

There are actually two versions of the form. The "3500" version is for voluntary reporting by healthcare professionals and the public and the "3500A" version is for mandatory reporting by manufacturers.

The FDA has published detailed instructions on its website for completing the voluntary 3500 MedWatch form at http://www.fda.gov/medwatch/REPORT/CONSUMER/INSTRUCT.HTM and the mandatory 3500A MedWatch form at http://www.fda.gov/medwatch/report/instruc_10-13-06.htm.

MEDWATCH PROGRAM

The FDA Safety Information and Adverse Event Reporting Program for healthcare professionals and the public. It was formed in 1993 by a consolidation of several adverse reaction reporting systems as MedWatch and was designed for voluntary reporting of problems associated with medical products to be filed with the FDA by healthcare professionals.

It provides important and timely clinical information about safety issues involving medical products, including prescription and over-the-counter drugs, biologics, medical and radiation-emitting devices, and special nutritional products (e.g., medical foods, dietary supplements, and infant formulas).

Medical product safety alerts, recalls, withdrawals, and important labeling changes that may affect public health are disseminated to the medical community and the general public via the MedWatch website and the MedWatch E-list. Reports, safety notifications, and labeling changes posted to the website since 1996 are available.

MedWatch also allows healthcare professionals and consumers to report suspected AEs on drugs and devices online, by phone, or by submitting the MedWatch 3500 form by mail or fax.

www.fda.gov/medwatch

Authors' note: This is the backbone of the postmarketing drug surveillance system in the US. It is based entirely on the goodwill of the reporters (healthcare professionals and patients). There is much ongoing activity to develop newer and more efficacious systems such as data mining in computerized health databases to pick up signals earlier to minimize morbidity and mortality. Whatever does come must do better than the MedWatch program, which remains the gold standard in the US.

MEDWATCH TO MANUFACTURER

The US government program in which the FDA sends copies of MedWatch reports of SAEs that they receive directly on newly approved NDAs to the manufacturer of the product. The drug must be a new chemical entity. This program lasts 3 years after NDA approval and is done at the request of the manufacturer. These reports do not have to be resubmitted to the FDA by the company unless additional information is obtained. See: http://www.fda.gov/medwatch/report/mmp.htm

ME

See Medication Error.

META-ANALYSIS

A form of systematic review of controlled studies (observational, experimental) involving the use of statistical methods, as opposed to a narrative review by experts. Odds ratios are frequently presented as a statistical parameter used to compare treatments. Data are extracted from all available studies (e.g., clinical trials, cohorts) fulfilling predetermined quality and quantity criteria, and then combined to get a maximum amount of statistical information. It is most useful when the individual studies are too small to allow meaningful or statistically significant results. Meta-analysis, however, may produce distortion by the selection process, by the heterogeneity of studies, and by the unpublished negative studies. The Cochrane Reviews (http://www.cochrane.org/reviews/clibintro.htm) are a highly reliable source of meta-analyses. Meta-analyses are now increasingly being used for safety studies (Nissen 2007).

Results are usually not considered definitive and good large clinical trials may be more reliable. (Lelorier 1997)

METRICS

Data that are objective, measurable, and, in theory, unbiased and are used to make decisions. Also known as "key performance indicators" (KPI). Very commonly used in industry to measure the effectiveness of some aspects of pharmacovigilance.

Some commonly used metrics:

- Number of on-time and late 15-day reports and PSURs/NDA periodic reports to the FDA and other health agencies.
- For late 15-day reports and PSURs, degree of lateness.
- AEs processed per medical professional.
- Cost of processing each AE.

MEYLER'S SIDE EFFECTS OF DRUGS

"International Encyclopedia of Adverse Drug Reactions and Interactions"—A standard in the field. The 15th edition (2006 Elsevier Science) contains monographs dealing with about 1,800 drugs in over 4000 pages. It covers prescription drugs, antiseptics, anesthetics, herbal medicines, and some devices. It is available in printed and electronic formats.

One of the rare standard references in the field of pharmacovigilance to be regularly updated. The authors cover the recently published new ADRs. Times to onset and predisposing factors for spontaneously reported ADRs are especially useful. An indispensable tool for teaching pharmacovigilance.

MHRA

See Medicines and Healthcare Products Regulatory Agency.

MINIMUM INFORMATION FOR REPORTABILITY

A reportable AE or ADR requires the following minimum information:

1. An identifiable healthcare professional reporter. The reporter can be identified either by name or initials, or address or qualifications (e.g., physician, dentist, pharmacist, nurse).
2. An identifiable patient who can be identified either by initials or patient number, or date of birth (or age information if date of birth is not available), or sex.
3. At least one suspected substance or medicinal product.
4. At least one suspected adverse reaction.

The minimum information is the smallest amount of information required for the submission of a report and every effort should be made to obtain and submit further information when it becomes available.

There is much discussion and controversy over what constitutes an identifiable patient. For example:

- A male patient (yes)
- A few patients (no)
- A few male patients (?no)
- Four patients (yes)
- The patient John Smith (yes)
- The patient JS (yes)
- An email address with no other information (?)
- A 60-year-old (yes)
- Someone in Chicago (?)

MINISTRY OF HEALTH, LABOUR AND WELFARE–JAPAN (MHLW)

The Japanese Health Authority responsible for, among other things, drug safety. The ministry has been a member of the ICH from its onset in 1989. The English language website is www.mhlw.go.jp/english/index.html.

MINOR OR OTHER FINDING (AUDITS AND INSPECTIONS)

From the British MHRA: "A deficiency in pharmacovigilance systems, practices, or processes that would not be expected to adversely affect the rights, safety, or well-being of patients."

Another definition in use is "findings other than critical or major ones such as non-adherence to internal SOPs or requirements."

See Critical Finding, Major Finding.

MISSION STATEMENT OF DRUG SAFETY DEPARTMENTS

The mission of the drug safety group, whether in a company or a health agency, is first and foremost to protect the public health by maintaining accurate, up-to-date, and complete safety information on company or national products, respectively.

Medical analyses must be done with patient safety in mind, not only for "product protection." Secondary goals within a company's safety department relate to such corporate functions as the preparation of regulatory reports (NDA periodic reports, Periodic Safety Update Reports, IND annual reports, etc.) for submission to health authorities and consultation within the company on safety issues.

MISUSE

In its wider meaning the "proper use," from the prescriber to the patient, involves several conditions. The prescriber must make a diagnosis and make a good one, and choose a sensible therapeutic objective. He or she must decide which type of intervention is appropriate after considering the medical and pharmaceutical history; if a pharmacologic approach is best, one must choose the right class; the best product; the proper route, dose, and duration; and add a minimum of information for safe usage. The pharmacy must deliver the right product and information. In a hospital, the nursing staff must administer correctly. For long-term treatments, the prescriber must check for compliance, efficacy, and ADRs; for newly emerging comorbidity and comedication; and reconsider the benefit:risk analysis, the diagnosis, and the objectives as necessary. All ADRs stemming from an unnecessary or improper prescription are ipso facto avoidable and unacceptable.

This term "misuse" is not always clear or well defined for practical use in drug safety reporting. It generally means the improper use of a drug by a patient or healthcare professional. For example, it may be used at the wrong dose or in the wrong patient population or for an inappropriate indication by the prescriber. Similarly the patient may use it incorrectly or without medical advice. In these situations, "less proper" use is usually intentional; if it were not it would more properly be a medication error.

MODERNIZATION ACT OF 1997 (FDA)

This Act reauthorized in 1997 the Prescription Drug User Fee Act of 1992 and mandated the most wide-ranging reforms in agency practices since 1938. Provisions included measures to accelerate review of devices, regulate advertising of unapproved uses of approved drugs and devices, and regulate health claims for foods.

This act produced a highly politicized situation with many attacking the bill for allowing pharmaceutical companies to pay money (as fees) to their regulators, implying some quid pro quo. Others felt that as the fees could not be spent for safety matters, safety was compromised. Advocacy groups were afraid it would lead to "regulatory capture." The controversy continued throughout the life of the bill. A major revision and new law went into effect in late 2007. *See* FDA Revitalization Act.

MOIETY (OR ACTIVE MOIETY)

Usually synonymous with "active ingredient." It refers to the chemical in a drug that produces the desired pharmacologic effect when administered to a patient. In chemistry it means the whole or part of a molecule. It is often used in contradistinction to an excipient which is, in theory, inactive or without pharmacologic effect. Generic products contain, in theory, the same moiety as the branded products, but not the same excipients. This is the basis for the claims that generic products may be substituted without issue for branded products. However, the safety profiles may differ because the excipients (which may produce ADRs) differ.

MONITORED ADR

This term usually refers to AEs/ADRs that a health authority or pharmaceutical company wishes to track in a more directed manner than the usual passive spontaneous AE collection system. It may involve a clinical trial or epidemiologic study or a call from a health authority to all practitioners to report cases of a particular AE/ADR seen with a drug or group or class of drugs. It usually involves an attempt to investigate a signal or potential signal (in other words, an ADR "under surveillance").

MONOGRAPH PRODUCT

Regulations published by the FDA starting in 1972 for various over-the-counter (OTC) drugs that covered various therapeutic categories of products rather than specific drugs: cold products, antacids, laxatives, contraceptives, analgesics, and others. The monographs list the active ingredients, the required product labeling, dosage forms, warnings, and directions for use by consumers without medical intervention and in some cases packaging and testing information. A company may market a product without additional studies, data, or health authority approval if it follows the OTC monograph. No FDA review or approval is required. NDA regulations do not apply to these products. There is no marketing exclusivity and all similar drugs must be labeled in the same way.

Drugs that meet these requirements were determined primarily by panels of experts established by the FDA to review proposed OTC products and determine if they are "Generally Recognized as Safe and Effective (GRASE)." Those that were determined to be GRASE are included in the monographs. There are now other ways to add products to the monographs (including "citizen's petition" and "time and extent applications").

Authors' note: Do not confuse Monograph Product with Product Monograph, the name given in Canada to the Labeling (USA) or the SPC (EU).

MORBIDITY AND MORTALITY WEEKLY REPORT (MMWR)

A weekly publication from the US Department of Health and Human Services' Centers for Disease Control and Prevention in Atlanta. This publication carries statistics, detection and prevention alerts, regulatory actions, and other information concerning vaccinovigilance, maternal pharmacovigilance, toxicovigilance, and occasionally pharmacovigilance. Its primary focus is the global aspect of public health in the US. It is available as a podcast and an RSS feed. See the website http://www.cdc.gov/mmwr/.

MOTHERISK PROGRAM

A program at The Hospital for Sick Children affiliated with the University of Toronto, Canada, including clinical, research, and teaching dedicated to antenatal drug, chemical, and disease risk counseling. Created in 1985, *Motherisk* provides evidence-based information and guidance about the safety or risk to the developing fetus or infant, of maternal exposure to drugs, chemicals, diseases, radiation, and environmental agents.

There are excellent sections (in both the consumer and healthcare professional sections of the website) on the safe (or unsafe) use of drugs in pregnancy in which publications from the *Motherisk Program* and others are listed. Actual recommendations on classes of drugs or specific drugs are noted. There are also similar sections on breastfeeding and drugs.

An excellent resource. www.motherisk.org/index.jsp

MUTUAL RECOGNITION AUTHORIZATION (EU)

One of the pathways to get a drug approved in one or more European Union countries. Identical drug dossiers requesting marketing authorization are submitted to the Reference Member State and the Concerned Member States. If the reference member state approves the drug, the other countries that received the application should mutually recognize the marketing authorization from the reference member state within 90 days.

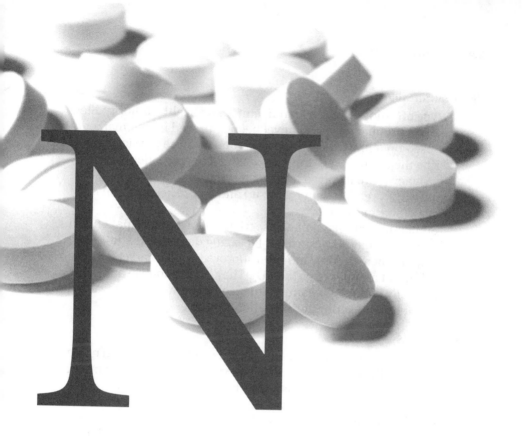

N OF 1 TRIAL

A type of controlled clinical trial in which the patient serves as his or her own control. The N of 1 trial assesses what is best for an individual patient but not for a population or group of patients with the same or similar problems. The patient undergoes two treatments, usually a drug and a placebo, given in random order and ideally under double-blind conditions. The pair of treatments may be repeated one or more times. There must be measurable markers and/or outcomes. Not all diseases (e.g., self-limited ones or diseases that wax and wane) lend themselves to this type of trial.

This design may be particularly useful for determining treatment-related ADRs as multiple periods (pairs) of exposure are a form of dechallenges and rechallenges; the use of blinding may help reveal a nocebo effect.

NAMED PATIENT PROGRAM

See Compassionate Use Programs.

NAMED PATIENT STUDY

A type of "study" where a manufacturer and health authority allow use of a product that has not yet been approved in that market to be used on a limited basis in which one or more physicians prescribe the unapproved drug to specific "named" patients. Usually pharmacists are involved for drug dispensing. The study must be done with careful patient follow-up and record keeping and must include pharmacovigilance.

Similar to a compassionate use trial, it allows very ill patients to obtain what may be a critical or lifesaving drug. These studies are common where the drug has been approved in one market (e.g., the US) but not another (e.g., the EU). They build goodwill and allow potentially lifesaving treatment to reach patients without waiting for a formal marketing authorization.

NAMES FOR DRUGS

Every drug has several names. Initially, a drug has a chemical name that is usually related to the molecular structure and is too complex to be useful in medical practice. A short version of the name may be used when a drug enters clinical trials usually with the company initials and a number (e.g., HOE760).

At approval the drug obtains a generic and a trade (brand, proprietary) name. For example, ranitidine is the generic name and Zantac® the brand name. In the US, the generic name is chosen by an official body, the United States Adopted Names Council (USAN). The trade name is chosen by the company.

Names should, in general, be simple and not confused with other drug names, especially when a prescription is handwritten.

Outside the US similar bodies exist. This poses problems as drugs may have different generic and different trade names from country to country or region to region. For example, acetaminophen is also known as paracetamol.

Other name problems, in addition to multiple names, exist:

- Drug names change.
- A drug with the same trade name may have different formulations in different countries.
- Spelling varies, and some languages do not use our alphabet.
- Combination drugs have multiple names.
- Combination drugs may have names that do not reflect what is in the product. For example, many cough and cold products with multiple ingredients contain acetaminophen. If a patient takes more than one product he may not realize that both con-

tain acetaminophen. This could produce an overdose and drug toxicity if too much of a product is unknowingly taken.
- Drugs may be very similar, varying only in the salt. They may have the same names or totally different names.

In global pharmacovigilance it is necessary for the healthcare professionals collecting the data to be aware that the source of the product must be carefully noted. The name and country of sale or origin should be recorded and then the actual chemical contents verified in the product labeling or a reference source (e.g., Martindale's).

NARRATIVE, ADVERSE EVENT

In an individual case safety report, a concise summary of the patient's adverse event(s), medical history, reason for taking the product, clinical course, and outcome. Also called a capsule summary (though this may be a shorter version of the narrative in some cases). The narrative appears on the MedWatch and CIOMS I forms as well as in E2B transmissions. The narrative allows the reader to rapidly understand the essence of the case.

Unfortunately it is not available on CIOMS line listings or in the WHO databases. (MedWatch forms with narratives may be obtained from the FDA under the Freedom of Information program, but this is complicated and takes quite some time.)

When an important new signal is the subject of a safety investigation, it is generally good pharmacovigilance practice to review the narratives to examine the exact wording used by the healthcare professionals to describe the suspected ADRs.

NATIONAL APPROVAL

The permission to legally market a drug in a particular country. In the US this would be the equivalent of the FDA's approval of an NDA, ANDA, or BLA. In the EU, a country may issue a marketing authorization (MA) for a product. In addition in the EU, there are other mechanisms to gain approval (mutual recognition authorization and central approval). See these terms.

NATIONAL LIBRARY OF MEDICINE (NLM)

From their website (http://www.nlm.nih.gov/): The NLM is located on the campus of the National Institutes of Health in Bethesda, Maryland and is the world's largest medical library.

The Library published the Index Medicus®, a monthly subject/author guide to articles in 4000 journals. This information, and more, is today available in the database MEDLINE®, the major component of PubMed®, freely accessible via the Internet. PubMed has more than 16 million MEDLINE journal article references and abstracts going back to the mid-1960's with another 1.5 million references back to the early 1950's. The NLM has created a special Web site, MedlinePlus, to link the general public to many sources of consumer health information.

NATURALISTIC SETTING

A clinical environment that closely mirrors routine practice or normal life.

NCE

See New Chemical Entity.

NDA

See New Drug Application.

NDA ANNUAL REPORT

See NDA Periodic Report.

NDA PERIODIC REPORT

After NDA approval by the FDA, the sponsor must submit update reports every three months for three years and then yearly thereafter.

All "adverse drug experiences" not submitted as 15-day alert reports must be submitted in the NDA periodic report. Each report must be submitted 30 days after the close of the quarter for quarterly reports and 60 days after the close of the anniversary date for yearly reports. Thus the company has 30 or 60 days to prepare the report. Each periodic report must contain the following:

- A narrative summary and analysis of the information in the report and an analysis of the 15-day alert reports submitted during the reporting interval.
- A MedWatch form (3500A) for each US adverse drug experience not reported as a 15-day expedited report.
- A history of actions taken since the last report because of adverse drug experiences (e.g., labeling changes or studies initiated).

The narrative summary and analysis of the information in the postmarketing periodic report and an analysis of the 15-day reports (i.e., serious, unexpected, adverse experiences) submitted during the reporting period must be provided and should include the following:

Section 1

- The number of non-15-day initial adverse experience reports and the number of non-15-day follow-up reports contained in this periodic report and the time period covered by the periodic report.

- A line listing of the 15-day reports submitted during the reporting period. This line listing should include the manufacturer report number, adverse experience term(s), and the date the 15-day report was sent to the FDA.

- A summary tabulation by body system (e.g., cardiovascular, central nervous system, endocrine, renal) of all adverse experience terms and counts of occurrences submitted during the reporting period.

- Any nonserious, expected, adverse experiences not submitted to the FDA but maintained on file by the applicant. Drug interactions should be identified in the tabulation.

- A summary listing of the adverse experience reports in which the drug or biologic product was listed as one of the suspect products but the report was filed to another NDA, Abbreviated NDA, or BLA held by the applicant.

- A narrative discussion of the clinical significance of the 15-day reports submitted during the reporting period and of any increased reporting frequency of serious, expected, adverse experiences when, in the judgment of the applicant, it is believed the data reflect a clinically meaningful change in adverse experience occurrence. This narrative should assess clinical significance by type of adverse experience, body system, and overall product safety relating the new information received during this reporting period to what was already known about the product. The narrative should also state what further actions, if any, the applicant plans to undertake based on the information gained during the reporting period and include the time period for completing the actions.

- The narrative discussion should indicate, based on the information learned during the reporting period, whether the applicant believes either that (1) no change in the product's current approved labeling is warranted, or (2) there are safety-related issues that need to be addressed in the approved product labeling. If changes in the approved product labeling are under consideration by the FDA, the applicant should state in the narrative the date and number of the supplemental application submitted to address the labeling changes.

Section 2

A narrative discussion of actions taken must be provided, including any labeling changes and studies initiated since the last periodic report. This section should include:

- A copy of current US product labeling.
- A list of any labeling changes made during the reporting period.
- A list of studies initiated.
- A summary of important foreign regulatory actions (e.g., new warnings, limitations in the indications and use of the product).
- Any communication of new safety information (e.g., a "Dear Doctor" letter).

Section 3

An index line listing of FDA Form 3500As or Vaccine Adverse Event Reporting System (VAERS) forms must be provided. The line listing should include:

- Manufacturer report number.
- Adverse experience term(s).
- Page number of FDA Form 3500A or VAERS form as located in the periodic report.
- Identification of interacting products for any product interaction labeled as an adverse experience.

Section 4

FDA Form 3500As or VAERS forms must be provided for serious and expected, nonserious and unexpected, and nonserious and expected AEs that occurred in the United States during the reporting period.

The FDA is moving, following ICH proposals, toward the use of PSURs instead of NDA periodic reports. Sponsors are encouraged to request permission to submit PSURs instead of NDA periodic reports. At some point PSURs will become obligatory.

NESTED CASE-CONTROL STUDY

In epidemiology, this is a type of case-control study that obtains patients (AE cases and non-AE controls) from a cohort that has already been followed over time, such as in a health database. Thus the cohort at the beginning of the study has exposure information and, over time, some patients will develop the adverse event in question (cases) and some will not (controls).

The investigator will then compare exposure frequencies in cases and in controls just as in a regular case-control study. This type of study decreases recall bias compared to a nonnested case control study and is usually faster and less expensive to perform than cohort studies. They may be quite useful in the detection of adverse events, provided that the limitations of the database are accounted for.

NEURAL NETWORK DATA MINING

A technique used to generate and analyze signals from a spontaneous reports database. The Uppsala Monitoring Center is a prime example of a group using neural network data mining.

A technique known as the Bayesian Confidence Propagation Neural Network (BCPNN) has been developed. The technique uses a neural network architecture to search for dependencies between drugs and adverse reactions within the WHO database. The BCPNN can be used to detect unexpected patterns in the data and to examine how such patterns vary over time. The BCPNN uses a measure of disproportionality called the Information Component (IC), which is a measure of the strength of the dependency between a drug and an ADR. A positive IC value indicates that a particular drug–ADR combination is reported to the database more often than expected from the rest of the reports in the database. An IC value of zero means that there is no quantitative dependency while a negative IC value indicates that the combination is occurring less frequently than statistically expected in the database. The higher the value of the IC, the more the combination stands out from the background. The IC does not give any information about the qualitative causality of a drug–ADR combination.

For the causality determination, clinical judgment and a signal analysis need to be done. See their website: http://www.umc-products.com/DynPage.aspx?id=3563

NEUROLEPTIC MALIGNANT SYNDROME

A syndrome consisting of fever, confusion, disorientation or other cognitive function changes, muscle rigidity, profuse sweating, and autonomic instability such as tachycardia. Increased creatine kinase is frequent. This syndrome is generally drug induced. It may be caused by neuroleptics and by antipsychotics (even the newer atypical ones).

NEW CHEMICAL ENTITY (NCE)

A drug whose active component (moiety, entity) is new and not previously approved for use. It represents a chemical/biological innovation, frequently a pharmacological innovation (new mechanism), and hopefully a therapeutic advance. In general, these products tend to get more rapid review by health authorities for approval because they may represent a therapeutic innovation. The safety profiles are obviously less well characterized when approval is accelerated and particular attention must be paid to these matters before and after launch.

NEW DRUG APPLICATION (NDA)

A dossier submitted to the FDA requesting approval to market a new drug for human use in interstate commerce. The application must contain, among other things, data from specific technical viewpoints for FDA review, including chemistry, pharmacology, medical, biopharmaceutics, statistics, and, for anti-infectives, microbiology. Information leading to safe usage should be transparent, complete, and explicit.

From the FDA website (www.fda.gov):

For decades, the regulation and control of new drugs in the United States has been based on the New Drug Application (NDA). Since 1938, every new drug has been the subject of an approved NDA before U.S. commercialization. The NDA application is the vehicle through which drug sponsors formally propose that the FDA approve a new pharmaceutical for sale and marketing in the U.S. The data gathered during the animal studies and human clinical trials of an Investigational New Drug (IND) become part of the NDA.

The goals of the NDA are to provide enough information to permit the FDA reviewer to reach the following key decisions:

- Whether the drug is safe and effective in its proposed use(s), and whether the benefits of the drug outweigh the risks.
- Whether the drug's proposed labeling (package insert) is appropriate, and what it should contain.
- Whether the methods used in manufacturing the drug and the controls used to maintain the drug's quality are adequate to preserve the drug's identity, strength, quality, and purity.

The documentation required in an NDA is supposed to tell the whole story about the drug, including what happened during the clinical tests, what the ingredients of the drug are, the results of the animal studies, how the drug behaves in the body, and how it is manufactured, processed, and packaged.

NEW MOLECULAR ENTITY (NME)

See New Chemical Entity.

NEW PRODUCT

In the regulatory context, the notion of a new product is more than just that of a new active ingredient or new chemical entity. It also includes:

- New preparations and presentations: dose, galenic formulation, route of administration.
- New indication.
- New population approved for use: pediatrics, geriatrics, etc.

In some countries new products get intensified surveillance, such as in the UK where the Black Triangle system is in effect. (*See* Black Triangle.)

In many countries, the use of the word "new" in advertising and publicity is limited to a fixed period of time after approval or launch (e.g., six months). In the context of pharmacovigilance, this is important to know because it is possible that there will be an increase in AE/ADR reporting during this period. (*See* Weber effects)

NEW ZEALAND INTENSIVE MEDICINES MONITORING PROGRAMME (IMMP)

A program in the University of Otago, Dunedin, New Zealand, in which prospective observational cohort studies on selected new drugs are carried out; the methodology is not too different from Prescription-Event Monitoring (PEM). *See* Prescription Event Monitoring. See also http://carm.otago.ac.nz/index.asp?link=immp.

NGO

See Non-Governmental Agency.

NNTH OR NNH

See Number Needed to Harm.

NO OBSERVED AE LEVEL (NOAEL)

The highest tested dose of a substance that has been reported to have no adverse effects on people or animals. In other words, the dose (single or multiple) at which no AEs are observed. A fraction of this dose found in animals may be used to determine the lowest dose to start using in human volunteers during phase I trials.

NOCEBO EFFECT

This is harm or an adverse effect of a drug due to the power of suggestion or belief that it is harmful and not due to its pharmacodynamic or specific properties. The expression may apply to medical practice and to drug trials. (Nocebo in Latin means "I will harm.")

The opposite is the placebo effect. Adverse events observed in the placebo arm of drug trials are attributed to the nocebo effect or to the natural course of the disease or possibly excipients in the placebo.

NON-GOVERNMENTAL AGENCY (NGO)

An organization, usually nonprofit, that is not part of a government institution. Some are involved in drug safety. Examples include the Uppsala Monitoring Center (UMC), the MedDRA Service Organization (MSSO), and the Institute for Safe Medicine Practices (ISM).

NONPRESCRIPTION PRODUCT

Products available without a prescription by a medical professional. These products are, in general, used to treat symptoms rather than diseases and do not require a diagnosis by a medical professional. The doses are usually lower than those of similar (or chemically identical) products sold by prescription. Adverse events are theoretically milder with these products. However, many nonprescription products can cause ADRs (e.g., NSAIDs, aspirin) even at these lower doses, especially if used with other products that might contain the same chemical (unbeknownst to the consumer) or that might interact with prescription medications a person is already taking.

In general, the labeling of nonprescription products is minimal.

There are two types of nonprescription products in most countries:

Over-the-counter (OTC): These products are freely available to consumers on the shelves of pharmacies and, in some countries, supermarkets, convenience stores, etc. No medical advice or intervention is required (or even available).

Behind-the-counter: These products are available without a prescription, but the consumer must request the product from the pharmacist who keeps them "behind" the counter so that they are not freely available. The goal is that the pharmacist will counsel the consumer on the need and use for the product.

Due to the vagaries of regulations around the world, a product may be prescription in one country, behind-the-counter in another, and over-the-counter in a third.

NONSERIOUS AEs

Adverse events that do not meet the criteria for serious AEs. *See* Serious Adverse Event.

NUMBER NEEDED TO HARM (NNTH)

Also called Number Needed to Harm One. The number of patients that must be exposed to a drug to produce any AE/ADR or a specific AE/ADR in one patient. Exposure may, for example, be one course or one year of treatment. For example, an inception cohort study of 252,460 patients treated with various statins and fibrates between 1998 and 2001 revealed that the number of patients needed to treat for one year to produce one case of severe rhabdomyolysis was roughly as follows:

- 23,000 for monotherapy with atorvastatin, pravastatin, or simvastatin.
- 3,500 for monotherapy with a fibrate.
- 2,000 for monotherapy with cerivastatin.
- 1,500 for fibrate plus a statin other than cerivastatin and only about 10 for fibrate plus cerivastatin.

(Source: Graham 2004)

NUMBER NEEDED TO BENEFIT (NNTB)

Also called Number Needed to Treat (NNT). The number of patients that must be exposed to a drug to get a beneficial effect or to prevent a negative event in one patient. Exposure may, for example, be one course or one year of treatment. For example, if the NNTB for a drug is 10, one must treat 10 people to get a beneficial effect or prevent a negative event in a single patient. When preventing a negative event (reducing risk) is the outcome measure, the NNTB is the inverse of the Absolute Risk Reduction (ARR). For example, NNTB = 1/ARR.

NUTRACEUTICAL

A blend of "nutrition" and "pharmaceutical." A food or food component that is claimed to have medical benefits and is marketed as a pharmaceutical product. It could be applied to dietary supplements, vitamins, etc. Although generally innocuous, safety problems may arise from abuse by consumers or from quality problems (contamination, counterfeit). Efficacy is uncertain because they are not tested and regulated as drug products are.

NUTRITIONALS—ADVERSE EVENT MONITORING SYSTEM

The US FDA's monitoring system for special nutritional products that are defined as dietary supplements, infant formulas, and medical foods; established in 1993 and ended in 1999. Reporting was voluntary and cases came from a variety of sources, including the FDA's MedWatch program and field offices; other federal, state, and local public health agencies; and letters and phone calls from consumers and healthcare professionals. However, few cases were reported.

In August 2002 the FDA's Center for Food Safety and Applied Nutrition (CFSAN) announced the plan to develop the new CFSAN Adverse Events Reporting System (CAERS), with a pilot due in 2003. There is no notation on CFSAN's home page about reporting food safety problems. However, there is a site http://www.foodsafety. gov/~fsg/fsgprobs.html that gives information on where to report illnesses and product complaints about food:

Foodborne illness is reported to the Center for Disease Control (CDC)

Meat, poultry, and egg product issues are reported to the Food Safety and Inspection Service of the US Department of Agriculture (USDA)

Seafood, fruits, vegetables, and other nonmeat food product issues are reported to the FDA

Food away from home (e.g., from caterers, restaurants, community picnics) issues are reported to the state or local health department

Advertising and fraud complaints are reported to the Federal Trade Commission

Bottled water issues are reported to the Food and Drug Administration

Ground water and drinking water issues are reported to the Environmental Protection Agency

Authors' note: This website and AE reporting in general is not easily found on the FDA's CFSAN website. The foodsafety.gov website is more helpful but also not easily found and reporting is not simple. Obviously this is a situation that calls for simple, "one-stop" reporting for industry and consumers alike.

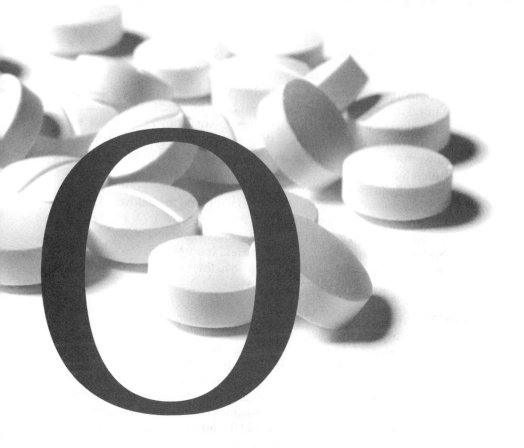

OBSERVATIONAL STUDY

In drug safety, an epidemiological study in which a group of patients is observed for their exposure to certain treatments (preventive or therapeutic) and for the occurrence of certain adverse events. They may be prospective (the cohort type) or retrospective (the case-control type).

From simply descriptive, an epidemiological study becomes analytical when a control group is included that permits comparison with unexposed patients (in the cohort type) or with noncases (in the case-control type).

Contrary to an experimental clinical trial, intervention maneuvers in an observational study are determined not by the investigator but by the patient or the prescribers, such as in the course of normal medical practice. The investigator exerts no control on the allocation of treatments.

There are more biases in observational studies than in experimental trials since control measures such as randomization to treatments, double blinding, etc., are not possible. However, the number of patients and their heterogeneity make the study population more representative than the selected samples used in clinical trials. The number of patients may be much greater than in clinical trials and may lead to more statistical power to detect adverse events. In this respect, the case-control approach is more powerful than the cohort approach but also has more biases to watch for.

In some jurisdictions, informed consent may be required.

The application of the observational method to health databases (Medicare, Kaiser Permanente, Canadian provinces, etc.) is increasingly useful in the field of pharmacovigilance, provided that biases stemming from secondary data (computerized claims for medical care and drug treatments have their own biases) are fully recognized.

OCCURRENCE RATES OF AEs

The number of AEs that truly happen in a defined number of patients receiving a drug. This number can be precisely counted in clinical trials where there is close follow-up of patients to see how many develop which AEs. The (true) occurrence rate can never be obtained from spontaneously reported data as the number of reports of the AE is always below the true number (some patients or healthcare professionals do not report the AEs) and the number of patients actually taking the drug is also not precisely known. This is called the reporting rate (not to be confused with the occurrence rate).

OCULOMUCOCUTANEOUS SYNDROME

See Practolol Syndrome.

ODDS RATIO

Also known as estimated or approximate relative risk. In case-control studies concerning drug safety, the ratio between the rate of exposure to a suspect drug in a group of cases (with the AE) and the rate of exposure in a group of noncases (controls without the AE). Like relative risk from cohort studies, the odds ratio is a useful estimation of the strength of cause-effect relationships. This parameter is often used in meta-analyses.

OFF-LABEL USE

The use of a drug that does not conform to the health authority (e.g., FDA, EMEA) approved indication, dosage form, prescribing regimen, or target population. That is, a use that does not fully conform to the officially approved prescribing information (e.g., the labeling). In most jurisdictions off-label use by the prescribing physician is not illegal though it may entail medical and legal risks if problems occur. Manufacturers are not allowed to promote off-label use.

OFFICE OF SAFETY POLICY AND COMMUNICATION STAFF (IN CDER)

In the Center for Drug Evaluation and Research (CDER) of the FDA, a section that includes MedWatch and the Drug Safety Oversight Board. This group is separate from the Office of Surveillance and Epidemiology and includes the Division of Drug Risk Evaluation; the Division of Surveillance, Research and Communication Support; and the Division of Medication Errors and Technical Support.

OFFICE OF SURVEILLANCE AND EPIDEMIOLOGY (IN CDER)

This office in the FDA has three divisions:

(1) Division of Drug Risk Evaluation (DDRE), which evaluates the safety of marketed drugs, reviews adverse drug event reports with the Office of New Drugs, recommends appropriate actions, estimates the public health impact of safety signals, performs epidemiologic research on drug safety issues, reviews epidemiologic study protocols and results, and provides recommendations on risk management programs.

(2) Division of Medication Errors and Technical Support (DMETS), which evaluates and provides recommendations on proprietary names from a safety perspective to minimize medication errors; identifies error-prone aspects of labels, labeling, and packaging of drug products; provides recommendations to minimize user error; reviews postmarketing medication error reports; recommends appropriate actions to prevent further errors; and provides information technology support to the Office of Drug Safety (specialized database searches, websites, desktop support).

(3) Division of Surveillance, Research, and Communication Support (DSRCS), which reviews medication guides and patient labeling; consults on drug utilization databases such as IMS Health, Caremark, and Premier; oversees the MedWatch program; conducts pharmacoepidemiological analyses; reviews epidemiological studies; handles data resources, risk communication, and outcomes/effectiveness research components of drug safety risk management programs; and analyzes social science research on risk communication issues.

OFFICER, DRUG SAFETY

In a pharmaceutical company, a person (usually a healthcare professional) with drug safety responsibilities. The term may refer to:

• Individuals who work in the drug safety department.

- Individuals who work in other departments (e.g., regulatory, legal, subsidiaries, affiliates) whose responsibility is to identify and convey AEs to the drug safety department.
- The Chief Drug Safety Officer.

OFF-SHORING OF PHARMACOVIGILANCE

In pharmaceutical companies, the moving of some or all safety functions to an area of the world where there is a greater availability of medical personnel and lower costs. The countries in question either have English as the native language or as a major second language such that the English language abilities of the personnel are at a very high level. Usually the personnel are employees of the pharmaceutical company (not employees of a CRO or other company). Countries where this is done include (so far) India and the Philippines.

Off-shoring of pharmacovigilance should be distinguished from outsourcing of pharmacovigilance (see this term).

Care must be taken to ensure that quality is maintained and that all regulations are followed both of the "original" country and of the new host country.

It is expected that other major languages with global distribution will be off-shored too (e.g., French, Spanish).

ONCOVIGILANCE

In drug safety, the area of pharmacovigilance that consists of the surveillance of unexpected AEs in cancer patients exposed to new antineoplastic agents. New ADRs may be uncovered, as well as new interactions. This differs from the routine surveillance by the treating oncologist of patients undergoing standard chemotherapy. In this "hard medicine" specialty a close surveillance of the patients exposed to potent and risky products is essential to ensure their optimal usage.

Experience shows that oncologists are more prone to report new signals to their peers (specialty meetings and journals) than to national spontaneous reporting systems such as MedWatch.

Authors' note: Since cancer patients are usually quite ill and the chemotherapeutic agents used are often quite toxic, the threshold for spontaneous AE/ADR reporting by oncologists is unfortunately fairly high. Their reasoning for reporting only very severe or unusual AEs is that all of their patients have AEs and ADRs and some practical selectivity must be used in reporting.

ORGANIZATION OF TERATOLOGY INFORMATION SERVICES (OTIS)

An organization created in 1990 to stimulate and encourage the dissemination of knowledge, education, and research in the field of clinical teratology and teratovigilance, and to improve the abilities of teratology information services to provide accurate and timely information about prenatal exposures with the overall objective of improving pregnancy outcomes. The organization includes 35 Teratology Information Services (TIS) in the US and Canada.

See their website: www.otispregnancy.org.

ORPHAN ADR

Refers to an isolated unlabeled adverse event that is associated with the drug (i.e., a suspected ADR) but without any meaningful effect on public health or on the benefit:risk assessment of the product, even if the signal was to be confirmed later. By "isolated" it is meant that the ADR has been reported (and/or published) once without being considered an important safety signal and without being reported elsewhere. It is usually single in number and may only be weakly associated with the drug (i.e., causality is not strong). The inability to ascribe a strong causality may be due to confounding factors (e.g., comedications or concomitant diseases), insufficient information (quite common), uncertain plausibility, or unreliable medical information.

Authors' note: An orphan ADR may occur either because the product in question is rarely used or because the true incidence of the AE/ADR is very low. An orphan ADR does not justify an alert because it has no impact on public health. It is, of course, of importance to the individual patient who should not be reexposed to the suspect product. The event must be kept in the pharmacovigilance database since additional cases could always be reported, making this no longer an orphan.

Thus an orphan is a type of signal which, for the moment, is merely a curiosity but nevertheless could ultimately contribute to the safety picture and help explain the mechanism(s) of the drug's toxicity. On the other hand, should the patient in question experience the event a second time without having taken the suspect drug or should the reporter uncover further evidence that the original observation was not valid, the signal is proven false.

ORPHAN DRUG

A regulatory term used to designate a new product indicated for a very rare disease (defined to be less than 200,000 cases in the US) and which is intended to motivate its research and development by the pharmaceutical industry. There are about 5,000 diseases that affect only 1 in 1,000 people. In order to promote the commercialization of efficacious products that are often off-patent and for which there are few patients to treat, the Orphan Drug Act of 1983 offers incentives for development. These incentives include a smaller number of patients studied, more rapid review by the FDA, and monetary benefits.

The EU adopted similar legislation in 2000 defining an orphan drug as one that could treat a disease with a prevalence of less than five per 10,000 of the population.

By decreasing the requirements for approval, the number of patients and treatment duration in controlled clinical trials are decreased. This decreases the likelihood of the detection in phase III trials of ADRs that are rare, have long latency periods, are of type B, or are due to drug–drug interactions. In other words, if the preapproval study of the drug is truncated, the postapproval pharmacovigilance study of the drug becomes even more critical. In such cases, health authorities may impose certain phase IV postapproval requirements, such as cohort studies of the first patients exposed after approval.

Authors' note: An orphan ADR is NOT an AE/ADR seen with an orphan drug. See Orphan ADR.

OTC PRODUCT

See Over-the-Counter Product.

OTIS

See Organization of Teratology Information Services.

OUTCOME

In drug safety, the final consequence, in terms of seriousness, of an ADR that occurred in a patient. The outcome must be listed on the MedWatch or CIOMS 1 form. The usual choices are death, life-threatening situation, hospitalization (initial or prolonged), disability or permanent damage, congenital anomaly/birth defect, required intervention to prevent permanent impairment or damage (devices only), and other serious (important) medical events. Other less negative outcomes are considered nonserious.

In medical jargon, the final result, consequence, or course of a medical illness, ADR, or treatment in a patient (gradual recovery, residual disability, total resolution, etc.).

For pregnancy cases (with or without an accompanying AE): The result of the pregnancy (e.g., healthy live birth, abortion, etc.).

OUTREACH PROGRAM

In drug safety, a program to track patients to help them stay on their course of therapy to the end in order to obtain maximal clinical efficacy (and sell more product). These programs are usually created and supported by the manufacturer of the product in question. Such programs usually employ nurses or other healthcare professionals to periodically contact patients taking a treatment for an extended length of time (e.g., for hepatitis) where ADRs are relatively frequent. Also known as "coaching."

The goal is to give support, encouragement, and assistance to the patients without interfering with the treating physician's role and function. In particular, side-effect management by trained healthcare professionals may allow patients to complete their prescribed course of therapy. Any AEs/ADRs noted must be reported to the pharmaceutical company (and usually the treating physician) for entry into the company's database and reporting to health authorities.

Advocacy groups are afraid that coaching may be financed for boosting sales of branded products and represents, in a sense, a form of direct-to-consumer promotion.

OUTSOURCING OF PHARMACOVIGILANCE

In pharmaceutical companies, the hiring of an external company (or vendor) to handle some or all safety functions. This may be done in the country where the original safety group is located or in another country. It may be done for cost reasons or to meet acute needs during a drug safety crisis (e.g., a product recall or withdrawal) where the in-house staff is insufficient. Outsourcing of pharmacovigilance should be distinguished from off-shoring of pharmacovigilance (see this term).

Care must be taken to be sure that all regulations are met and that quality is maintained.

OVER-THE-COUNTER PRODUCT

A drug or device for which a prescription, medical intervention, diagnosis, and advice are not needed. The patient makes a "self diagnosis" and decides him- or herself on the treatment. This should be distinguished from "behind-the-counter" products for which a prescription is not needed but for which the patient must ask the pharmacist for the product not visible on the shelves (i.e., "behind-the-counter"). The pharmacist is expected to ask the patient, at the least, why the product is needed and to give advice where appropriate.

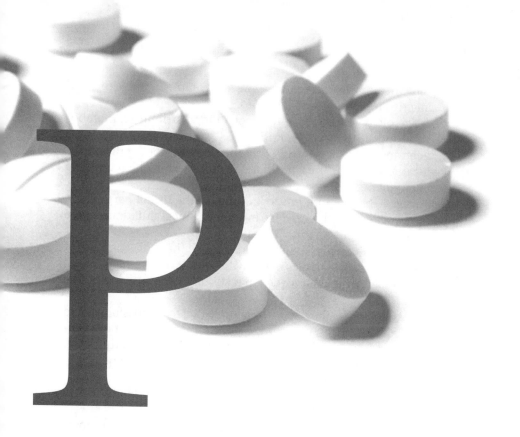

PACKAGE INSERT (PI)

In the US, the medical and scientific documentation included with the manufacturer's packaging of a drug. It is the official FDA-approved labeling for the drug and is also known as the professional labeling, direction circular, and package circular.

The basic components of labeling in the US for prescription drugs include: boxed warning (if applicable), indications and usage, dosage and administration, how supplied, contraindications, warnings, general precautions, drug interactions, drug/laboratory test interactions, laboratory tests, information for patients, teratogenic effects, nonteratogenic effects, labor and delivery, nursing mothers, pediatric use, geriatric use, carcinogenesis, mutagenesis, impairment of fertility, adverse reactions, controlled substance (if applicable), abuse, dependence, overdosage, description, clinical pharmacology, animal pharmacology/toxicology, clinical studies, and references.

Some of the key sections for the clinician:

Description—the chemical name of the drug, the chemical formula and diagram of the structure, the formulation and the route of administration (e.g., oral, intravenous, etc.). Active and inactive ingredients are included.

Pharmacology—describes the absorption, distribution, metabolism, and elimination (ADME).

Indications and usage—the FDA-approved uses for the drug.

Contraindications—the conditions or diseases for which the drug must not be used.

Warnings—this section draws attention to the risk of particularly noteworthy or severe adverse events or clinical situations where particular attention must be paid.

Precautions—information on the safe use of the drug, such as not taking the drug with alcohol or with certain other drugs.

Drug interactions—other drugs that should not be used with this drug.

Adverse reactions—the adverse reactions (felt to be possibly due to the drug) as well as, in some cases, adverse events (felt not necessarily related to the drug but noted in patients using the drug). Generally all AEs seen in clinical trials and most from postmarketing use are listed here.

Drug abuse and dependence—included if abuse and habituation or dependence are likely to occur.

Overdosage—information on the occurrence, signs, and symptoms and treatment of overdosage.

Dosage and administration—information on approved dosages. They may vary by disease or indication, age group, etc.

How supplied—describes how the product looks and the packaging, along with special storage instructions if appropriate (e.g., "do not freeze").

The FDA enacted new regulations effective in 2006 changing the package insert somewhat in order to help manage the risks and to reduce medical errors; in other words, the regulations make the insert more "prescriber and user friendly."

A new "highlights" section includes the most commonly used information in the label:

- The date of the approval of the original product.
- A summary of any "black box warning."
- Recent major changes made within the last year regarding black boxes, indications and usage, dosage and administration, contraindications, and warnings and precautions.
- Adverse reactions: most frequent adverse reactions that are important for reasons other than frequency.
- AE reporting contact information for both the FDA and the manufacturer.

- Drug interactions.
- Use in specific populations.

There are also format (use of XML) and reordering changes.

Risk information is consolidated with the AE section after the warnings and precautions section.

In other countries, similar documents exist and go under a variety of names including the Summary of Product Characteristics (SPC or SmPC) in Europe and the Product Monograph in Canada.

The official labeling of drugs in the US is available online on the FDA's website and the manufacturers' websites (in most cases), as well as in various compendia put out by non-governmental organizations such as the AMA's drug guide, the Physicians' Desk Reference® (PDR) in the US; the Vidal® in France, the Compendium of Pharmaceuticals and Specialties® (CPS) in Canada, and the Rote Liste® in Germany.

PACKAGING

Broad definition: The actual packaging (box, container, bottle, etc.), plus the galenic formulation (capsule, tablet, gelule, injection, suspension, inhalation product, etc.), and the labeling.

Narrow definition (most common usage): Primary and secondary presentation. The primary presentation concerns the actual container (bottle, blister package, watertight container, etc.). The secondary presentation includes the packaging (outer box; label; accessory for administration, such as an eye dropper or a metered dosage aerosol; etc.). Packaging problems can lead to administration errors, which in turn can lead to adverse drug reactions.

In examining packaging during an AE investigation, it is necessary to keep in mind that there may in fact be three (or even more) packagings to consider:

- The trade packaging, which refers to the container that the manufacturer ships out. For example, this might be bottles of 500 or 1000 tablets destined for the pharmacy or wholesaler.
- The pharmacy packaging, which refers to the packaging the pharmacy uses at the retail level. This might involve transferring 30 tablets to a small vial that is given to the patient.
- The patient packaging, which refers to the container the patient uses in his or her home or travels. The patient might, for example, transfer a few tablets to a small pill-box, tissue, etc., for use later.

Each time the drug is moved from one package to another storage conditions are altered and stability problems with drug products could be produced, which may lead to adverse events or loss of efficacy.

PACKAGING-RELATED PROBLEM

See Product Quality Problem.

PAPER STORAGE ISSUES

In health agencies as well as in pharmaceutical companies the masses of paper generated by submissions, adverse events, clinical trials, emails, etc., have produced significant storage issues for these documents. With the FDA and some large companies receiving hundreds of thousands of AEs per year, the number of pages needed to be securely stored, catalogued, and indexed has become a major problem. There is thus a movement to the "paperless office," with all information stored and transferred electronically.

In drug safety, the use of the E2B protocol for electronic transfer and storage of AEs promises to be part of the answer to this problem. This has produced new issues that need to be resolved, such as what constitutes an acceptable source document or what is legally useable in court or other hearings.

In the situation of electronic storage there is not yet an accepted standard for the media on which documents are stored, as the technology is rapidly evolving and documents stored on one medium (e.g., 5-1/4″ floppy disks) may no longer be useable as the hardware that can read such disks is no longer made.

PARADOXICAL ADR

The situation in which a drug produces an adverse drug reaction that is similar to the problem being treated. For example, beta-2 agonists used in asthma for bronchodilation have, in some situations, been associated with more asthmatic deaths. The experimental drug FIAU (see next page), which was intended to treat hepatitis, actually worsened hepatitis.

The antiarrhythmics encainide and flecainide, when they were used to prevent future cardiac arrests by controlling rhythm problems in survivors of cardiac arrest during a myocardial infarction, were found to actually increase arrhythmias (a pharmacologic paradox) and sudden death (a therapeutic paradox), discovered thanks to the landmark publicly-funded CAST clinical trial.

Some SSRI antidepressants have been associated with suicidality, although they are prescribed to depressed patients and depression may lead to suicidality.

The antivitamin-K oral anticoagulant warfarin is efficacious in the prevention of thromboembolism, but very rarely can induce thrombosis of peripheral venules and capillaries, as well as cholesterol micro-emboli.

Fialuridine (FIAU), a pyrimidine nucleoside analogue, was studied in the early 1990s as an antiviral treatment for hepatitis B. In 1993 a clinical trial was stopped by the investigators when it became apparent that one of the patients may have suffered liver damage due to the drug. Of 15 patients treated, eight experienced minor or no adverse effects but seven patients developed progressive hepatic failure and five died. The conduct of the trial produced much controversy. The paradox here is that the drug worsened the patients' liver status rather than improving it. The diagnostic difficulty revolved around the question of whether the worsening liver tests were due to the worsening of the underlying liver disease (hepatitis) or the drug.

PASSIVE POSTMARKETING SURVEILLANCE, PASSIVE REPORTING

The system currently in place in most countries in which adverse events suspected to be drug induced are spontaneously reported to health authorities and manufacturers by healthcare professionals and patients. Passive reporting is really spontaneous and entirely voluntary. Such reports are screened for important and urgent alert AEs, then entered into a safety database and analyzed periodically for signals and trends.

This method is passive, meaning that the health authorities and manufacturers must wait for reports to arrive. AEs are not sought out. Specific drugs are not pointed at. This method is felt to be useful, effective, sensitive, and fairly inexpensive to perform. History has largely justified this view.

However, it has been criticized for missing important AEs and for taking too long to allow enough data to be collected to make meaningful medical judgments and take action to prevent other patients from suffering from drug-induced morbidity and mortality.

There is now a push to develop and implement new mechanisms of active, prompted, intensified surveillance in which AEs to new and/or specific drugs are sought out by the health authorities and manufacturers. Such techniques include patient registries, epidemiologic studies, sentinel sites (e.g., medical centers enlisted to be on the lookout for AEs with newly approved drugs), postapproval clinical trials (phase IV), "calls to report" in newsletters (electronic and printed) to health professionals, and more.

PAST ADR HISTORY

The previous episodes of an ADR when a drug was taken or the pertinent negative that no ADR occurred when the drug was taken.

Authors' note: When a clinician questions a patient about his or her past medical history during the causality assessment of a suspected ADR, it is necessary to inquire about all past ADRs as well as the one in question.

It is necessary to distinguish between past history of ADRs in general and the specific history of prior occurrence of the ADR under suspicion. This distinction is necessary because the simple fact of having already experienced one or more ADRs constitutes by itself a nonnegligible risk factor for experiencing further ADRs even if the past ADRs are somewhat different from the current one in question and even if the drugs that produced the past ADRs are different from the current suspect drug. Relative risks ranging from 1.5 to 3.6 have been reported, confirming the old adage that "this patient doesn't tolerate drugs very well."

The specific history of the ADR in question is obtained by determining which of four possibilities has occurred, regarding the patient's previous exposure to the suspect drug ("prechallenge") and whether the ADR in question has ever occurred without drug exposure. All ADR reports should contain this information or indicate that it is unavailable. The four possible results are:

- A positive prechallenge—The ADR in question occurred when the patient was exposed to the suspect drug in the past.
- A negative prechallenge—The ADR in question did not occur when the patient was exposed to the suspect drug in the past.
- The ADR in question occurred without a prior exposure to the drug. In this case, then, the ADR was actually an AE.
- The AE in question did not occur in the past, and the patient has never been exposed to the suspect drug.

PATIENT DIARY

A technique for measuring patient compliance to medication, in which the patient is instructed by his physician to note in a diary (sometimes specially formatted and supplied by the physician or pharmaceutical company) the times he or she takes the drug in question (and any other drugs taken) along with all other noteworthy events that occurred during the day. In particular, the patient should note adverse events or problems that occur.

This technique is used in clinical trials where it is critical that the patient's symptoms (i.e., subjective) must be recorded in real time to draw meaningful medical conclusions. For example, a patient with heart disease taking a new cardiac medication might record the time and circumstances of all episodes of chest pain and shortness of breath as well as possible AEs such as dizziness, faintness, nausea, etc. A similar technique may be used by physicians in normal practice to track efficacy or adverse events after prescribing a newly marketed drug prescribed for the first time in one of his patients. Diaries may be paper or electronic.

PATIENT EXPOSURE

In drug safety, this term refers to the actual use by a patient of a drug. Thus, a patient is "exposed" to a drug for a particular length of time. Patient exposure must be ascertained, not just assumed, since compliance is often less than optimal. Adverse events cannot be suspected to be drug induced unless the drug has been taken.

PATIENT IDENTITY

One of the four minimal pieces of information needed for a valid adverse event report for regulatory purposes. One must be sure that the patient actually exists. Such information may include initials, name, sex, age, date of birth, etc. *See* Validated Report.

PATIENT INFORMATION LEAFLET (PIL)

Information that is written in nontechnical language so that patients are able to understand how to use the drug properly and safely. The information may parallel the contents of the approved labeling for the product (e.g., the package insert, the SPC) but is shortened and simplified for lay use. It may not contain all information that is listed in the labeling for the healthcare professional and thus the PIL will direct the patient to the physician or provider for further information if issues occur.

Such leaflets are obligatory in various countries for some or all drugs.

PATIENT SAFETY NEWS (PSN)

The FDA's monthly video news show for healthcare professionals. It covers significant new product approvals, recalls, and safety alerts, and offers important tips on protecting patients at http://www.fda.gov/psn. The video is available for viewing online or as an RSS feed or podcast.

Many of these PSN stories contain video footage and demonstrations that may be especially useful to educators in healthcare facilities and academic institutions.

PAUL-EHRLICH-INSTITUTE

The primary health authority in Germany. The Paul-Ehrlich-Institute is an institution of the Federal Republic of Germany reporting to the

Ministry of Health. It has multiple duties. In regard to drug safety it is responsible for the collection and evaluation of reports of adverse reactions to medicinal products and, if necessary, the taking of appropriate measures, such as changing the instructions for use ("package leaflet"), introducing a warning message, recalling a batch, or revoking the marketing authorization.

Safety is handled by the Safety of Medicinal Products and Medical Devices division, which includes a pharmacovigilance section and a clinical trial section.

See www.pei.de/EN/home/node-en.html?__nnn=true for the website in English.

PDR

See Physicians' Desk Reference.

PDUFA (PRESCRIPTION DRUG USER FEE ACT)

From the FDA website: In 1992, Congress passed the Prescription Drug User Fee Act (PDUFA). This was reauthorized by the Food and Drug Modernization Act of 1997 and again by the Public Health Security and Bioterrorism Preparedness and Response Act of 2002. PDUFA authorized the FDA to collect fees from companies that produce certain human drug and biological products. Any time a company wants the FDA to approve a new drug or biologic for marketing, it must submit an application along with a fee to support the review process. In addition, companies pay annual fees for each manufacturing establishment and for each prescription drug product marketed. Previously, taxpayers alone paid for product reviews through budgets provided by Congress. In the new program, industry provides the funding in exchange for FDA agreement to meet drug-review performance goals, which emphasize timeliness. http://www.fda.gov/oc/pdufa/overview.html

The current user fee program expired in September 2007 and was replaced by the FDA Revitalization Act. *See* FDA Revitalization Act.

Authors' note: Some advocacy groups are afraid that any incentive to accelerate examination of NDA dossiers and their approval may jeopardize the proper evaluation of the safety profile and lead to an increase in black box warnings and market withdrawals.

PEDIATRIC TESTING AND EXCLUSIVITY

Children are a special group because they are not simply "small adults" but rather may be (depending on age and other factors) biologic beings who absorb, distribute, metabolize, and excrete drugs differently from adults.

Historically, however, the testing of drugs in children has been a neglected area for many reasons—primarily involving the perception that the risks were too great to test most drugs in children.

A series of initiatives by the US federal government to encourage the testing of drugs in children started in December 1998 when the FDA issued a final rule entitled, "Regulations Requiring Manufacturers to Assess the Safety and Effectiveness of New Drugs and Biological Products in Pediatric Patients." This rule requires that every new product contain a pediatric assessment or a deferral or waiver of this assessment. It also allows the FDA to require pediatric studies and requires a pediatric section in New Drug Application periodic reports.

In September 1999 the FDA issued a Guidance for Industry entitled, "Qualifying for Pediatric Exclusivity Under Section 505A of the Food, Drug and Cosmetic Act," which allowed the FDA to request, before approval of a drug, that pediatric clinical trials be done. As an industry incentive to do this, a six-month additional period of "exclusivity" (patent protection) could be granted.

Additional guidances and documents have been issued by the FDA since then, including the "Guidance on Clinical Investigation of Medicinal Products in the Pediatric Population (ICH)," which notes that because children differ from adults in having still-developing body systems, "long term studies or surveillance data, either while patients are on chronic therapy or during the post-therapy period, may be needed to determine possible effects on skeletal, behavioral, cognitive, sexual and immune maturation and development. . . Normally the pediatric (safety) database is limited at the time of approval. Therefore, post-marketing surveillance is particularly important. In some cases, long term follow-up studies may provide additional safety and/or efficacy information for subgroups within the pediatric population or additional information for the entire pediatric population."

The guidance also addresses the question of the definition of a "child," noting the following possible categories and describing the issues in safety and efficacy of each:

- Preterm newborn infants
- Term newborn infants (0–27 days)
- Infants and toddlers (28 days to 23 months)
- Children (2–11 years)
- Adolescents (12–16 or 18 years depending on region)

Other initiatives continue because there is still the perception that not enough is known about drugs in children, especially concerning safe dosages and adverse reactions.

PERIODIC NDA REPORT

See NDA Periodic Report.

PERIODIC SAFETY UPDATE REPORT (PSUR)

The Periodic Safety Update Report is a summary of the safety of a marketed drug. The contents and format were originally described in the ICH E2C document and have been adopted with some relatively minor modifications by many countries (EU, Japan, Canada, Australia, and elsewhere) and is encouraged and accepted by the FDA in the US. They are submitted at 6 month, 1 year, 3 year or 5 year intervals.

The general principles are as follows:

- One report for one active substance. The PSUR should cover all dosage forms, formulations, and indications. There may be separate presentation of data for different dosage forms or populations if appropriate. The PSUR should be a "standalone" document.
- For combination products also marketed individually, safety information may be done as a separate PSUR or included in the PSURs prepared for one of the components with cross-referencing.
- The report should present data for the interval of the PSUR only except for regulatory status information, renewals, and serious unlisted ADRs, which should be cumulative.
- The report should focus on ADRs. All spontaneous reports should be assumed to be reactions (i.e., possibly related). Reports should be from healthcare professionals. For clinical trial and literature reports, only those cases believed by the reporter and sponsor to be unrelated to the drug should be excluded.
- Lack of efficacy reports (which are considered to be AEs) should not be included in the tables but should be discussed in the "other information" section.
- Increased frequency reports for known reactions should be reported if appropriate.
- If more than one company markets a drug in the same market, each marketing authorization holder (MAH) is responsible for submitting PSURs. If contractual arrangements are made to share safety information and responsibilities, this should be specified.

- Each product should have an international birth date (IBD), usually the date of the first marketing authorization anywhere in the world. This date should be synchronized around the world for PSUR reporting such that all authorities receive reports every six months or multiples of six months based on the IBD.
- The report should be submitted within 60 days of the data lockpoint.
- The reference document for expectedness ("listedness" as opposed to "labeledness," which refers to national data sheets such as the US package insert) should be the company core data sheet (CCDS), the safety section of which is known as the company core safety information (CSI).
- The verbatim reporter term as well as standardized coding term (i.e., MedDRA, which was approved after E2C was finished) should be used.
- ADR cases should be presented as line listings and summary tabulations. That is, individual CIOMS I or MedWatch forms are not included.

The sections of a PSUR are as follows:

- Introduction.
- Worldwide market authorization status.
- A table with dates of market authorization and renewals, indications, lack of approvals, withdrawals, dates of launch, and trade names.
- Update of regulatory authority or MAH actions taken for safety reasons.
- Changes to the reference product information:
  - The version of the CCDS in place at the beginning (or end) of the PSUR interval as the reference document. If there is a time lag between changes to the CCDS and local labeling, this should be commented on when submitting to that local health authority.
- Patient exposure:
  - The most appropriate method should be used and an explanation for its choice provided. This includes patients exposed, patient-days, number of prescriptions, and tonnage sold.
- Presentation of individual case histories from all sources (except nonmedically confirmed consumer reports):
  - Follow-up data on previously reported cases should be presented if significant.

- Literature should be monitored and cases included. Duplicates should be avoided. If a case is mentioned in the literature, even if obtained also as a spontaneous or trial case, the citation should be noted.
- If medically unconfirmed cases received from consumers are required to be submitted in the PSUR, they should be submitted as addenda line listings and summary reports.
- Line listings should include each patient only once. If a patient has more than one adverse drug experience/ADR, the case should be listed under the most serious adverse drug experience/ADR with the others also mentioned there. If appropriate, it may be useful to have more than one line listing for different dosage forms and indications. The headings for the listings are:
  - MAH reference number.
  - Country where the case occurred.
  - Source (trial, literature, spontaneous, regulatory authority).
  - Age and sex.
  - Daily dose, dosage form, and route of suspected drug.
  - Reaction onset date.
  - Treatment dates.
  - Description of the reaction (MedDRA code).
  - Patient outcome at the case level (resolved, fatal, improved, sequelae, unknown).
  - Comments (e.g., causality if manufacturer disagrees with reporter, concomitant medications, etc.).
  - Line listings should include the following cases:
    Spontaneous reports: all serious reactions, nonserious unlisted reactions.
    Studies or compassionate use: all serious reactions (believed to be serious by either the sponsor or investigator).
    Literature: All serious reactions and nonserious unlisted reactions.
    Regulatory authority cases: All serious reactions.
    If nonserious, listed ADRs are required by some authorities, they should be reported as an addendum.
- Summary tabulations:
  - Each line listing should have an aggregate summary that will normally contain more terms than patients. It may be broken down by serious and nonserious and listed and unlisted as well as other breakdowns as appropriate. There should also be a summary for nonserious listed spontaneous reactions.
  - Data in summary tabulations should be noncumulative except for ADRs that are both serious and unlisted and for which a cumulated figure should be provided in the table.

- MAH analysis of individual case histories
  - This section may contain brief comments on individual cases. The focus here is on individual cases (e.g., unanticipated findings, mechanism, reporting frequency, etc.) and should not be confused with the overall safety evaluation as described below.
- Studies:
  - All completed studies (nonclinical, clinical, epidemiologic), planned or in-progress studies, and published studies yielding or with potential to yield safety information should be discussed.
- Other information:
  - Lack of efficacy information should be presented here.
  - Late-breaking information after database lock should be presented here.
- Overall safety evaluation. The data should be presented by system organ class and should discuss:
  - A change in characteristics of listed reactions.
  - Serious unlisted reactions, placing into perspective the cumulative reports.
  - Nonserious unlisted reactions.
  - Increased frequency of listed reactions.
  - New safety issues.
  - Drug interactions.
  - Overdose and its treatment.
  - Drug misuse or abuse.
  - Pregnancy and lactation information.
  - Experience in special patient groups.
  - Effects of long-term treatment.
- Conclusion:
  - This section should indicate which safety data do not remain in accord with the previous cumulative experience and with the company CSI.
  - Any action recommended or initiated.
- Appendix: Company Core Data Sheet (CCDS).

PERSISTENT DISABILITY

One of the criteria for an AE to be called serious. The concept is not actually defined clearly but implies a problem associated with an AE that does not go away. *See* Disability.

PHARMACEUTICAL EDUCATION AND RESEARCH INSTITUTE (PERI)

Founded in 1989, this nonprofit US corporation is dedicated to the continuing education of scientists in the pharmaceutical industry and offers open courses, workshops, in-house training, and distance education. See www.peri.org.

PHARMACEUTICAL MEDICINE

The medical field devoted to the research, discovery, development, evaluation, and registration of new drugs; the surveillance of marketing, prescribers, and consumers; and communications regarding drugs, biologics, and devices. Most people engaged in pharmaceutical medicine are in the pharmaceutical industry; others work for health authorities and universities. Pharmacovigilance is part of this field.

The Drug Information Association and its publication the Drug Information Journal are devoted to this field in the US and abroad. See their website at www.diahome.org/DIAHome/.

The UK Royal College of Physicians in London recognizes this "specialty" through a "Faculty" of Pharmaceutical Medicine and a Society of Pharmaceutical Medicine (actually it is an association of professionals), both of which are associated with ADIS, the publisher of the *International Journal of Pharmaceutical Medicine (IJPM)*. See their website at http://www.rcplondon.ac.uk/specialty/Pharmaceutical.asp.

PHARMACEUTICAL RESEARCH MANUFACTURERS OF AMERICA (PhRMA)

The organization promoting the interests (and lobbying) of the innovative pharmaceutical industry in the US. It describes itself as the industry association representing "the country's leading pharmaceutical research and biotechnology companies, which are devoted to inventing medicines that allow patients to live longer, healthier, and more productive lives. PhRMA's mission is winning advocacy for public policies that encourage the discovery of life-saving and life enhancing new medicines for patients by pharmaceutical/biotechnology research companies."

See their website: http://www.phrma.org/.

PHARMACISTS

Health professionals in the "front line" of adverse event reporting. Patients may more readily complain of AEs/ADRs to pharmacists than to physicians who are harder to reach. Pharmacists have been by far the most frequent reporters of AEs to the FDA. The reporting is motivated by altruism and concern for public health since the time spent in gathering the information and reporting it to the FDA or manufacturer is not financially compensated. Schools of pharmacy are more likely than schools of medicine to include some pharmacovigilance in their curriculum.

PHARMACOBEZOAR

This term refers to the localized accumulation of an orally ingested pharmaceutical product that has mixed with digestive secretions to form a mass. It can produce an obstruction anywhere along the digestive tract as well as producing pain, ulceration, or bleeding, particularly in the stomach. There is also the danger of sudden release of the active ingredient, producing a drug overdose.

Nondrug bezoars can also consist of hair (trichobezoars) or vegetable material (phytobezoars). Although gastroscopy may be useful to remove the latter types of bezoars when located in the stomach, surgical removal may be necessary, particularly for pharmacobezoars, where the sudden release of excess amounts of the active ingredient is a risk.

Guar gum is an example of a pharmacobezoar. This hydrophilic compound was sold as a weight loss product. In 1989 a 39-year-old male patient presented to the emergency room noting that several hours after ingesting three tablets he was no longer able to swallow his saliva. Rigid esophagoscopy was required but the esophagus was torn during the procedure, requiring surgical repair. Several days later the patient died of a pulmonary embolus. Examination of the FDA database revealed 17 other cases of esophageal retention, though none serious. The product was withdrawn from the market. (FDA 1998)

PHARMACODEPENDENCE

The dependence on a pharmaceutical product is an ADR of a behavioral nature. The patient is not able to do without daily consumption of the suspect product and stopping abruptly may lead to withdrawal symptoms. The patient may not realize that he is dependent until he or she tries to stop. Some authors use the words physical dependence. The dependence on a drug is by definition inherently caused by the drug.

Authors' note: There is a trend toward differentiating dependence (e.g., on nicotine) and addiction, with the latter involving behavioral harm; the entire life of the addicted may become focused on consuming and buying the product (e.g., cocaine, heroin, amphetaminics, alcohol), harming himself and his dependents. This is a controversial and evolving area.

PHARMACODYNAMIC DRUG INTERACTION

A situation in which the pharmacologic effect of one drug is increased (additive) or diminished (antagonistic) by the pharmacologic effect of another drug.

There may be clinical consequences, such as an exaggeration of the desired effect, accompanied by type A reactions, as when two drugs prolong the QT interval on the EKG and lead to arrhythmia.

Antagonism can be beneficial for opposing an adverse type A reaction: thiazides and ACE inhibitors have opposing effects on potassium excretion, a desired consequence.

Pharmacodynamic interactions are less frequent than pharmacokinetic drug interactions (see this term).

PHARMACODYNAMICS

The study of the effects of a drug on the functions of the body. Equivalent to pharmacologic effects. The study of mechanisms of action belong to the domain of pharmacodynamics.

By contrast, pharmacokinetics study the fate of a drug once it is administered; i.e., what the body does to the drug and what dose is required to achieve the target tissue concentration. Dosages are adjusted according to pharmacokinetic and dynamic properties.

PHARMACOECONOMICS

The branch of health economics devoted to the study of cost-benefit, cost-utility, cost-minimization, and cost-effectiveness analyses. Observed or predicted costs of ADRs, in terms of quality of life and costs for preventing, detecting, and treating them, must be taken into account in these analyses.

PHARMACOEPIDEMIOLOGY

A medical science applied to interactions between marketed medications and the population. From the Greek *pharmakon* (poison), *epi* (concerning), and *demos* (people). It applies the methods of classic and clinical epidemiology as well as the technologies of modern communication to that of clinical pharmacology and pharmacotherapy. The first use of the term in a medical journal dates back only to 1984. It represents the last phase in the evaluation of a medication in development and is absolutely essential to complete the full picture of a new product to ensure effective, safe, rational, and cost-effective use. The main subjects of interest are:

- Benefit—obtained by completing the evaluation of efficacy (clinical trials) with observational studies of effectiveness in clinical practice, outcomes research analyses, etc.
- Safety—obtained by pharmacovigilance.
- Use—obtained by drug utilization reviews.
- Value—obtained by pharmacoeconomics (efficiency, etc.).

PHARMACOGENETICS

The field of genetics and pharmacology that examines the influences of genetic variations on differing responses to drugs, focusing on a single gene or a few genes, especially those related to drug metabolism leading to variations in blood levels of drugs and consequences on efficacy and safety.

PHARMACOGENOMICS

The study of how the genotype affects the response to drug treatments, desired or adverse. This new field promises to improve drug development, reduce adverse reactions by identifying the intolerants, and maximize drug efficacy by identifying the responders.

PHARMACOKINETIC DRUG INTERACTION

The situation in which the use of a drug produces changes in the absorption, distribution, metabolism, or elimination of another drug. Such interactions are of clinical importance if they compromise the efficacy or increase the toxicity of the affected drug.

In particular, there may be an alteration by one of the drugs on the cytochrome P450 enzyme system producing *induction* of one or more of the enzymes. This may result in increased metabolism of the other drug with a reduction in that drug's efficacy or with the production of toxic metabolites. Enzyme induction may also *reduce* efficacy if the other drug is a prodrug requiring activation by the enzyme.

Conversely, there may be enzyme *inhibition* by one drug, producing toxicity from the other drug if its metabolism into less toxic metabolites is slowed. Enzyme induction may also produce decreased efficacy if the other drug is a prodrug requiring activation by the enzyme.

See Prodrug.

PHARMACOKINETICS

The study of what the body does to the drug in comparison to pharmacodynamics, which is the study of what the drug does to the body. Pharmacokinetics concerns the absorption, distribution, metabolism (biotransformation), and excretion (elimination) of the drug from the body (ADME).

PHARMACOTRANSPARENCY

The presentation of unbiased, complete, impartial, and uncensored data in regard to drug efficacy, effectiveness, efficiency, safety, cost, and appropriateness of use.

Authors' note: Advocacy groups have been asking for the public availability of premarketing clinical dossiers (phase I, II, and III) submitted to drug agencies, reasons behind regulatory decisions (approval, nonapproval, withdrawal from the market, restrictions of use), user-friendly and timely access to ADR reports in national agencies' databases and other data that they feel should be in the public domain. The opposite is opacity, secretiveness.

PHARMACOLOGY

The biomedical science applied to molecules developed and/or used as potential or actual medications. It describes and explains their interactions with the living organism.

PHARMACOTHERAPY

A therapeutic approach based on the use of pharmaceutical products that produce a pharmacologic effect, as opposed to other modes of therapy such as radiotherapy, psychotherapy, surgery, medical devices, and "watchful waiting."

PHARMACOVIGILANCE

Also known as postmarketing drug surveillance and postmarketing drug safety monitoring. A public health activity whose purpose is the promotion and collection of AE/ADR spontaneous reports; the identification of signals; and the quantification, evaluation, and prevention of risks associated with marketed medicinal products. It includes passive and active (prompted, stimulated) surveillance. In a broad sense, it includes both the organization of spontaneous reporting of suspected ADRs and of structured pharmacoepidemiology studies. Inversely, some authors use pharmacoepidemiology to cover both spontaneous reporting and structured phase IV studies, both observational and experimental.

"The science and activities relating to the detection, assessment, understanding and prevention of adverse effects of drugs, biologics and other medical products, or any other possible product-related problems." From the Erice Manifesto (see this term).

PHARMACOVIGILANCE DATABASE

A collection of safety information stored on a computer in a defined and structured form, allowing addition of new information and retrieval of older information in a variety of formats and reports. Health authorities and manufacturers must maintain databases of adverse events on drugs for periodic review, analysis, and reporting.

PHARMACOVIGILANCE INVESTIGATION

Also called a signal or safety investigation. *See* Signal Investigation or Workup.

PHARMACOVIGILANCE PLAN

In the context of risk management, the development of methodology to study and track adverse events and other safety issues associated with a drug, in particular a new drug. This should be a specific series of steps or actions that will track, record, and analyze safety issues that arise in the use of a drug. The plan is usually reviewed periodically to examine whether it is achieving its stated goal. If it is not, then alternatives and changes are proposed.

Such plans have been proposed by ICH and are now required by the FDA and EMEA and other health agencies. *See* Risk Minimization Action Plan.

PHARMACOVIGILANTE

Better known as Drug Safety Officer. Health scientist responsible for drug safety in a drug industry, a regulatory agency, an academic center, an advocacy group, a professional association, an international institution, a contract Research Organization, etc. Except in an ironic or jocular sense, the term is seldom used in North America because of the negative political connotation of the word "vigilante."

PHASE 0 STUDY

The FDA is considering the approval of Exploratory IND "phase 0 studies" in which healthy volunteers can be given microdoses of experimental drugs even before animal studies are completed.

Sometimes used to refer to a preclinical (nonclinical) study not carried out in human subjects.

PHASE I STUDY

The first human beings to be exposed to a new drug are (usually paid) healthy volunteers and the study is called a phase I trial. When the new drug is considered dangerous, such as those for cancer and HIV, the first humans exposed are volunteers suffering from the disease. The main objective is to establish tolerance. Small groups are given a very small single dose of the drug, observed for adverse reactions, then a higher dose is used in another group and so on until determination of the maximum tolerated dose. The secondary objectives are the measures of efficacy (if applicable) and pharmacokinetics (plasma concentration, metabolites, etc.).

PHASE IIA TRIAL

Phase II trial specifically designed to assess dosing requirements in volunteer patients while assessing efficacy and toxicity. Includes dose-ranging studies.

PHASE IIB TRIAL

Phase II trial specifically designed to study efficacy.

PHASE III TRIAL

Large-scale comparative clinical trial conducted to look at safety and efficacy. Frequent and predictable (type A) ADRs are usually, but not always, detected during these trials. The results are usually clear and easily understandable with the calculation of an absolute risk difference between groups being possible. For example, if the group receiving drug A had a 6% incidence of AEs and the placebo group a 2% incidence of AEs, the difference is 4% or 0.04. The NNTH (Number Needed To Harm) can be calculated as the reciprocal of the absolute rate; in this example it would be 50 because $1/0.04 = 50$.

PhRMA

See Pharmaceutical Research Manufacturers of America.

PHOCOMELIA

A congenital malformation (dysmorphology) that affected thousands of babies born in the early 1960s after in utero exposure to thalidomide. The almost total absence of the upper limbs gave the impression that the victims had seallike flippers (hence the name derived from phoque, which is "seal" in French). The national health agencies played an active role in this drama and in many countries the laws and regulations were strengthened in response to it.

PHOTOSENSITIVITY

An exaggerated cutaneous response to ultraviolet radiation. It is familiarly described as an exaggerated "sunburn" whether induced by a drug or not. There are two clinical and pathophysiologic forms: phototoxicity and photoallergy.

PHYSICIANS' DESK REFERENCE (PDR)

A widely used compendium of many, but not all, of the labels for prescription drugs sold in the US. It is about 3,000 pages long and has photos of many of the products as well as the product information. It is published yearly. This is the main source consulted by

US physicians, nurses, and pharmacists to find out whether an ADR is currently labeled as well as other key information on drugs. There are other editions for OTC products, veterinary products, and so on. An electronic version is available free to medical professionals at www.pdr.net.

PHYTOCEUTICAL

Plant nutrients with properties that are claimed to have medical benefits.

PHYTOVIGILANCE

Postmarketing surveillance of the adverse events seen with plant-based products (also known as *herbal medicines, traditional medicine*). Although perceived as benign and harmless in the eyes of the public, major sequelae and even deaths have been reported. Phytovigilance is being recognized as an area well worth medical attention, and the Uppsala Monitoring Centre (UMC) has engaged the services of an expert in the field.

PINK SHEET

A widely read US bulletin in the field of pharmaceutical and biotechnology medicine published by F-D-C Reports, Inc. There is a daily and weekly edition. It covers news topics in the areas of drug safety, marketing, FDA news, patents, and business matters. See http://www.thepinksheet.com/fdcreports/pink/showHome.do.

PLA

See Product License Application.

PLACEBO

An inactive formulation (e.g., tablet, capsule, liquid, etc.) that has, in theory, no biological activity at all. Thus it should produce no beneficial effects or adverse events. Placebos are products used in clinical trials to compare the effects of an active drug to its placebo and distinguish between the pharmacologic effects and the confidence inspired by confidence in the experimental drug.

In reality, placebos may produce beneficial results (*see* Placebo Effect) or adverse events (*see* Nocebo Effect) due to the power of suggestion, and adverse events (extrinsic) due to excipients. Historically, lactose was often used as a filler in placebos and produced diarrhea in highly sensitive lactase-deficient patients.

"The ethics of placebo use are a complex issue and were addressed by the World Medical Association in comments amended to the Declaration of Helsinki in 2002 stating the following: The

WMA hereby reaffirms its position that extreme care must be taken in making use of a placebo-controlled trial and that in general this methodology should only be used in the absence of existing proven therapy. However, a placebo-controlled trial may be ethically acceptable, even if proven therapy is available, under the following circumstances:

Where for compelling and scientifically sound methodological reasons its use is necessary to determine the efficacy or safety of a prophylactic, diagnostic, or therapeutic method; or

Where a prophylactic, diagnostic, or therapeutic method is being investigated for a minor condition and the patients who receive placebo will not be subject to any additional risk of serious or irreversible harm."

http://www.wma.net/e/policy/pdf/17c.pdf

PLACEBO EFFECT (OR RESPONSE)

Beneficial, desirable effect of any treatment due to the power of suggestion but not due to the pharmacodynamic or other specific properties of a drug product. The expression may apply to self medications, alternative medicine procedures (herbs, manipulations, etc.), and mainstream medicines used during medical practice and drug trials. It may even apply to experimental sham surgical operations.

In daily practice, the confidence in the product can be strengthened by positive feelings of the physician and pharmacist as well as by publicity in the media, popular belief, and personal experience with the product.

In comparative clinical trials, the placebo effect can be reinforced by the surroundings and ambiance, as well as by the attention and enthusiasm of the research team.

PLACEBO STUDY

Clinical research in which a comparison group of patients receives an inactive product (without active ingredient) instead of the active product under study. The study is necessarily blinded.

PLAUSIBILITY

Also known as "biologic plausibility." This term is used in regard to the evaluation of causality of adverse events in relation to the drug in individual case safety reports and in signal interpretation. An AE or signal is said to be plausible (likely related to the drug in question) if it is consistent with the established mechanism of action of the drug and with current medical knowledge.

For example, in a patient given a nitrate to treat cardiac ischemia, fainting and loss of consciousness are consistent with the nitrate's pharmacologic effects of vasodilatation and lowering of the blood pressure. The attribution of the fainting to the nitrate is said to be biologically plausible.

Time to onset should be examined when looking at plausibility since the time may be so short or so long as to make an AE implausible as an ADR.

PODCAST

A new word ("portmanteau word") created from iPod® and broadcasting. Audio (and sometimes video) transmissions are loaded as files onto the Internet, from which the files may be downloaded to an MP3 player (e.g., the iPod® or Zune®) for later listening or viewing. Users may download files ad hoc or may subscribe and receive regular downloads. They are usually free (to date). In drug safety, there are now podcasts available from the FDA (http://www.fda.gov/cder/drug/podcast/default.htm) and more are to be expected from other sources in the near future. The CDC also puts out a podcast covering the *Morbidity and Mortality Weekly Report* (www.cdc.org).

POISON CONTROL CENTER (PCC)

Organizations set up around the US, Canada, Europe, and many other countries staffed by medical personnel expert on poisoning and the ingestion or exposure to toxic agents. A physician acting as a clinical toxicologist is usually its chief officer.

Toxics include overdosed prescription and OTC drugs, biologics, and other products such as household and industrial agents and products. The Centers maintain large databases with information on such agents and products. They are usually available 24/7 by telephone and are able to recommend treatments for overdoses, poisoning, etc., to healthcare practitioners as well as consumers.

In terms of drug safety they are able to give product information obtained from the official labeling as well as product monographs and other sources. The centers keep detailed records of all cases and are an important source of safety and overdose information for pharmacovigilance. Unfortunately many of these reports do not reach the health authorities or the manufacturer.

Some manufacturers establish contractual arrangements for poison control centers to receive AEs and to supply information to the public and healthcare practitioners on their products when the companies are closed (after working hours, weekends, and holidays).

Authors' note: These Centers should collaborate closely with national or, even better, regional pharmacovigilance centers, since they are in a unique position:

- *To see cases of accidental or suicidal poisoning attempted by ingesting old or new drugs;*
- *To evaluate the efficacy of antidotes;*
- *To observe suicidal ideations suspected of being caused by products prescribed according to label or off-label;*
- *To receive cases of therapeutic overdose in susceptible patients or from drug–drug interactions (type A reactions); and*
- *To note errors in drug administration.*

They should become regular reporters of suspected ADRs and mutually exchange information with their national pharmacovigilance center.

POISSON FORMULA

A statistical distribution used to calculate probabilities of rare events. It has been used in data mining and increased frequency analyses for rare adverse events. It is useful to determine the statistical power of detection of ADRs; for example, when 0 occurrences of an AE are observed in a population under study or in subjects of a clinical trial, the formula allows the calculation of the upper limit of the confidence interval around zero.

For example, if the number of occurrences of hepatitis observed among 300 subjects exposed to an experimental drug is 0 (zero), it can be inferred with 95% confidence that the true incidence of drug-induced hepatitis is less than 1%. *See* Rule of Threes.

If one desires a 99% confidence for ruling out a 1% hepatitis incidence rate, the Poisson confidence interval would show that 460 treated subjects must be free of hepatitis.

POLYPHARMACY

The use of multiple drugs by a patient. Important drug safety issues arise here as the drugs may be prescribed by multiple physicians, each unaware of what the other is prescribing. The risk of drug interaction is increased—some say "exponentially," to emphasize the situation. In addition, if the patient is unable to be compliant to the dosing regimen of each product, there is a risk of making mistakes. This situation is common in the elderly and in those who have trouble reading.

Polypharmacy is a recognized source of ADRs. In drug safety and signal analysis, it may be very difficult to ascribe causality to a particular drug if multiple drugs are being used simultaneously.

POSSIBLY RELATED

One of the many terms used in pharmacovigilance causality or relatedness. There is no standardized terminology yet in the drug safety world for causality. In spontaneous reporting regulations, all reports are considered to be "possibly related" or attributable to the drug in question ("implied causality") because the consumer or healthcare professional has taken the time and effort to report the case.

In the clinical trial situation for regulatory reporting of a serious, unlabeled AE, the manufacturer and the clinical investigator must make a determination of causality. This is, in practice, a dichotomy: "not related" vs. "possibly related." The first is that the drug is clearly not related to the AE and thus not reportable as a 15-day expedited report. The second is that there is some level of possibility that the drug and the AE are related and thus reportable. So, the choice boils down to unrelated vs. possibly related.

POSTAPPROVAL DATA MANAGEMENT (ICH)

The ICH E2D document of May 2004. See http://eudravigilance. emea.eu.int/human/docs/ICH%20E2D.pdf. This document describes the definitions and methodology for the collection and reporting of individual case safety reports (expedited reports) for products after they have been put on the market. This methodology has largely been adopted in the US, EU, Canada, Japan, and elsewhere. *See* E2D.

POSTMARKETING AEs/ADRs

Adverse events that occur after a drug has been marketed in comparison to AEs from the premarketing phase (clinical trial AEs). They are usually spontaneously reported. Postmarketing AEs may differ from the clinical trial AEs, as many more patients and different patient groups are exposed than in the clinical trial phases. Rarer AEs/ADRs as well as drug interactions may only first be seen with postmarketing AEs/ADRs.

Authors' note: A drug, in the course of its life cycle, may be marketed in one country and still unmarketed and in clinical trials in another country. Thus this product will lead to both postmarketing ADR reports and clinical trial AEs. Care must be taken to differentiate them.

POSTTREATMENT STUDY VISIT

In a clinical trial, when a patient returns to see the clinical investigator at the study site for a follow-up visit after the treatment (study drug, placebo, etc.) has been stopped. At this visit, an assessment of AEs/ADRs that occurred and persisted during the study are evaluated to see if they have disappeared after treatment was stopped (dechallenge) or whether AEs have occurred off study medication that might either be due to residual effects of the medication or to the power of suggestion. An AE that occurs well after the study is completed and no drug is present in the body is not likely to be due to the treatment (except for teratogenic disorders).

POTENTIAL MEDICATION ERROR

As defined in the FDA's proposed 2003 regulations ("The Tome"), an individual case safety report of information or complaint about product name, labeling, or packaging similarities that does not involve a patient.

This is in comparison to an "actual ME," which involves an identifiable patient whether the error was prevented before administration of the product or, if the product was administered, whether the error results in a serious SADR, nonserious SADR, or no SADR. *See* Medication Error.

PRACTOLOL SYNDROME

Also known as the Oculomucocutaneous Syndrome. It was seen with the drug practolol (one of the first beta blockers) and represented one of the first pharmacovigilance disasters after thalidomide and the creation of national pharmacovigilance systems that followed. The syndrome is characterized by conjunctivitis sicca, xerophthalmia due to lacrymal gland fibrosis, psoriasiform rashes, otitis media, sclerosing peritonitis, and a lupus-like syndrome. The signal was very difficult to discover and required good acumen from astute clinicians, especially ophthalmologists. Intestinal occlusions from sclerosing peritonitis led to fatalities. The drug was withdrawn from the market. This is not a class effect since subsequently developed beta-blockers were free of this ADR.

PRECAUTION

In drug labeling in the US, an advisory to the healthcare professional to consider before prescribing the drug. The FDA changed US drug labeling in 2006 creating a new category known as "Warnings and Precautions" to be used in all drug labeling.

The FDA issued a draft guidance on what the contents of the newly created "Warnings and Precautions" section of the drug label should contain.

The "Warnings and Precautions" section should include:

- Certain adverse reactions observed in association with the use of a drug for which there is reasonable evidence of a causal association between the drug and the adverse reaction, or when the product interferes with a laboratory test.

- Adverse reactions that can be expected to occur with a drug, despite not having been observed with that drug, or with other members of the drug class or animal studies.
- Certain adverse reactions associated with unapproved uses (off-label use).
- Known or predicted drug interactions with serious or otherwise clinically significant outcomes.
- Any laboratory tests helpful in following the patient's response or in identifying possible adverse reactions (liver enzymes level, white blood cells count, etc.).

Further information can be found at http://www.fda.gov/cder/guidance/5538dft.htm.

PRECHALLENGE

Refers to the previous administration of a suspect drug. It is an important item of the medical and pharmaceutical history of a patient in which a suspected ADR is being observed and analyzed for causality. The exposure of the suspect drug prior to the actual AE being investigated is referred to as the "prechallenge" and the exposure during the AE under investigation the "challenge." If the patient is later reexposed to the suspect drug, it becomes a "rechallenge."

In Pharmacotherapy: A conscientious physician who prescribes a product must inquire as to whether there were prechallenges (previous administrations) and whether any AEs were associated with them. This should be noted in the patient's chart and on the AE report.

Negative Prechallenge: The absence of the AE/ADR during a previous administration of the suspect product. On a spontaneous report form this information should be included in the past drug history. Several points must be kept in mind:

- A negative prechallenge is not always an absolute argument against a drug etiology for the AE/ADR. If the mechanism of the event is immunologic the (negative) prechallenge may have played a sensitizing role and is thus an argument in favor of drug etiology and not an argument against!
- A negative prechallenge done with a low dose of the drug does not exclude the drug as the cause of the AE/ADR if the mechanism is dose-dependent.
- A negative prechallenge when the drug was given by mouth does not exclude the possibility of an ADR when the drug is given by another route (e.g., intravenously).

- A negative prechallenge with a drug that had the same active ingredient but which was manufactured by a different company or manufactured by the same company but in a different formulation (e.g., tablet instead of capsule) does not exclude the possibility of an ADR when a different brand or formulation with the same active ingredient is administered. The ADR may be due to an excipient in the second drug that was not involved in the prechallenge.

Positive Prechallenge: The occurrence of an AE/ADR during a previous administration of the suspect product. On a spontaneous report form this information would be included in the past drug history. A positive prechallenge may be "specific" (same drug, same ADR) or "nonspecific" (similar drug, similar reaction). A positive prechallenge is a risk factor for that specific patient and supports a drug etiology for the AE. A positive prechallenge to halothane (fever, jaundice) is an absolute contraindication to its reuse.

Sensitizing Prechallenge: This term can be applied to a negative prechallenge if it is believed that the mechanism of the ADR that occurs on the next exposure is immunologic. This phenomenon is seen in particular in vaccinovigilance: Cases of arthritis have appeared after the second or third vaccination of hepatitis B vaccine. (Pope 1998)

PREDICATE RULES

Refers to the various set of rules, regulations, and guidelines in the US covering Good Manufacturing Practice (GMP), Good Laboratory Practice (GLP), Good Clinical Practice (GCP), and Good Pharmacovigilance Practice (GPVP or GVP). They are collectively known as "GXP" or "the predicate rules."

PREFERRED TERM (PT)

In MedDRA, the fourth-highest level of codes that is just below the High Level Terms (HLTs) and just above the Lowest Level Terms (LLTs). There are approximately 17,000 PTs. These terms are more "granular" (specific) than HLTs but less granular (specific) than LLTs. They are usually used in reporting adverse events to regulatory agencies (particularly the FDA) in expedited and periodic reports. Some agencies require LLTs for reporting. The E2B file for electronic transmission is capable of holding both LLTs and PTs for an individual case safety report. *See* MedDRA.

PREGNANCY

Although prescribing to a pregnant woman is not considered an adverse event, most health authorities require that manufacturers track all women known to be pregnant and taking a company's product through the outcome of the pregnancy. The results should be tracked, and any AEs, congenital malformations, etc., also noted and should be tracked as a signal and reported in periodic reports.

PREGNANCY RATING OR CATEGORIES OF DRUGS

There is no consistently used or standardized methodology for rating drug risk in pregnancy. The FDA scale is as follows:

- *Category A:* Adequate, well-controlled studies in pregnant women have not shown an increased risk of fetal abnormalities to the fetus in any trimester of pregnancy.
- *Category B:* Animal studies have revealed no evidence of harm to the fetus; however, there are no adequate and well-controlled studies in pregnant women. OR Animal studies have shown an adverse effect, but adequate and well-controlled studies in pregnant women have failed to demonstrate a risk to the fetus in any trimester.
- *Category C:* Animal studies have shown an adverse effect, and there are no adequate and well-controlled studies in pregnant women. OR No animal studies have been conducted, and there are no adequate and well-controlled studies in pregnant women.
- *Category D:* Adequate well-controlled or observational studies in pregnant women have demonstrated a risk to the fetus. However, the benefits of therapy may outweigh the potential risk. For example, the drug may be acceptable if needed in a life-threatening situation or serious disease for which safer drugs cannot be used or are ineffective.
- *Category X:* Adequate well-controlled or observational studies in animals or pregnant women have demonstrated positive evidence of fetal abnormalities or risks. The use of the product is contraindicated in women who are or may become pregnant.

In the EU, the Summary of Product Characteristics should include, with respect to clinical data, comprehensive information on relevant adverse events reported in the embryo, the fetus, neonates, and pregnant women, when appropriate. The frequency of such events (for example, the frequency of birth defects) may be specified when available. The section should specify the extent of the human experience if no adverse events have been reported in pregnancy (no experience, limited experience).

Consequently, the paragraph should include:

a) Clinical data from human experience in pregnancy with the frequency when appropriate.

b) Conclusions from developmental studies, which are relevant for the assessment of the risk associated with exposure during pregnancy. Only malformative, fetotoxic, and neonatal effects should be mentioned in this paragraph.

c) Recommendations on the use of the medicinal product during the different periods of gestation. A sentence should provide the reason(s) for these recommendations.

d) Recommendations for the management of exposure during pregnancy when appropriate (including relevant specific monitoring such as fetal ultrasound and specific biological or clinical surveillance of the neonate).

PRESCRIPTION DRUG USER FEE ACT

See PDUFA.

PRESCRIPTION EVENT MONITORING (PEM)

A type of prospective noninterventional observational cohort technique applied to patients exposed to selected products recently marketed in the UK. The application of this epidemiologic technique was developed and is being used by the Drug Safety Research Unit (DSRU) at the University of Southampton using data collected from UK general practitioners.

"The PEM technique is most applicable for new drugs intended for long term widespread use. PEM is a hypothesis generating technique; the large database with data on 900,000 patients can be used for hypothesis testing.

The technique relies upon the collection of individual prescriptions once these have been issued to the patients and dispensed by pharmacists. The DSRU collects details of the prescriptions for the drugs it is monitoring and thereby records information on the first 20,000–50,000 patients given the new drug.

This information provides the exposure data. After a suitable interval the doctors who prescribed the drug being monitored are sent green form questionnaires on which they are asked to record medical events reported by the patient subsequent to the initial prescription. The information on these green forms provides the outcome data."

The AEs in question are the medical events recorded in the patients' files during the normal course of their visit with the doctor, not recorded as a suspected ADR. The frequency of these medical events during drug treatment is then compared after stopping the drug. Their website is www.dsru.org/pem2002.html. *See also* Drug Safety Research Unit (DSRU).

PRESCRIRE INTERNATIONAL & LA REVUE PRESCRIRE

La Revue Prescrire is a French language journal published monthly in Paris, presenting critical reviews of drugs and indications newly released in France, of new knowledge in pharmacovigilance, and of current and forthcoming European and French drug policies. This journal is independent of industry and government, is financed solely by its 30,000 subscribers, and is a leading member of the International Society of Drug Bulletins (ISDB). The editorial team is made of general practitioners, specialists, and pharmacists, backed by a wide variety of numerous outside reviewers; editors are trained in-house and are required to sign a no-conflict-of-interest declaration annually.

Both the French and English editions are published by a nonprofit organization, Association Mieux Prescrire, that initiated a sales representative monitoring network and has been advocating a widening use of generic names by prescribers, more public health-oriented laws, more transparency in regulatory agencies, and stricter control of drug promotion.

Prescrire International, the concise English language version of *La Revue Prescrire,* is a unique source in Europe of independent comparative information on drugs and other therapeutic interventions. The New Drugs section provides comparative assessments of new drugs and new indications. The Reviews section presents assessments of therapeutic interventions as well as treatment guidelines selected to promote patient care based on the best available unbiased evidence. The Adverse Effects section gives a balanced view of the latest suspected or confirmed ADR data collected from both published and unpublished wordwide sources. Subscribers to the printed version will benefit from an English version of the website scheduled for 2008.

http://www.prescrire.org/signature/productions/international.php.

PREVALENCE RATE

The number of occurrences of an AE or a disease in a population at a particular point in time. *See* Incidence Rate.

PRIMARY LEGISLATION (EU)

A regulatory term. European Union "primary legislation" represents treaties and agreements among the member states. This includes the Single European Act (1987), the Maastricht Treaty (1992), and the Treaty of Amsterdam (1997). "Secondary legislation" derives from the treaties (directives, regulations, and recommendations). *See* Secondary Legislation.

PRIVACY

See Data Privacy.

PRODRUG

A drug that is usually inactive in the body until it is transformed, usually by metabolism, into an active, therapeutic form. Examples include L-dopa, which is transformed into the active dopamine; enalapril, which is converted to enalaprilat; and codeine, which is demethylated into morphine.

PRODUCT DATA SHEET

Primarily an EU term. It is, in essence, the drug labeling. A standardized document containing essential scientific information on the reference medicinal product for its dissemination to healthcare professionals by the marketing authorization holder. It is approved by the competent health authorities granting the marketing authorization.

There are several synonyms or variants used to refer to product labeling:

- In the US, this would refer to the "package insert" or FDA-approved "labeling."
- The "Core Safety Data Sheet" (CDS) as defined in CIOMS II (see this term) is: A document prepared by the manufacturer containing all relevant safety information, including adverse drug reactions.
- In the EU it is also known as the Summary of Product Characteristics (SmPC or SPC) and/or the Product Monograph. This usually covers a product in all of the EU countries where the product is marketed.
- In Canada it is called the Product Monograph.
- There are also national data sheets, which may vary from country to country, containing the essential scientific information.

PRODUCT LABELING

See Labeling.

PRODUCT LIFE CYCLE EFFECT

See Weber Effect.

PRODUCT LICENSE APPLICATION (PLA)

A submission to the US FDA for permission to market a biotechnology substance. It is the biotechnology equivalent of an NDA (New Drug Application). For certain substances (e.g., plasma-derived products), the FDA will now accept a Biologics License Application (BLA) instead of a PLA and an Establishment License Application (ELA). Safety reporting for PLAs and BLAs is similar to that required for NDAs.

PRODUCT QUALITY PROBLEM

An issue relating to the manufacture, packaging, storage, tampering, etc., that may produce adverse events or other problems with the product. It is to be distinguished from adverse events due to the active moiety (drug product) itself. Sometimes the quality problem is quite evident (two different drugs mistakenly put in one package, discoloration or visible impurities, etc.) but sometimes it is not.

In practice it may be very hard to distinguish an AE/ADR due to quality issues compared to the active moiety itself. A high level of suspicion for product quality problems and excipient problems is needed to make this distinction. Clues to a product quality issue may be seen from a clustering of similar AEs from a particular lot or geographic area.

PROOF OF CONCEPT STUDY

A clinical trial, usually small, meant to test the pharmacologic concept behind a new drug or new indication or new patient population. It is done in patients under tightly controlled conditions, usually in phase II. The results may produce a "go-no-go" situation whereby a negative result ends that line of investigation of the drug.

PROPORTIONAL REPORTING RATES

A technique for signal detection using large databases of AEs. For each AE, the calculation of the proportion of that AE as a function of all AEs reported for a drug is calculated and compared with the proportion of that AE for all other drugs in the database. If the proportion for the drug is greater than that for the database as a whole, this is suggestive of a signal.

PSEUDOMEMBRANOUS COLITIS

An iatrogenic disease associated with the prior use of antibiotics (which has a characteristic colonoscopic appearance) and should not be confused with a simple diarrhea. Pseudomembranous colitis has been defined by the following three criteria:

- The *severity* of the diarrhea,
- the presence in the stool of the cytotoxin of *Clostridium difficile*, or
- the presence of pseudo-membranes on sigmoidoscopy.

PSUR

See Periodic Safety Update Report.

PUBLIC CITIZENS HEALTH RESEARCH GROUP (PCHRG)

A US nonprofit "watchdog" organization that promotes research-based, system-wide changes in healthcare policy and provides oversight concerning drugs, medical devices, etc. Its members work to ban or relabel unsafe or ineffective drugs and medical devices. They publish a book entitled *Worst Pills, Best Pills* and maintain a website with critical reviews of certain medications. They sometimes initiate lawsuits against the FDA. See their website: http://www.citizen.org/hrg/about/.

PUBMED

An excellent and free online resource for medical literature. From their website, http://www.ncbi.nlm.nih.gov/entrez/query.fcgi?db=PubMed:

"PubMed is a service of the U.S. National Library of Medicine that includes over 16 million citations from MEDLINE and other life science journals for biomedical articles back to the 1950s. PubMed includes links to full text articles and other related resources." For example if you enter "Drug Safety", you will find (as of this writing) 2,272 titles of articles on the subject, some with the abstract; you will also find 1,136 titles concerning "Pharmacovigilance" (at this mid-2007 writing).

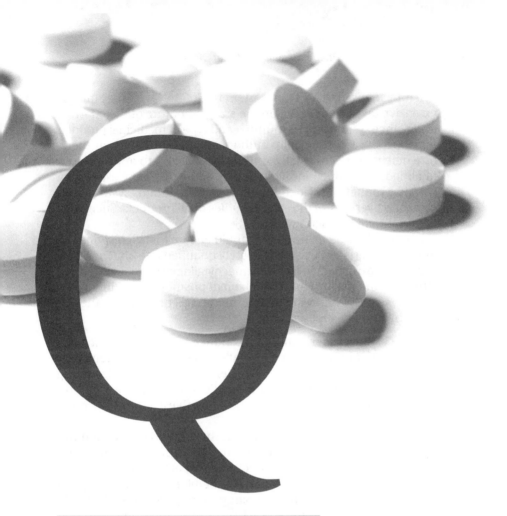

QUALIFIED PERSON FOR PHARMACOVIGILANCE (QP OR QPPV)

The Qualified Person for Pharmacovigilance refers to a person situated in the European Union who is responsible for pharmacovigilance. The role is complicated and was redefined in the 2007 version of Volume 9A. Because of its critical role in the EU, extensive excerpts from the appropriate section on the QP are given here: http://eudravigilance.emea.eu.int/human/docs/vol9A_2007-04.pdf.

The QPPV is responsible for

- Establishing and maintaining/managing the Marketing Authorisation Holder's pharmacovigilance system.
- Having an overview of the safety profiles and any emerging safety concerns in relation to the medicinal products for which the Marketing Authorisation Holder holds licenses.
- Acting as a single contact point for the Competent Authorities on a 24-hour basis.

It is recognised that this important role of the QPPV may impose extensive tasks, depending on the size and nature of the pharmacovigilance system and the number and type of medicinal products for which the company holds authorisations. The QPPV may therefore delegate specific tasks, under supervision, to appropriately qualified and trained individuals, e.g. acting as safety experts for certain products, provided that the QPPV maintains system oversight and overview of the safety profiles of all products. Such delegation should be documented.

In case of absence, the QPPV should ensure that all responsibilities are undertaken by an adequately qualified person. The QPPV should have oversight of the pharmacovigilance system in terms of structure and performance and be in a position to ensure in particular the following system components and processes, either directly or through supervision:

- The establishment and maintenance of a system which ensures that information about all suspected adverse reactions which are reported to the personnel of the Marketing Authorisation Holder, and to medical representatives, is collected and collated in order to be accessible at least at one point within the EU.
- The preparation for Competent Authorities of the Member States, where the medicinal product is authorised and in case of centrally authorised products the preparation for the Agency and Competent Authorities of the Member States of the reports including Individual Case Safety Reports (ICSRs), Periodic Safety Update Reports (PSURs), and reports on company-sponsored post-authorisation safety studies.
- The conduct of continuous overall pharmacovigilance evaluation during the post-authorisation period.
- The ensuring that any request from the Competent Authorities for the provision of additional information necessary for the evaluation of the benefits and the risks afforded by a medicinal product is answered fully and promptly, including the provision of information about the volume of sales or prescriptions of the medicinal product concerned.
- The provision to the Competent Authorities of any other information relevant to the evaluation of the benefits and risks afforded by a medicinal product, including appropriate information on post-authorisation studies.

The oversight referred to above should cover the functioning of the Marketing Authorisation Holder's pharmacovigilance system in all relevant aspects, including quality control and assurance procedures, standard operating procedures, database operations, contractual arrangements, compliance data (e.g. in relation to the quality, completeness and timeliness for expedited reporting and submission of Periodic Safety Update Reports), audit reports and training of personnel in relation to pharmacovigilance.

The QPPV should also act as the Marketing Authorisation Holder's contact point for pharmacovigilance inspections or should be made aware by the Marketing Authorisation Holder of any inspection, in order to be available as necessary.

The Marketing Authorisation Holder should adequately support the QPPV and ensure that there are appropriate processes, resources, communication mechanisms and access to all sources of relevant information in place for the fulfilment of the QPPV's responsibilities and tasks.

The Marketing Authorisation Holder should ensure that there is full documentation covering all procedures and activities of the QPPV and that mechanisms are in place to ensure that the QPPV may receive or seek all relevant information. The Marketing Authorisation Holder should also implement mechanisms for the QPPV to be kept informed of emerging safety concerns and any other information relating to the evaluation of the risk-benefit balance. This should include information from ongoing or completed clinical trials and other studies the Marketing Authorisation Holder is aware of and which may be relevant to the safety of the medicinal product, as well as information from sources other than the specific Marketing Authorisation Holder, e.g. from those with whom the Marketing Authorisation Holder has contractual arrangements.

The Marketing Authorisation Holder should ensure that the QPPV has sufficient authority:

- To implement changes to the Marketing Authorisation Holder's pharmacovigilance system in order to promote, maintain and improve compliance.
- To provide input into Risk Management Plans and into the preparation of regulatory action in response to emerging safety concerns (e.g. variations, urgent safety restrictions, and, as appropriate, communication to Patients and Healthcare Professionals).

The Marketing Authorisation Holder should assess risks with potential impact on the pharmacovigilance system and plan for business contingency, including back-up procedures (e.g. in case of non-availability of personnel, adverse reaction database failure,

failure of other hardware or software with impact on electronic reporting and data analysis).

QUALITY ASSURANCE

This term refers to actions taken *during* the process of handling safety data to ensure that the work is correct and complete. For example, during the preparation of a MedWatch or CIOMS I form for submission to a health authority by a pharmacist, the QA might be done by his or her supervisor.

Drug safety organizations should have both quality assurance and quality control functions in place. During the processing and analysis of safety data, QA should be performed at the appropriate stages in the process. After the work is done, a review or an audit may be done on selective cases routinely or periodically (e.g., monthly) to see that the entire process is done correctly. The goal is standardized and consistent methodologies and workflow as well as use of best practices.

Many safety departments in companies have a yearly audit done by the quality group (separate from the drug safety group). And, of course, the FDA and other health authorities (particularly the MHRA in the UK) do periodic pharmacovigilance audits to check the quality of the safety department's work. *See* Quality Control.

The FDA announced various measures in late 2006 in the field of safety, including one regarding Quality Assurance. (*Source:* The Future of Drug Safety—Promoting and Protecting the Health of the Public: FDA's Response to the Institute of Medicine's 2006 Report http://www.fda.gov/oc/reports/iom013007.html):

"Applying a quality systems approach to improve drug adverse event detection.

"We are strengthening and standardizing the process used by safety evaluators in OSE. These safety evaluators critically review adverse event reports that have been submitted to the Agency's AERS reporting system by sponsors of approved applications, healthcare professionals, consumers, and other sources. The goal of this initiative to strengthen the safety evaluation process is to identify best review practices and develop a quality assurance system including standardized methodologies, training and mentoring, workload prioritization, and management tools to optimize the use of resources to ensure efficient risk management."

QA

See Quality Assurance.

QUALITY CONTROL (QC)

This term refers to a review of the (final) deliverable of the work done handling safety data in a safety department, such as preparing a CIOMS I form or a PSUR or NDA Periodic Report. This work is done to ensure that the deliverables were correctly and completely prepared and that no data are lost or changed along the way. Quality control may include formal audits by third parties from outside or inside the company or organization. Such audits are routinely done at the end of the process. The difference from quality assurance is that this review is usually done after the case is completed.

Quality control in a drug safety department includes internal auditing and review of the department's performance against regulations, their internal SOPs and good pharmacovigilance practices, to track key performance indicators (metrics) such as on-time expedited reports, PSURs, and NDA periodic reports, to give feedback on errors, to identify training needs, etc.

See Quality Assurance.

QC

See Quality Control.

QPPV OR QP

See Qualified Person.

QT/QTC PROLONGATION

An adverse cardiologic event, often drug-induced, sometimes leading to the dangerous arrhythmia called *Torsades de pointes*. The QT interval refers to the period of ventricular depolarization and repolarization as observed on the electrocardiogram. The QTc interval is the QT interval corrected for the rate ($QTc = QT/\sqrt{R\text{-}R}$ interval). In general, QTc intervals greater than 0.44 sec in men and 0.46 sec in women are felt to be abnormal.

Although the interval may be elongated due to various reasons, including the inherited "Long QT Syndrome," the most common cause is drug therapy. It is felt to be due to blockage of the hERG channel and may lead to severe cardiac arrhythmias (including *Torsades de pointes*), which may be fatal.

Screening for QT interval prolongation is often carried out in animal preparations as part of the preclinical safety pharmacology evaluation of selected drugs in development.

QUALITATIVE SIGNALS OF RISK

This refers to the historical method of having medical professionals skilled in pharmacovigilance review safety data (individual case
safety reports, case series, line listings, etc.) to try to "pull out" signals and safety information based on nonquantitative clinical judgment ("global introspection"). Currently, attempts are being made
to look at quantitative methods of screening for signals or potential signals which are then evaluated by the pharmacovigilance
professionals.

*Authors' note: Clearly a skilled pharmacovigilance medical pro-
fessional who can tease out signals and meaningful safety data from
a large mass of complex and scattered safety data is worth his or her
weight in gold. However, this leads to the obvious issues of inconsis-
tency of quality and availability of such professionals as well as the
lack of any way to measure such skills. In addition, some reviewers
will "jump" on an early signal and others will wait until more data
or additional cases are available, particularly in equivocal situations. Many now feel that initial computerized data mining (quantitative review) of safety data followed by human analysis will
become a preferred methodology since medical databases (claims
from HMOs, etc.) and ADR databases are becoming large enough
for useful data mining.*

QUALITY OF SAFETY DATA

It should go without saying that the better the quality of data obtained, the better the possibility for making a causality assessment.
For this reason, corroborative data (lab tests, hospital reports, etc.)
serve strongly to validate a safety report. Adverse events reported
by patients without medical validation may be particularly hard to
evaluate. Although given with entirely good intentions, the use of
certain terminology by patients may give false or misleading information to the drug safety reviewer. For example, the lay person's
use of the term "heart attack" or "shock" is not necessarily the same
as that of a medical professional. Where possible, medical validation should be sought. In some situations this is impossible.
Adverse events reported to over-the-counter products in which the
patient did self-diagnosis and self-treatment without the intervention of any medical professional (e.g., pharmacist, physician)
may produce reports that are very hard to interpret.

QUANTITATIVE SIGNALS OF RISK

See Data Mining and Proportional Reporting Rates.

QUESTIONNAIRES FOR AEs

Over the years various questionnaires have been created to collect adverse events. They have been used in clinical trial and postmarketing settings. They may be filled out by the patient or by a medical or nonmedical professional asking the questions.

There has been a lively debate over whether the use of such a questionnaire or checklist is superior to a more open-ended method of data collection ("So how are you today?" or "Did any problems occur since you were last here?").

The advantages include the possibility of asking "embarrassing" questions more easily, less physician time is needed, very clear and precise questions can be asked, a complete review of systems can be obtained, the questions can be customized to the drug and/or patient in question, etc.

The disadvantages include more paper (or computer screens) and more data to analyze, the suggestion of adverse events to the patient possibly causing an overcall of AEs, etc. Data may be lost if the patient's verbatim narrative account of symptoms is not captured for interpretation by a healthcare professional. Forcing a complex story into a checklist or yes/no questions may lose data. Some feel that too much data is collected overestimating adverse events with questionnaires. The use of control groups (particularly placebo) allows the reviewer to interpret the data in context.

In general, a nonspecific questioning of the patient for AEs is favored in clinical trials. However, safety-specific trials looking for particular AEs do include directed questions.

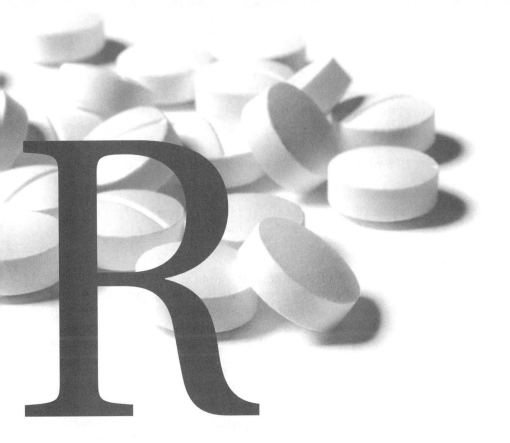

RANDOMIZED CLINICAL TRIAL (RCT)

A trial is an experimental study; i.e., the experimenter rather than the personal physician or the patient chooses the treatments to be compared and the method for allocating patients to the compared treatments. As a result, the treatment is determined without bias using a method that prevents preselection, usually a table of random numbers. The experimental protocol may differ from the normal practice of medicine. Randomization is the best control measure available for equalizing known and especially unknown prognostic factors among the compared treatment groups.

It may be single-blinded (the patient does not know what the treatment allocation is) or double-blinded (neither the patient nor the investigator knows what the treatment allocation is). These trials are often multicenter and costly. They represent the gold standard of research for testing efficacy: the double-blind, randomized, controlled trial. They are usually done during phase III of drug development and for many reasons (ethical, availability of patients, etc.) may not be feasible after the drug is marketed. Meta-analysis of RCTs is increasingly being used for studying drug safety.

Frequent and predictable (type A) ADRs are usually, but not always, detected during large phase III trials.

RAPS

See Regulatory Affairs Professionals Society.

RARE (AE/ADR FREQUENCY)

Under the CIOMS III definition, rare refers to an AE/ADR that occurs from 0.01% to 0.1% of the time (1/10 000 to 1/1000).

RATE

Ratio in which the numerator is the number of patients with a particular characteristic (the *cases*) and the denominator is the total number of patients capable of having this characteristic. It is given in the form of a decimal between 0.0 and 1.0 or as a percentage between 0% and 100%. In a 2 × 2 table of type **abcd** the rate is the number of cases divided by the total for that row or column; thus **a/[a + b]** and **a/[a + c]** are rates.

This term may refer to the number of occurrences of an AE per patient exposed or per unit of time. Careful attention should be paid to the use of this word in postmarketing drug safety where "reporting rate" refers to the number of new reports of an AE per unit of time (e.g., per year) received by the manufacturer or health authority.

This must be distinguished from the (true) "incidence rate," which is the number of new AEs that actually occur in the population in question over this time period and in relation to the number of patients exposed. The issue here is that many if not most of the AEs never get reported by the patient or healthcare professional to the manufacturer or health authority. Thus the true incidence rate is always greater than the reporting rate by an unknown and variable amount. It has been estimated roughly that only 10% of all AEs that occur are actually reported though this number is unknown for most categories of adverse events, as well as their seriousness, and for most indications and drugs. When there is no suspicion by clinicians the reporting rate is 0. Finally, the "background" rate refers to the incidence rate of the AE in question in the general population not taking the drug being examined.

In clinical trials, where the study is done under careful supervision, the likelihood of an AE being missed or not reported is much lower and the reporting rate in the study should equal the incidence rate.

RATIO

Quantitative relationship of two magnitudes of the same dimension. It may be expressed with a colon, such as 2:3 (spoken "two to three ratio") or as a fraction or its conversion in percentage, such as 2/5 (spoken "two out of five") or 40% (forty per hundred).

Authors' note: In drug safety, the terms "benefit/risk ratio" or "risk/benefit ratio" are sometimes used. This is, strictly speaking, incorrect since there are no numbers or values to compare. Neither overall risk nor overall benefit can be reduced to a single risk and a single benefit; risks and benefits are usually multiple and must be weighted, and some remain qualitative in their evaluation. Thus a ratio is an improper simplification. Better terms are "benefit/risk analysis," "assessment," or "balance."

REACTIONS WEEKLY

A bulletin published by ADIS. This weekly publication provides an accessible and up-to-date summary of clinical observations and regulatory information published in the major pharmacovigilance and other medical journals. It is available in print or electronically. It is indispensable to anyone working in the field of pharmacovigilance. See their website: www.adis.com.

REACTIVE METABOLITE

The metabolism or bioactivation in the body of a drug to another chemical (metabolite) that is more likely to produce toxicity than the original chemical. A classic example of this is the cytochrome P450-dependent oxidation in the liver of acetaminophen (paracetamol) to N-acetyl-p-benzoquinone imine, a toxic metabolite. Overdose may be fatal.

REBOUND EFFECT (OR PHENOMENON)

The return or worsening of symptoms being treated, after a drug given to treat those symptoms is withdrawn. This may be seen with many drugs after their pharmacologic effects wear off. In some cases this is a return to the baseline symptom levels (e.g., decongestants for nasal stuffiness or analgesics for pain), whereas in other cases the return of symptoms may be more severe than before treatment (gastric acid production after calcium containing antacids, hypertension crisis after stopping a beta blocker abruptly).

Authors' note: The prescriber must inform the patient of three salient points:

1. *The way in which a rebound effect can be prevented; i.e. by the gradual withdrawal of the drug rather than an abrupt cessation.*
2. *How to recognize the symptoms of the rebound effect.*
3. *How to treat the symptoms: restarting the medication at a lower dosage, substituting another drug, or using a nonpharmacologic approach.*

RECALL

According to the FDA, "action taken by a firm to remove a product from the market. Recalls may be conducted on a firm's own initiative, by FDA request, or by FDA order under statutory authority." Removal means physical removal from drugstore, hospital pharmacies, etc. See http://www.fda.gov/oc/po/firmrecalls/recall_defin.html.

The FDA-classified recalls are available online as Recalls and Field Corrections under the heading of a weekly Enforcement Report and cover drugs, biologics, and devices. (http://www.fda.gov/opacom/Enforce.html, accessed April 2006)

Medical device

"A safety alert is issued in situations where a medical device may present an unreasonable risk of substantial harm. In some cases, these situations also are considered recalls."

Minor violation; tampering

"A market withdrawal occurs when a product has a minor violation that would not be subject to FDA legal action. The firm removes the product from the market or corrects the violation. For example, a product removed from the market due to tampering, without evidence of manufacturing or distribution problems, would be a market withdrawal."

Recall, Class I

"A situation in which there is a reasonable probability that the use of or exposure to a violative product will cause serious adverse health consequences or death."

Recall, Class II

"A situation in which use of or exposure to a violative product may cause temporary or medically reversible adverse health consequences or where the probability of serious adverse health consequences is remote."

Recall, Class III

"A situation in which use of or exposure to a violative product is not likely to cause adverse health consequences."

A company needs to have a recall strategy which the FDA defines as "a planned specific course of action to be taken in conducting a specific recall, which addresses the depth of recall, need for public warnings, and extent of effectiveness checks for the recall." 21CFR7.3(l)

A recall may be instituted by a health authority if there is a major safety risk; it may be instituted by a pharmaceutical company if they discover a safety issue and wish to withdraw the drug immediately to protect the public (and the company) or, as is often the case, under intense pressure from the health authority to remove the drug from the market before the authority forces the issue ("staying one step ahead of the sheriff"). The recall may, in theory, be definitive or temporary. In reality, most are definitive with a reappearance on the market being rare. Thalidomide is an unusual case. It was withdrawn due to terrible birth defects in the offspring when taken by pregnant women to prevent morning sickness and as a sleeping pill. It was recently reintroduced in the US market as a treatment for leprosy.

In practice the words "recall" and "withdrawal" are used quite loosely. A recall is usually used to refer to a lot or formulation that is removed from the market usually for safety or product quality reasons whereas a withdrawal usually implies the definitive removal from the market of the product. *See* Withdrawal.

Authors' note: Withdrawal from the market is surely one of the most severe actions a company or health authority can take. In extreme cases, the recall may be an emergency and one or more media can be used: television; the Internet; radio; and letters to doctors, pharmacists, and patients. Pharmacists and physicians may need to contact their patients if the recall goes down to the patient level. Large recalls are exceedingly difficult and expensive. Once a drug has left the middleman (wholesaler) it may already have been distributed to thousands or even hundreds of thousands of pharmacies in many countries.

RECALL BIAS

An error or flaw in a clinical trial, an observational study, or in data collection of AEs, due to the incomplete or inaccurate remembering of something in the past. A patient may forget the exact dates that medications were taken or forget that an OTC product was taken that was relevant to the safety issue under investigation.

This type of measurement error or bias can produce incorrect results in studies that rely mainly on patients' recall without objective verification of the data collected.

RECENTLY MARKETED MEDICINAL PRODUCT

Any medicinal product that is within its first years of marketing. In some countries the limit is two years, as this is the time period when the reporting of suspected adverse reactions is usually the highest. For example, in Australia drugs of current interest normally remain on the list for two years. In the UK the "black triangle" scheme (*see* Black Triangle) is used for new medications to call attention to the fact that experience with the product is limited. After two years (usually) an assessment is made of the drug's safety and a decision as to whether to continue or remove the black triangle is made.

RECHALLENGE

The reintroduction of a medication after its withdrawal and disappearance of the AE (positive dechallenge) in a patient presenting with an adverse event.

For example, if one wishes to determine whether a drug produced diarrhea after its use, one may withdraw the drug from the patient to see whether the diarrhea stops. If yes (a positive dechallenge) after a drug-free interval, the product may be reintroduced (rechallenge) to see if the diarrhea recurs. If yes (a positive rechallenge) this is very strong evidence that the drug is the cause of the diarrhea. Rechallenges should be medically necessary and ethically acceptable.

RECORD LINKAGE

This refers to finding information on a patient from two different databases (e.g., drug reimbursement and hospitalization databases). In drug safety this is used as an epidemiologic surveillance technique (pharmacoepidemiology).

In some areas, countries, or regions, particularly those with a single-payer health scheme, one may go into the claims database of, say, all hospitalizations and compare the data on these patients with the prescriptions filled for a particular drug by these patients found in a separate database. By comparing the hospitalizations (and the reasons for them) with the drugs given prior to or during the hospitalization one may look for associations of AEs/ADRs and drugs.

Authors' note: These studies are possibly biased by the mechanism of data input into the claims database; that is, there may be bias or error in the claims data compared to the original medical records. The claims data are secondary data; primary data can only be accessed when the epidemiologist is allowed to go back to the original patients' files. Quality, standardization, access, and completeness may also present issues. However, this is still a useful and increasingly used method of doing drug surveillance.

RECOVERY; RECOVERED

This term is one of the possible outcomes in a spontaneous AE report. It refers to a cure or a return to the patient's baseline or original condition before the event occurred.

REFERENCE RANGE

The normal values of a laboratory test. These normals may differ from laboratory to laboratory, day to day, test kit/reagent to test kit, etc. Also note that the units of measurement may differ from one laboratory to another. Thus if one receives, say, a report of phosphorus level of 159, it is not clear what this means and whether it is high, low, or normal unless one knows the units and reference range. This is something to remember when suspecting a drug of being the cause of what seems to be an abnormal value.

In other situations, a reference range may refer to a series of levels in a test that determine severity. For example:

SGOT: Normal (10-40 IU), Mild elevation (40-120 IU), Moderate (120-400 IU), Severe (>400 IU).

REGIONAL DATA ENTRY

In pharmaceutical companies, this refers to the databasing of drug safety information in a small number of centers where expertise, quality, and the efficiency of higher volumes may be developed. This is in contrast to entering the data at each point of collection.

For example, for postmarketing AEs that are collected in each affiliate or subsidiary of a multinational pharmaceutical company, the data might be entered into the corporate safety database in one center in North America, one in Europe, one in Asia, and one in South America, rather than in the 80 or more affiliated companies.

In clinical trials, this refers to entering the safety data at one or two data entry sites rather than having each investigational site enter data (remote data entry).

REGIONAL PHARMACOVIGILANCE CENTER

A system for drug surveillance used in various countries.

In France there are over 30 drug safety centers located at regional university hospitals and medical schools (usually in the departments of pharmacology) around the country that play an active role in signaling, signal investigations, pharmacovigilance, drug information, poison control, drug addiction, and teratovigilance, in addition to undergraduate and graduate teaching of drug safety to medical students, pharmacists, midwives, and other health professionals. They work in cooperation with the central health authority, the Agence Française de Sécurité Sanitaire des Produits de Santé. This very interesting system allows a much wider national involvement in drug safety by local physicians, pharmacists, pharmacologists, toxicologists, and academics, compared to the US system, which is largely centered around the FDA in the Washington, DC, area.

In Spain, the regional unit is defined as the functional unit linked to the public health system, designated by the body competent in pharmacovigilance of each region, responsible for implementation of the official pharmacovigilance programs in its region: scheduling; coordination; collection; evaluation; and coding of, and database entry, training, and information on adverse drug reactions. Its technicians must be accredited by the Spanish Pharmacovigilance System before they can carry out its functions.

In Sweden, the postmarketing AE surveillance system in the health authority is linked with regional centers in departments of clinical pharmacology in academic medical centers around the country, with links to drug information centers, allowing rapid communication of safety information to the media.

In Canada there are seven offices that serve as regional points-of-contact to collect reports submitted by health professionals and consumers. These offices are no longer embedded in an academic and/or healthcare environment, as some of them had been for a few years. The reports are forwarded to the National Adverse Reaction Centre in Ottawa for analysis along with information from postmarketing surveillance around the world, as part of its determination as to whether the benefits of a drug outweigh the risks.

REGISTRY

A form of observational prospective follow-up (cohort) of a population with specified characteristics.

As defined by the FDA in its March 2005 Risk Management guidance: "an organized system for the collection, storage, retrieval, analysis and dissemination of information on individual persons exposed to a specific medical intervention who have either a particular disease, a condition (e.g., a risk factor) that predisposes [them] to the occurrence of a health-related event, prior exposure to substances (or circumstances) known or suspected to cause adverse health effects." A control or comparison group should be included where possible. They may be used when such data are not available in automated databases or when collection is from multiple sources (e.g., medical doctors, hospitals, pathologists, etc.) over time. The FDA suggests that all registries have written protocols describing objectives; a literature review; plans for systematic patient recruitment and follow-up; methodology for data collection, management, and analysis; and registry termination conditions. Again, the FDA suggests collaboration between the sponsor and agency in the development of the registry.

CIOMS V has noted that "a registry is not a study. Cases should be treated as solicited reports (causality assessment required)."

Authors' note: Registries are commonly used for collecting disease specific information (e.g., AIDS), especially about rare or unusual diseases, as well as for pregnancy and teratology information. A registry may also be a collection of consecutive patients exposed to selected products or of consecutive cases presenting the AE of interest. It is a form of noncomparative observational study.

REGULATION

In the US the FDA, like other federal agencies, is empowered to create regulations. Regulations are rules issued by government authorities and have the force of law. To create a regulation, the FDA publishes the proposed version of the new or amended regulation in the Federal Register. A period is defined during which time the public may send written comments on the proposal to the FDA. After review, a final regulation is published in the *Federal Register* and in the Code of Federal Regulations. A long period may elapse between first publishing the draft and the final regulation; also, the draft regulation may be withdrawn.

In the European Union, the meaning of "regulation" is somewhat different. Regulations are issued out of Brussels for the whole of the EU and are directly applicable and binding in all EU member states without the need for any additional national implementation legislation. That is, the regulation as it is published is, word for word, the law in each of the member states. Note that this is different from the use of the word "regulation" in the United States.

The bottom line, however, is the same. Regulations have the force of law and must be obeyed.

REGULATIONS FOR HUMAN SUBJECT PROTECTIONS

Rules revised in 1981 by the FDA and the Department of Health and Human Services, based on the 1979 Belmont Report, which had been issued by the National Commission for the Protection of Human Subjects of Biomedical and Behavioral Research. The revision provided for wider representation on institutional review boards and they detailed elements of what constitutes informed consent.

Authors' note: A step forward to better inform human volunteers about the known and unknown risks associated with experimental drugs, biologicals, or devices.

REGULATORY AFFAIRS UNIT

In pharmaceutical companies, the group that handles interactions with the drug agency and other health authorities. They are also usually the corporate experts on the regulations involved in all pharmaceutical issues from manufacturing, marketing, drug safety, dossier submissions, etc.

In terms of drug safety, the regulatory affairs unit may handle the submissions to the health authorities of documents (periodic reports, PSURs, etc.) and any interactions (phone contacts, meetings, product withdrawals, etc.).

REGULATORY AFFAIRS PROFESSIONALS SOCIETY (RAPS)

Although not directly involved with drug safety per se, the organization does cover regulatory aspects of drug safety, in particular postmarketing surveillance.

It is devoted to the health product regulatory profession, with more than 11,000 individual members from industry, government, research, clinical, and academic organizations in more than 50 countries. RAPS develops professional standards for knowledge, competency, and ethics, and is a leading source of information on the scope of practice of regulatory professionals and their critical roles in the health sector.

Founded in 1976, RAPS advances learning and fosters knowledge exchange in regulatory, scientific, business, legal, and other areas essential to effective product development and regulation. RAPS administers a credential for the profession—the Regulatory Affairs Certification (RAC).

http://www.raps.org/s_raps/index.asp

REGULATORY CLOCK START DATE

See Clock Start Date.

RELATEDNESS

See Causality Determination.

RELATIVE RISK

In a trial or in an observational cohort, the ratio between the rate of an outcome (beneficial or adverse) in a group exposed to a treatment and the rate in a control group. It is a measure of the strength of a cause–effect relationship. Its application to clinical practice is justified only when the baseline risk is taken into account to calculate the risk difference and when other relevant information affecting internal and external validity of the trial are taken into account.

In an observational case-control study, the odds ratio is accepted as an estimate or approximation of the relative risk under certain conditions. The absolute risk difference cannot be derived.

See also Odds Ratio.

REMOTE DATA ENTRY

Also called Electronic Data Capture (EDC). In clinical trials, the entering of patient data in real time into the clinical trial database (or a "holding area" that allows data to be examined before being put into the database) at the investigational sites. This is in contrast to shipping the data (paper case report forms) to a regional or central site for manual data entry at a later date.

There are advantages and disadvantages to remote data entry. The advantages include data entry immediately (or nearly so) at each patient's visit. The data is available immediately in the database and it is no longer necessary to have a large data entry team at the central site awaiting the receipt of paper copies of case reports. Safety data is available immediately and serious events may be picked up and investigated with minimal delay, allowing cessation of the study or changes in the protocol for safety reasons more quickly. Disadvantages include maintaining quality at multiple sites around the country or world, turnover in data entry people, lack of written source documents, as well as more complex computer and IT issues: network maintenance, privacy and data protection, maintenance of a complex computer network/website to collect the data, etc. There are now third-party vendors selling systems for remote data entry. This methodology is now replacing paper case reports especially in large trials.

REPORT, AE/ADR

Also known as a pharmacovigilance report or an individual case safety report (ICSR). A communication to a pharmacovigilance unit (industry, regulatory, etc.) made by a health worker or a patient, by any means (email, phone, letter, etc.) of a suspected adverse reaction to a medicinal product, a medical device, a biologic product, or in fact to any therapeutic product. It includes publications of AE reports in the medical literature as well as in the lay press.

REPORTABILITY

This refers to the obligation—whether ethical, medical, or regulatory—to report the observation to the competent authorities.

For the Clinician in Daily Medical Practice

Unless the reporter is a researcher (clinical investigator) in a clinical trial where reporting is obligatory, the reporting of an AE or suspected ADR is voluntary and the determination of whether to report or not is the clinician's choice. A healthcare professional is a privileged witness. It is his or her sense of duty that provides the impetus to the observer of an AE/ADR, representing a potentially important signal, to report it to the manufacturer or health agency. There are few countries that make such notification a legal obligation and in those countries the law does not seem to be applied with any force or regularity. In France, reporting rates did not significantly increase after the passage of such a law in 1984.

For the Manufacturer

In most countries in North America and Europe as well as Japan, Australia, New Zealand, and elsewhere, AE/ADR reporting is mandatory and well established in law and regulation for drugs. Severe penalties are applied for persistent failure to report. Reporting is generally optional for other products, such as over-the-counter drugs, nutraceuticals, food supplements, etc. In the US, AE/ADR reporting for over-the-counter products was made mandatory in 2007 and the trend toward reporting is continuing around the world.

For the Patient or Consumer

Reporting is voluntary. They may report the incident to their health provider (physician, pharmacist) and, in a growing number of countries, to their drug agency.

REPORTABILITY CRITERIA

See Minimum Information for Reportability.

REPORTER

An AE reporter is a healthcare professional who suspected a drug to be related to an adverse event and has reported it to the pharmacovigilance unit of the health authority or manufacturer or, rarely, an academic institution. It also applies to the author of an ADR report published in a medical journal.

A reporter may also be a consumer or patient who reports it to the health authority or manufacturer. In general, a report from a nonmedical professional should be validated by the treating or prescribing physician, pharmacist, or healthcare professional.

REPORTER IDENTIFIABILITY

The minimum information needed to satisfy the criterion for a valid reporter. Any information that ensures that the reporter exists is sufficient. The reporter may be a healthcare professional, consumer, or patient.

The information could be name, initials, email address, phone conversation (whether male or female should be noted), profession, license number, etc.

REPORTING FORM

See MedWatch Form and CIOMS I Form.

REPORTING GUIDE, ADR

Instructions for health professionals. For example, the British Medical Association published a guide available since May 2006 on their website www.bma.org.uk/ap.nsf/content/home. Australia has *How to report problems* instructions on their website at http://www.tga.gov.au/problem/index.htm.

The FDA has published detailed instructions on its website for completing the voluntary 3500 MedWatch form (http://www.fda. gov/medwatch/REPORT/CONSUMER/INSTRUCT.HTM) and the mandatory 3500A MedWatch form (http://www.fda.gov/ medwatch/report/instruc_10-13-06.htm).

REPORTING RATE

See Rate.

REPORTING RATE DETERMINANTS

See Appendix 2.

REPORTING, PROMPTED

Also called stimulated reporting. These reports are not spontaneous but rather occur after something has been done to prod the healthcare professional, consumer, or patient to report a case.

Stimulated reporting may occur in certain situations, such as a notification by a "Dear Healthcare Professional" letter following a signal that needs confirmation, a publication in the press, or questioning of healthcare professionals by company representatives.

Many companies have patient support programs in which company representatives or outside representatives (e.g., nurses, physicians) contact patients to encourage them to continue to take their medications (coaching). During the course of discussions, AE reports may be obtained. If the company is involved in these support programs, a mechanism must be created to ensure that the SAEs reach the company in a timely manner. Other programs such as speaker programs (prominent physicians given "stipends" to speak to other physicians about the product and disease being promoted), named-patient programs, and compassionate use may also stimulate or prompt reports.

RESIDUES FROM MANUFACTURING PROCESS

A problem related to product quality. In the course of manufacturing a product, residues or intermediate products may be created. These products either disappear from the final marketed product or are of a nature and level as to be, in theory, nontoxic. Drug manufacture is tightly regulated (Good Manufacturing Practices) so that any such products are identified and quality controlled. Any changes in process must be documented and, in certain cases, approved by the health authority.

That said, it is still possible that residues occur that are unexpected due to errors, problems with process or ingredients, machine failure, human failure, etc.

The drug safety officer should always keep in the back of his or her mind the possibility that an AE is due not to the active ingredient but to one of the excipients or residues and that the problem is one of quality and manufacture rather than a classic adverse reaction to an active ingredient.

RESPONSIBILITY AND LIABILITY

In the EU, Volume 9A clearly states (Introduction, Section 3.1):

"The Marketing Authorisation Holder must ensure that it has an appropriate system of pharmacovigilance and risk management in place in order to assure responsibility and liability for its products on the market and to ensure that appropriate action can be taken, when necessary."

and in Part 2, Section 1.4:

"The Marketing Authorisation Holder should ensure that a Qualified Person for Pharmacovigilance (QPPV) is permanently and continuously available and that an appropriate system of pharmacovigilance is in place in order to ensure responsibility and liability for marketed products to ensure that appropriate action can be taken, in accordance with the legal requirements."

In the US, there are similar responsibilities for the NDA holder in laws, regulations, and guidelines. The topic is exceedingly complex and beyond the scope of this entry.

The manufacturers of drugs have a "duty to warn" about any known or possible adverse events or safety issues involving their products. They are, in general, not expected to warn healthcare professionals or the public about any unknown dangers. In general, for prescription products, the manufacturer warns the pharmacist and physician who in turn warn the patient or consumer. For OTC products, the warning must be on the package or box in the "drug facts" labeling. Manufacturers are expected to make efforts to remain up to date about their products and change the warning (labeling) as new knowledge is acquired.

Unlike many other products sold on the market, some drugs are known to be "unavoidably unsafe" but may still be sold. These are drugs that produce known serious and possibly fatal ADRs (e.g., anticancer drugs, antiHIV drugs, antivitamin K blood thinners) but have major beneficial effects. That is, though there are serious ADRs, the benefit/risk assessment is still positive in favor of the drug. Such drugs, with FDA approval and the appropriate labeling, may, in general, be sold without incurring greater liability for selling a known "unsafe" product.

RESTARTING REPORTING CLOCK FOR PSURs

In theory, the PSUR clock for an older drug on a 1-year, 3-year, or 5-year schedule should be reset to every 6 months if a new indication, formulation, or patient group is approved. In practice, the resetting of the clock is usually negotiable with the health authorities (the reference member state in the EU) if the change is minor and the increased risk negligible.

RETENTION RULES FOR SAFETY DATA

See Data Retention and Storage.

RISK

In drug safety, the possibility or probability of adverse or toxic effects due to a drug product in patients exposed to the drug. Its definition is complex because risks are determined not only by the "intrinsic" properties of the active chemical moiety but also by "extrinsic" factors such as the excipients, the packaging, the mode and rate of delivery, the doses (under-, over-) used, the non-compliance with the dosing regimen, etc., as well as host factors (age, sex, previous exposure, allergies, other medications being taken, nutrition, concomitant diseases, physiological conditions, weight, etc.).

RISK ASSESSMENT

In drug safety, the attempt to measure and quantify the dangers and toxicity of drugs. This concept has been heavily addressed in the last several years. In 2005 the FDA put forth three guidances on risk.

The first covered premarketing risk assessment. (See the document at http://www.fda.gov/cder/guidance/6357fnl.htm.) This guidance is not intended for use on all products but rather only on those that "pose a clinically important and unusual type or level of risk." The adequacy of assessment of risk depends on quantity (number of patients studied) and quality ("the appropriateness of the assessments performed, the appropriateness and breadth of the patient populations studied, and how results are analyzed"). Providing detailed guidance on what constitutes an adequate safety database for all products is impossible. Each product must be weighed on its own merits.

Some of the critical aspects examined are size of the safety database, whether long-term controlled safety trials were performed, the diversity of the patients studied, measurement of dose-effects and drug interactions, comparators with placebo and active drugs, whether "large simple safety studies" (see this term) were done, long term follow-up, and other investigations to determine the safety of the drug before large scale marketing to the public.

The second document (http://www.fda.gov/cder/guidance/6358fnl.htm) covered risk minimization action plans, covered the postmarketing phase of risk assessment, and looked at such items as signal identification, developing case series, data mining, the decision on which signals to study further, epidemiologic studies, and the development of an action plan. (*See* Risk Management.)

The third document covered good pharmacovigilance practices (http://www.fda.gov/cder/guidance/6359OCC.htm).

Similarly, the EU and other governmental health authorities have put forth similar documents summarizing the need for risk assessment as an ongoing function during the entire life of the drug as well as the need for action plans and continued surveillance.

The topic of risk assessment is large and growing daily as new ideas, concepts, and techniques are developed.

RISK, ATTRIBUTABLE

See Risk Difference.

RISK–BENEFIT RATIO, ANALYSIS

See Ratio and Benefit–Risk Assessment.

RISK DIFFERENCE

Also called attributable risk. In clinical pharmacology, the difference between the rate of an outcome (whether beneficial or adverse) in a group exposed to an experimental drug and the rate in a control group. Its application to clinical practice is justified provided that other relevant information affecting internal and external validity of the trial are taken into account.

If the risk difference is known, the "Number Needed To Benefit" (NNTB, formerly NNT) or "Number Needed To Harm" (NNTH, formerly NNH) may be calculated as its reciprocal.

Risk difference is to be distinguished from the relative risk, and the latter should not be applied to medical practice decisions unless the baseline risk is known and used to calculate the risk difference.

RISK FACTOR, ADR

In drug safety, a risk factor is a variable that is associated with the probability of occurrence of an adverse event or bad outcome in a patient exposed to a drug product. It may also apply to other therapeutic products.

Some risk factors associated with the suspect drug are:

- The pharmacologic class. Some classes are more likely to produce a particular ADR, such as statins and rhabdomyolysis, NSAIDs and GI bleeding.
- The specific characteristics of the product.
- The total or daily dose administered, which can be "normal" or above normal (overdose). Overdoses may occur by error, negligence, accident, or intention.
- The duration of treatment.
- The route of administration.
- The rate of administration.
- The time of administration (before sleep; before, with, or after meals; interval between doses, etc.).
- Method of swallowing (with or without sufficient fluid), posture after swallowing (upright or lying down).

Other risk factors associated with the patient's medical status are:

- Past history: positive prior challenges ("prechallenges") to the same product or to the same class of products.
- Comorbid conditions.
- Demographics: age, sex, country, race, etc.
- Physiological factors: weight, pregnancy status.
- Chronic medical conditions: immunodeficiency (HIV), allergies, renal, cardiac, hepatic, pulmonary insufficiency, etc.
- Acute medical conditions: shock, dehydration, fasting.
- Concomitant medications.
- Concomitant conditions or habits: alcohol or tobacco use, exercise, heatwave, diet, specific foods.
- Genetic predisposition.

RISK MANAGEMENT

The efforts made to limit toxicity, adverse events, and bad outcomes seen with use of the drug once the possible dangers and toxicities of a drug are understood or suspected.

The FDA put forth its views on risk management in a series of guidances in 2005 looking at both risk assessment and risk management. The European Union and others have also developed concepts of risk management.

See Risk Minimization Action Plans (RiskMAPs) and Risk Assessment.

RiskMAPs

See Risk Minimization Action Plan.

RISK MINIMIZATION ACTION PLAN (RiskMAP)

In its 2005 Guidance on Risk Minimization, the FDA described the concept of Risk Minimization Action Plans (RiskMAPs) to minimize identified product risks. The guidance addresses:

- The selection and development of tools to minimize those risks.
- Evaluation of RiskMAPs and monitoring tools.
- Communication with the FDA about RiskMAPs.
- Components of a RiskMAP submission to the FDA.

Risks may be at the individual or population level. The FDA notes that the usual product labeling is sufficient in most cases to minimize risk. There are some cases in which a RiskMAP might be needed. The FDA "recommends that RiskMAPs be used judiciously to minimize risks without encumbering drug availability or otherwise interfering with the delivery of product benefits to patients." The FDA defines a RiskMAP as a strategic safety program designed to meet specific goals and objectives to minimize known risks while preserving the product's benefits.

A RiskMAP may be developed anytime during a product's life cycle. It may be done by the company or proposed by the FDA. It should include:

- The types, magnitude, and frequency of risks and benefits.
- The populations at greatest risk and/or those likely to derive the most benefit.
- The existence of treatment alternatives and their risks and benefits.
- The reversibility of the adverse events observed.
- The preventability of the adverse events in question.
- The probability of benefit.

As examples, the FDA recommends that all schedule II controlled substances (especially extended-release or high-concentration opiates) for pain control have a RiskMAP aimed at minimizing overdose, abuse, and addiction. Teratogens should also have a RiskMAP as well as drugs requiring specialized healthcare skills, training, or facilities to manage the therapeutic or adverse effects of a drug.

Various tools for risk minimization are described including targeted education and outreach, reminder systems to double check consent forms, enrollment of patients in tracking systems, limiting the amount of the product dispensed, etc. Whatever systems are put in place must be evaluated in an objective manner to see if risk reduction and bad outcomes have been reduced. If not, the system should be reexamined and changed in order to minimize risk.

Examples include informed consent and the requirement to use two forms of contraception for drugs that are known teratogens. By following the number of pregnancies that are reported (in a pregnancy registry) one can measure the effectiveness of the tools used.

ROTE LISTE

The German language compendium of drugs used in Germany. See the website http://www.rote-liste.de/.

RULE OF THREES

1. An application of the Poisson statistical distribution used to analyze rare events: to be 95% confident that a new drug does not cause a specific AE (hepatitis, for example) in more than 1/100 of patients, 300 exposed patients must be event-free. (See Appendix 3.)

2. An old concept that the labeling of a drug should list in a prominent place the three most common adverse events and the three most medically severe AEs.

RUN-IN PERIOD

In a clinical trial, the time before a patient actually begins the treatment phase of the study. Not all trials have run-in periods. When used they are often employed to validate entry criteria. For example, if a study of a new drug for poorly controlled angina pectoris required that a patient have 6–8 episodes of angina per week despite standard medical therapy, the patient may keep a diary to count and describe the number of episodes he or she has in a four-week run-in period. If a sufficient number of episodes do not occur the patient is not enrolled in the treatment phase of the study.

RX TO OTC SWITCH

The change in the legal status of a drug from requiring a prescription to being available over-the-counter (OTC) to the patient without any medical intervention. The patient then makes his or her own diagnosis and decides on treatment.

The OTC dose may be at the treatment dose used for prescription therapy or at a lower dose. The major way to determine this is to collect the safety data over a long period of time to show that the benefit-risk analysis is acceptable for patient use without medical intervention. It may be necessary to run additional clinical trials at the lower dose to validate the claim. An NDA (or equivalent marketing authorization request) must be submitted to the health authority in most cases. The indication may change. For example, H2 blockers at prescription doses are used to treat duodenal and gastric ulcers. At lower OTC doses they are used to treat heartburn.

Authors' note: It is surprising how the labeling of a drug changes when it moves from prescription to OTC status. Certain drugs that had extensive adverse event sections in the labeling for prescription usage including cardiac arrhythmias, severe hemorrhage, liver failure, etc. when used OTC carry minimal labeling (in the US, the labeling is the "drug facts," which use lay terms and have minimal ADRs labeled).

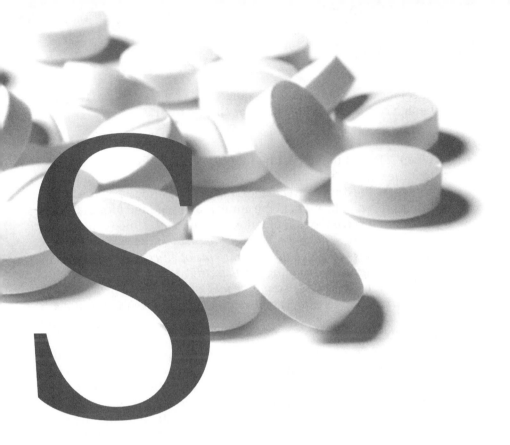

SADR

See Serious Adverse Drug Reaction.

SAE

See Serious Adverse Event.

SAFE, DEFINED

The dictionary definition of the word "safe" would be along the lines of "free from harm or danger."

In the context of drug safety it must be emphasized that, by the dictionary definition, no drug is totally "safe." That is, no drug is free from producing harm or danger or adverse drug reactions. In drug safety, safety is always judged in conjunction with efficacy and thus safety is always relative.

A drug that would be considered too dangerous ("unsafe") because of its AEs/ADRs for a benign condition might be considered quite acceptable for a life-threatening condition. The hair loss or decrease in platelets is an acceptable safety risk with certain oncology drugs but would, of course, not be acceptable to treat a benign condition like headache or allergic rhinitis.

SAFE AND EFFECTIVE

When it is said that a health authority has approved a drug and that the drug is "safe and effective," that actually means that the benefits of the drug outweigh the dangers of the drug when used for the approved indication, in the approved dosage and formulation in the approved patient population. It is not a guarantee of no risk.

Authors' note: The concept of "safe" as an absolute does not exist; safety (risk) is always evaluated in terms of efficacy (benefit). The use of this term is misleading, particularly to the lay public, which does not yet clearly understand the idea of "safety" and benefit:risk evaluation. However, its use is widespread and is likely to continue.

SAFE MEDICAL DEVICES ACT, FDA

This act, passed in 1990, requires nursing homes, hospitals, and other facilities that use medical devices to report to the FDA incidents that suggest that a medical device probably caused or contributed to the death, serious illness, or serious injury of a patient.

Manufacturers are required to conduct postmarketing surveillance on permanently implanted devices whose failure might cause serious harm or death and to establish methods for tracing and locating patients depending on such devices. The act authorizes the FDA to order device product recalls and perform other actions.

SAFETY DATA EXCHANGE AGREEMENT

See Data Exchange Agreement.

SAFETY INFORMATION AND ADVERSE EVENT REPORTING PROGRAM.

See MedWatch Program.

SAFETY INSPECTION

See Audit.

SAFETY INTELLIGENCE UNIT

A group within a pharmaceutical company whose mission is to track changes in regulations, laws, guidances, etc., regarding safety. The group may also track consumer groups, political lobbies, patient activist groups, the press and other media, FDA advisory committee meetings, etc., for trends and issues in the world of drug safety and pharmacovigilance. The goal is to keep the company in compliance by being up to date on the requirements for drug safety.

There may also be tracking of safety issues regarding specific products as well as more general pharmacovigilance issues.

The members of the group may also represent the company at international organizations such as ICH, CIOMS, PhRMA, etc.

SAFETY MONITORING COMMITTEE

See Data Monitoring Committee.

SAFETY SIGNAL

See Signal.

SAR

See Suspected Adverse Reaction.

SCANDAL

When certain unacceptable and serious ADRs occur and reoccur in spite of the fact that they are avoidable or if ADRs were known to a company or health authority and either kept secret, "buried," or not acted upon, a public scandal may ensue if four conditions are met:

- *Enormity:* The damage is clear, unequivocal, and dramatic. Its enormity does not allow room for any doubt.
- *Immorality:* The occurrence is incompatible with the moral values and norms of society.
- *Abuse of confidence:* The occurrence was unexpected and responsible people did not act in a manner expected of them.
- *Cover-up:* The occurrence was covered up or camouflaged in some form before it became public.

These conditions were met when HIV- and hepatitis C-contaminated blood products were transfused into patients in Japan, France, and Canada. The ensuing drama evolved into scandal, with some people going to prison. The former head of China's drug agency was sentenced to death in 2007 for accepting bribes and speeding the approval of drugs that were considered too risky.

Authors' note: This area is evolving rapidly. There are perceptions that:

- *Drugs are approved too quickly.*
- *Insufficient safety data is collected before marketing.*
- *Collection mechanisms for AEs/ADRs (e.g., spontaneous reporting) are inadequate or too slow to allow for discovery of signals.*
- *Companies and health authorities are too slow in responding to safety issues.*

- *Recommended postmarketing studies are not implemented.*
- *The governmental staff that approves drugs should not be the same that watches over drug safety.*
- *There are conflicts of interest slowing or preventing safety reporting.*
- *Money and profit impede drug safety and public health.*

It is likely that major changes will occur in the structure of corporate and governmental pharmacovigilance as well as the methodology of drug safety data gathering and analysis. A change in attitude of the medical establishment will hopefully follow.

SCRIBE FOR A HEALTH AUTHORITY INSPECTION

A somewhat jocular term for the person chosen among the group being inspected or audited (e.g., the company, the clinical investigational site) for taking copious notes during the inspection and helping to manage the requests for documents by the inspectors, their photocopying, etc. The scribe then issues minutes of the inspection.

SCRIP

A journal published by Informa Healthcare of the UK. Twice a week, *Scrip World Pharmaceutical News* updates subscribers on the key issues, companies, and personalities shaping the world pharmaceutical industry. http://www.scrip-news.com/

SCRIPT

In drug safety, a formal written text with the actual words to be said or a more general set of instructions for a drug safety officer to follow when taking a phone call from a patient or healthcare professional about an individual clinical safety report.

It is most commonly used in telephone call centers (which may not be staffed by medical professionals) to obtain a good level of medical and safety history. Ultimately, however, the AE report will have to go to a medical safety professional for review and probably follow-up in which directed and customized medical questions are asked of the reporter. Scripts should be written and/or reviewed by medical professionals. They may track diseases, symptoms, or AEs. For example, there may be a script for "diabetes" or "headaches" or "blood in the stool."

Some scripts take the form of "frequently asked questions" (FAQs), which the telephone center employee asks of the caller.

SEASONALITY OF AEs

Adverse events that are related to seasons of the year or to weather.

The relation may be due to an increased use of the drug in that season such as the use of more cough and cold products during flu season, more suncare and skin products in the summer, or allergy products during allergy season. The increased use of the products may produce more AEs simply because more people are using the products.

The relation may also be due to weather- (e.g., sun-) related effects, such as an increase in sun-induced skin sensitivity from non-sun drugs (e.g., antibiotics) during the summer compared to the winter, even though the usage of the drug does not increase or decrease with the season. The increase is due to more people taking the drug having sun exposure not due to more drug use.

AE trends and patterns must be examined over several years to see this relationship. Sales and usage data should also be examined.

Finally, it is possible that there is an increase in AEs due to other causes (e.g., a product quality defect in a lot) that coincides with seasonality.

SECOND GENERATION EFFECT

An ADR that manifests itself not in the patient taking the drug but in the offspring. The classic example is that of DES, which was taken by pregnant women whose daughters, in their teens and twenties, developed vaginal cancer (clear cell adenocarcinoma). *See* Diethylstilbestrol.

SECONDARY EFFECTS, CODING

See Cascade Effect. Also called "chaining."

The difficult question of whether an ADR that occurs as a consequence of another (primary) ADR should have a MedDRA code and be included in the case. For example, if a patient develops dizziness due to a drug and falls down, hitting his head and developed a fatal cerebral hemorrhage, what should be coded? Dizziness only or dizziness plus fall or dizziness plus fall plus cerebral hemorrhage plus death. A similar patient might develop dizziness without falling or simply fall onto his or her bed with no other adverse events. Falling follows dizziness if severe enough in susceptible individuals but remains partly accidental, and a cerebral hemorrhage is not a usual or physiological consequence of falling.

Thus the coding of this case will determine how the case is submitted to the health authority (expedited report or not) and whether it was fatal or not. The coding itself is difficult. What is the fatality related to: dizziness, the fall, or the cerebral hemorrhage? In the first case, it is possible that the drug labeling would include "fatal dizziness," which does not really convey the true sense of the case. The causal links are obvious, but partly accidental.

Another example would be a drug that produces anemia. There are many consequences of anemia, such as angina pectoris or myocardial infarction in susceptible individuals, dyspnea, etc. Should the labeling include myocardial infarction or dyspnea even though the drug has no direct cardiac effects?

One more example: If a drug causes fluid retention (due to a renal effect) that leads to congestive heart failure in susceptible individuals, should both AEs/ADRs be coded?

Authors' note: The answers to these questions are not obvious. In general, coding should be for AEs/ADRs that are felt to be directly related to the drug and for the secondary effects if they are a logical physiological consequence of the primary AE, such as in the last two examples given above.

On the other hand, it may be appropriate to warn the patient and healthcare professional about cascade effects, even if accidental, if they are severe, not obvious, or unusual.

SECONDARY LEGISLATION

Secondary legislation in the EU refers to regulations, directives, and recommendations that are derived from the primary or treaty law of the Union. There are several types of secondary legislation. The ones that touch most on pharmacovigilance are as follows:

- *Regulations:* Directly applicable and binding in all EU member states without the need for any additional national implementation legislation. That is, the regulation as it is published is, word for word, the law in each of the member states. Note that this is different from the use of the word "regulation" in the US.
- *Directives:* This legislation binds member states to the objectives of the legislation within a certain time period but allows each member state to create its own form of national law to so achieve it. That is, each member state may modify the wording and requirements of the directive as long as the objectives of the directive are met.
- *Recommendations, guidances and opinions:* Nonbinding and similar to FDA guidances.

See Primary Legislation.

SECULAR EFFECT

Also known as "temporal bias." This terminology reflects an increase in AE/ADR reporting for a drug or class of drugs following increased media attention, use of a medication by a celebrity, a warning from a health agency, etc. ADR reporting rates can be increased by external factors such as a change in a reporting system or an increased level of publicity attending a given drug or adverse reaction. It is to be distinguished from the Weber Effect (see this term).

SEEDING STUDY

A market-driven phase IV clinical trial. These types of studies are now forbidden in most parts of the world. These were pure marketing projects designed to encourage physicians to prescribe a particular product in place of a competitor's product. A very simple protocol was usually written (to justify calling the endeavor a study) but was often of poor quality. Results were not always collected by the sponsor and, if collected, often not analyzed. Prescribers were sometimes compensated.

SEIZURE

If a manufacturer fails to adhere to the US Quality System (QS) regulation (which describes current Good Manufacturing Practice) required by law, and failed to correct its problems despite several warnings from the FDA, the FDA may seize (take possession of) the product. This is usually done if there is an immediate threat to the public health from these products.

The United States Marshals Service may physically remove the products in question from the facility where they are found or may instead "seize them in place," meaning the manufacturer cannot remove, attempt to remove, or in any way interfere with the products at the facility without the prior written permission of the U.S. Marshal. The U.S. Marshal often seizes products in place when there are too many to move to another location or when removal would be impractical.

Authors' note: This is one of the most severe actions the FDA can take and often leads to litigation. It usually occurs after repeated interactions between the company and the FDA that fail to resolve the problem.

SELECTION BIAS

Selection bias refers to the choosing of particular patients in a clinical trial, which may introduce a systematic error into the trial. This may then influence the results and the (statistical) analysis, conclusions, internal validity, and external validity.

For example, choosing middle- and upper-income patients to participate in a trial because they are perceived to be more reliable and likely to take their study medications is a selection bias. Conversely, eliminating poor compliers by a run-in period can create selection bias. Still another example is excluding frail or older patients more prone to ADRs. In trials where high compliance is paramount for the efficacy of the tested drug while only average compliance is expected in the target population, biased selection may make quite a difference in evaluating efficacy. In trials involving mainly healthy patients, real safety problems may not be picked up.

Authors' note: Selection bias is hard to detect in a trial summary report; one must read the methodology section. And, of course, the bias may lead to less valid and less relevant conclusions, usually (but not always) in favor of the drug maximizing its efficacy and minimizing its problems and safety issues.

SEMIANNUAL REPORTS

Safety analyses done twice yearly or every six months. This usually refers to Periodic Safety Update Reports, which are done for new drugs every six months for the first several years after marketing approval.

SEMIAUTOMATED ANALYSIS OF AE DATA

See Data Mining.

SENSITIVITY

Used as a technical term in statistics or clinical trials, it refers to the ability of a test or trial or experiment to detect true positives. In a diagnostic test for disease, sensitivity is the likelihood of a positive test among patients with disease. This is in comparison to "specificity," which refers to whether a negative result only includes true negatives.

For example, the elevation of the enzymes AST and ALAT in a massive myocardial infarction are likely to be highly sensitive (heart attacks will very often show elevated levels), but the test is not specific because one may see such elevated levels with other diseases (e.g., hepatitis).

In the realm of drug safety (as in all of clinical medicine), one always searches for tests with high specificity and sensitivity so that patients with a particular AE are never missed and no patients without the AE are ever falsely claimed to have the AE.

SENTINEL SITE OF SURVEILLANCE

The use of a designated institution, hospital, physician, etc., to search for and report particular diseases or AEs. For example, in the early influenza season a few hospitals in each region of the US may be asked to report to the CDC all cases of influenza in order to get an early warning of an impending flu pandemic.

In the case of pharmacovigilance, after the release of a new drug, certain hospitals or physicians may be asked to report all cases of a particular AE that is under increased surveillance or is suspected of occurring. For example, a new statin might have some sentinel sites on the look-out for rhabdomyolysis. Also, certain hospitals may be chosen as sentinel sites for collecting all serious ADRs from all new drugs. This approach is used in Japan.

SERIOUS ADVERSE DRUG REACTION (SADR)

A noxious and unintended response to any dose of a drug or biologic product for which there is a reasonable possibility that the product caused the response, fulfilling the criteria for seriousness. In this definition, the phrase "a reasonable possibility" means that the relationship cannot be ruled out.

SERIOUS ADVERSE EVENT (SAE)

"A serious adverse event (experience) or serious adverse reaction is any untoward medical occurrence that at any dose:

- *results in death,*
- *is life-threatening,*
- *requires inpatient hospitalization or prolongation of existing hospitalization,*
- *results in persistent or significant disability/incapacity, or*
- *is a congenital anomaly/birth defect.*

"Medical and scientific judgment should be exercised in deciding whether expedited reporting is appropriate in other situations, such as important medical events that may not be immediately life-threatening or result in death or hospitalization but may jeopardize the patient or may require intervention to prevent one of the other outcomes listed in the definition above.

These should also usually be considered serious. "Examples of such events are intensive treatment in an emergency room or at home for allergic bronchospasm; blood dyscrasias or convulsions that do not result in hospitalization; or development of drug dependency or drug abuse".

Authors' note: Thus for reporting purposes, suspected adverse reactions that are judged to be medically important events will be con-

sidered serious, even if they do not meet the preceding, more rigid criteria.

SERIOUS ADVERSE REACTION (SAR)

Any adverse reaction which results in death, is life-threatening, requires inpatient hospitalization or prolongation of existing hospitalization, results in persistent or significant disability or incapacity, or is a congenital anomaly/birth defect. For reporting purposes, suspected adverse reactions that are judged to be medically important events will be considered serious, even if they do not meet the preceding criteria.

SERIOUS, DEFINED

See Serious Adverse Event.

The word "serious" is used in a specific regulatory manner in drug safety and must not be confused with "severe." The term "severe" is often used to describe the intensity (severity) of a specific event (as in mild, moderate, or severe myocardial infarction); the event itself, however, may be of relatively minor long-term medical significance (such as short-lived severe headache, severe urticaria). This is not the same as "serious," which is based on patient/event outcome usually associated with medical problems that pose a threat to a patient's life or functioning. Seriousness (not severity) is used for defining regulatory reporting obligations: postmarketing AEs must be serious and unexpected to be considered expedited reports.

SERVICE ORGANIZATIONS IN PHARMACEUTICAL INDUSTRY

Vendors that serve the pharmaceutical industry by doing certain functions that the company does not want or is unable to do itself. These organizations are commonly used by small or start-up companies to run clinical trials or collect safety data because the company is too small to do it by itself. Clinical/Contract Research Organizations (CROs) are a very common group of service organizations. They may be very specific, handling only, say, monitoring of clinical trials or they may be large international "full-service" organizations that are willing and able to do everything needed to submit an NDA or dossier to the health authority for approval, including preclinical studies and phase I, II, and III trials.

In drug safety, there are several service organizations that specialize in handling AE collection, databasing, analysis, and reporting.

SEVERE, DEFINED

See Serious, Defined.

SEX (GENDER)

In drug safety, sex refers to one of the criteria (identifiable patient) for a valid individual case safety report. *See* Minimum Information for Reportability.

Gender is also a risk factor for some ADRs and for ADRs in general. Women are slightly more likely than men to develop ADRs when exposed to pharmacotherapy for multiple reasons:

- Higher consumption rates.
- More frequent polypharmacy, leading to drug–drug interactions.
- Lower body weights.
- More very elderly women alive, with the ensuing diminishing renal function that comes with advanced age.

SGOT

Serum glutamic oxaloacetic transaminase, also called aspartate aminotransferase (AST). This is one of several enzymes present in various organs of the body, in particular the liver and heart, that is elevated when there is damage to one of those organs (e.g., hepatitis and myocardial infarction, respectively).

In drug safety, because liver problems are a very common ADR, an elevation in SGOT (and other "liver enzymes") should raise the suspicion of a drug related cause.

See Liver Function Tests and SGPT.

SGPT

Serum glutamic pyruvic transaminase, also called alanine aminotransferase (ALT). Very similar to SGOT in clinical use. *See* SGOT and Liver Function Tests.

SIDE EFFECT

A somewhat out-of-date popular term that generally should be avoided in medical and scientific usage. The better term is adverse event (AE) or adverse drug reaction (ADR) (see these terms). However, in discussions with patients the term "side effect" is still more widely used and recognized than "AE/ADR" and should be used if there is any doubt about the patient's understanding when questioned about AEs.

SIDE EFFECTS OF DRUGS ANNUAL

From their website: "*The Side Effects of Drugs Annual* was first published in 1977. It has been published continuously since then, as a yearly update to the encyclopedic volume *Meyler's Side Effects of Drugs*. Each new *Annual* provides clinicians and medical investigators with a reliable and critical yearly survey of new data and trends in the area of Adverse Drug Reactions and Interactions. An international team of specialists has contributed to the *Annuals* by selecting critically from each year's publications all that is truly new and informative, by critically interpreting it, and by pointing out whatever is misleading. The use of the book is enhanced by separate indexes, allowing the reader to enter the text via the drug name, adverse effect, or drug interaction. Special features of the *Annuals* are the Side Effects of Drugs Essay, usually written by a guest author, and the special reviews: short articles, within the different chapters, that give extra attention to topics of current interest. Current editor is Pr JK Aronson."

See http://www.elsevier.com.

SIGNAL

The WHO defines a signal as "reported information on a possible causal relationship between an adverse event and a drug, the relationship being unknown or incompletely documented previously.

It is a possible association considered important enough to investigate further. It may refer to new information on an already known association. Usually more than one report is required to generate a signal, depending on the seriousness of the event and the quality of the information."

It raises a hypothesis together with data and arguments and if important should lead to a safety or signal investigation. *See* Signal Investigation or Workup.

A signal may remain behind closed doors (agency, manufacturer) or divulged to the scientific community for discussion, as when *The Lancet* first published in 1961 that thalidomide was linked to birth defects. There is much debate on this topic and the value of public dissemination of early signals that may be real or may be disproven when all the data is in.

A signal may consist not only of a new suspected ADR, but also a new presentation or clinical feature of a known ADR, or a new severity (from enzyme elevation to fulminant liver failure, from QT prolongation to serious arrhythmia), a new outcome (death), or a new risk factor (drug interaction).

Authors' note: Less formally, one can describe a signal as a case or a series of cases that is noteworthy, unexpected either in type or frequency, that warrants a medical review by a healthcare professional skilled in pharmacovigilance and possibly further investigation since, if confirmed, it will have impact on public health and will require a change in labeling (or more) and communication to the public and the healthcare community.

SIGNAL

A publication edited and produced by the Uppsala Monitoring Centre (UMC) (see this term) to present information derived from the WHO database, containing summaries of case reports of suspected ADRs submitted by National Pharmacovigilance Centers in about half the countries of the world. A UMC Review Panel consists of international, experienced scientists usually associated with a governmental or academic institution or a pharmaceutical company, invited by the UMC. They assess under UMC responsibility the database for the occurrence of signals of possible importance for public health, drug regulation, and science.

The distribution is currently restricted to National Centers and regulatory staff and to international pharmaceutical companies, which can be identified as uniquely responsible for the drug concerned. National authorities and centers are responsible for deciding on further action including communicating the information in *SIGNAL*. (Edwards, 1994)

SIGNAL DETECTION

The study and analysis by medical professionals trained in drug safety and pharmacovigilance to uncover in safety databases potential new adverse events, increased frequency of adverse events, or the appearance of known adverse events in a new population associated with a drug.

SIGNAL FOLLOW-UP

See Signal Investigation or Workup.

SIGNAL INTERPRETATION

See Signal Investigation or Workup.

SIGNAL INVESTIGATION OR WORKUP

After a signal (see this term) or a potential signal is noted, it should be evaluated. The intensity and speed of the investigation depends upon many factors including the severity of the AE, the newness of the drug, the number of patients exposed, etc. The signal should be classified in a way as to account for the urgency and risk.

A signal may be found in the postmarketing setting or during a clinical trial before marketing approval.

The evaluation may be done by the pharmaceutical company or the health authority or both with or without collaboration.

The evaluation may have many components such as a review of all similar cases in the databases of the company, the FDA or another health authority, the Uppsala Monitoring Centre, poison control centers, teratolovigilance centers, etc., as appropriate. A case series should be gathered and evaluated by skilled drug safety medical professionals. Further studies (clinical trials, epidemiologic) may be done; registries may be established; animal data should be reviewed; other drugs in the class should be examined for similar signals or AEs/ADRs, etc.

The results of the investigations will determine what action a company or health authority will take. Corrective actions include continued surveillance of the signal, a change in the drug's labeling (restrictions of indications, black box warnings, etc.), withdrawal of the drug from the market, cessation or alteration of a study (if the drug is not yet marketed), etc.

Authors' note: There is an ongoing debate with regard to the level of transparency that should be maintained during the investigation. Some critics and advocacy groups say that the patients and the healthcare community should know about the signal—even if it is tenuous and unproven until the investigation gets underway—in order to factor that into their treatment decisions (in other words, the drug should be considered somewhat "guilty until proven innocent"). This means making the national databases of ADR reports publicly available in a user-friendly manner, following the example of the Drug Analysis Prints available from the UK pharmacovigilance.

Others say that an unproven signal, which may turn out to be disproven, should not be made public until there is some level of valid evidence to let all parties make an educated judgment. Premature judgment can cause bad treatment decisions to be made, as well as tarring the drug unfairly (in other words, the drug should be considered "innocent until proven guilty").

SIGNAL-TO-NOISE RATIO

Originally defined in communications for transmissions of radio, TV, etc. It refers to the amount of useful wave transmission (e.g., the radio program) compared to interference or extraneous noise.

This term has been used in drug safety to refer to the problem of the lack of sensitivity (see this term) or statistical power for many of the pharmacovigilance techniques used for safety surveillance. For example, the spontaneous reporting system receives many more reports of adverse events that do not add to the safety profile of the drug compared to those AEs that are new or unexpected that bring important new information. A similar concept is that of the "needle in the haystack." There is much extraneous information that must be examined to come up with the infrequent but critically important new safety information.

Authors' note: There is continued research to refine the techniques of pharmacovigilance to increase the signal-to-noise ratio so that less unimportant information is collected. Actual changes have been relatively few and far between (e.g., in the US not reporting nonserious expected AEs to the FDA in NDA periodic reports but still obliging the manufacturer to collect them and have them available). Given the exploding interest in drug safety and the limited resources devoted to it, there is a clear need to collect only the useful data and to avoid expending money, effort, and resources on meaningless or trivial information. How to best do this remains to be seen.

SIGNIFICANT MEDICAL EVENT

One of the criteria for "seriousness." *See* Serious Adverse Event.

SIZE OF THE SAFETY DATABASE

From the FDA's 2005 premarketing safety guidance (http://www.fda.gov/cder/guidance/6357fnl.htm).

The number of patients studied in safety trials done before or after marketing depends on the novelty of the drug, the availability and safety of alternate therapies, the intended population, the condition being treated, and the duration of use. Safety databases for life-threatening diseases, especially where there are no satisfactory alternate treatments, are smaller than the databases for products to treat less serious diseases where there are alternate treatments available.

The FDA does not give safety database size advice for products for short term (<6 months use) but does make suggestions for products aimed at treatment over 6 months. For these, the FDA and the International Conference on Harmonization (ICH) recommend 1,500 subjects in total with 300 to 600 exposed for 6 months and 100 exposed for 1 year using doses in the therapeutic range. Higher numbers of patients may need to be studied if:

- Specific safety issues arise from animal studies.
- Similar drugs or the class of drugs suggests a specific problem.
- Pharmacokinetic or pharmacodynamic properties of the drug are associated with certain adverse events (AEs).

- It is important to quantitate the occurrence of low frequency AEs.
- The benefit from the product is small and one wants to be very sure there are no rare AEs that will not be picked up unless large numbers of patients are studied.
- The benefit is experienced by only a fraction of the treated patients (i.e., the benefit is "rare" and thus the same reason as above to look for rare AEs).
- The benefit is unclear (e.g., surrogate endpoints used).
- Statistical power requires larger number of patients to show that an already high background rate of safety issues will not be unduly raised even more due to the drug.
- The proposed treatment is for healthy populations (e.g., preventive vaccines).
- A safe and effective alternate treatment is available.

Authors' note: Since the size of the safety database at the time of the first launch of a product is usually under 10,000 patients (usually fairly homogeneous patients) and often under 5,000 patients, the likelihood of detecting a rare serious ADR is low. These serious and rare ADRs are only found after the drug is used in very large numbers of patients in the general patient population (not the narrow test population looked at in premarketing drug development).

SKIPPED-GENERATION ADR

ADRs that do not appear in the patient taking the drug in question. Rather, the ADR appears in the offspring. *See* DES (Diethylstilbesterol).

SmPC

See Summary of Product Characteristics (SPC). This term is generally used now to refer to the official product labeling from the European Union. Compare to SPC.

SNOMED DICTIONARY

A very large global dictionary now being used primarily in the United States and the United Kingdom for AEs, medical history, diseases, pathology, etc. There is an initiative by the US Department of Health and Human Services to expand SNOMED's use to build "a national electronic health care system that will allow patients and their doctors to access their complete medical records anytime and anywhere they are needed, leading to reduced medical errors, improved patient care, and reduced health care costs." http://www.snomed.org/ or www.ithsdo.org

SOLICITED REPORT

An AE/ADR report that is received from disease management programs, patient support programs, and similar company or health authority initiatives. These AEs are then not truly spontaneous. In the US, they should be reported as 15-day reports to the NDA if they are serious, unexpected, and drug-related. It is the latter causality assessment that differentiates solicited reports from spontaneous reports (FDA Guidance for Industry, August 1997).

CIOMS V (2001): Solicited ADR reports arising in the course of interaction with patients should be regarded as distinct from spontaneous unsolicited reports.

- They should be processed separately and so identified in expedited and periodic reporting.
- To satisfy post-marketing regulations, solicited reports should be handled in the same way as study reports: Causality assessments are needed. Serious unexpected ADRs should be reported on an expedited basis.
- Serious expected and non-serious solicited reports should be kept in the safety database and reported to regulators on request.
- Signals may arise from solicited reports so they should be reviewed on an ongoing basis.

SOP

See Standard Operating Procedure.

SOURCE DOCUMENT

Original document related to an AE/ADR case report, particularly:

- A report of a telephone conversation.
- A letter or email from the reporter (patient, healthcare professional).
- An internal company note from a medical sales representative.
- An ADR report form (completed by the reporter or a drug safety officer).
- The results of supplementary tests or hospital discharges and follow-up and final reports, including their computer printouts.
- A published medical article.

The definition of a source document is less clear in the case of remote data entry in clinical trials or of telephone reports of AEs at a call center where there is no document from a hospital, physician, pharmacist, or patient. In these cases it may include working notes made by the caller and the receiver of the call as well as any forms filled in by the receiver. It may also be the computer data if that is the initial source of entry.

Authors' note: The source documents are crucial for establishing the validity of a case as well as documenting to internal and health authority auditors that safety data is being handled in a controlled, accurate, and proper manner. In general, source documents should not be written on or altered. Any data collected on a case should be considered source documents including working notes and draft reports. They should not be discarded. All source documents should be written in ink, not pencil.

SPANISH PHARMACOVIGILANCE COORDINATING CENTER

The Spanish national reference center on pharmacovigilance is located in the Division of Pharmacoepidemiology and Pharmacovigilance of the Subdirectorate General on Safety of Medicines. It harmonizes the tasks of the regional bodies competent in pharmacovigilance or Regional Pharmacovigilance Centers, administers the FEDRA database, coordinates the Technical Committees of the Spanish Pharmacovigilance System, and represents the Sistema Español de FarmacoVigilancia (SEFV) in official international forums.

SPC

See Summary of Product Characteristics. This term, in comparison to SmPC, is sometimes used to refer to the general concept of "product labeling." Thus various types of SPCs include the EU SmPC, the US package insert, etc.

Authors' note: Confusingly, many use SmPC and SPC synonymously for the EU labeling: the Summary of Product Characteristics. Although this seems to add a level of unneeded complexity, these terms appear to be gaining ground as standard terminology in the world of drug safety.

SPECIAL POPULATION GROUPS

Certain patients who are felt to be at particular risk for developing ADRs, such as the elderly, neonates, patients with renal or liver failure, pregnant women, etc. In the course of the development of new drugs, safety studies are often done in phase II with at-risk groups to determine whether the product can safely be administered to them. These studies may also look at dosing (dose-response) and efficacy.

SPECIFICITY

See Sensitivity. Specificity is the likelihood of a negative test among patients without disease. The higher the specificity the better. Used as a technical term in statistics or clinical trials, it refers to the ability of a test or trial or experiment to detect true negatives.

Authors' note: One always wants a test to have maximum specificity and sensitivity. Often, however, there is a trade-off. Excellent sensitivity (not miss people with the AE or disease one is testing for) may produce low specificity. That is, the need to test many patients without the AE or disease will produce false positives, which are accepted in order to find all those with the disease or AE.

SPEED OF MARKETING APPROVAL

The continuing controversy of whether drugs should be approved for marketing in a fairly rapid manner, making the drug available to the public but at the price of having a smaller safety database and less knowledge about the safety profile. In this situation, the postmarketing safety data is critical to complete the safety profile. The alternative is to take more time in the premarketing period in order to better characterize the drug's benefit/risk profile.

Authors' note: There is no correct answer to this conundrum. Most health authorities seem to take the position that truly new drugs that represent an advance in the treatment of serious disease should be marketed more quickly rather than less quickly. This is hard to judge, however, in advance: When severe patient morbidity and mortality occurs, it may be followed by drug withdrawal, lawsuits, and much suffering. Thus the search for better techniques to understand a drug's safety profile in the shortest possible time continues.

SPERM, DRUG EFFECTS ON

See Pregnancy and Pregnancy Rating or Categories of Drugs.

Drugs may affect the male reproductive system and the sperm. This is an area with little available information. Reproductive studies in animals are done to determine the effects of new drugs on the testes and sperm. Thus there are often animal data in regard to whether a drug is toxic to the male reproductive system. There are few data, however, on toxicity in the female and the fetus due to transfer of the drug into the female from the male's semen or other body fluids.

There are a few examples in the medical literature. Ribavirin is one. This drug, used for the treatment of hepatitis C in combination with with pegylated interferon, produces in exposed women certain embryocidal and teratogenic effects. In the male rat, it has been shown to produce sperm abnormalities.

Contraception should be used by couples in which either partner is taking ribavirin.

SPL INITIATIVE

See Structured Product Labeling Initiative.

SPLITTERS AND LUMPERS (AE CODING)

A potential problem in AE coding using MedDRA or another coding dictionary.

The issue is whether broad terms should be used in coding to cover several signs and/or symptoms or whether the specific signs and symptoms should be spelled out and coded individually.

Should one be "a lumper" or "a splitter"? The lumper will code "flu-like syndrome" while the splitter will code "fever," "malaise," "fatigue," "muscle aches," "headache," "chills," and "runny nose." The difference may not matter for such AEs as "flu-like syndrome" but would matter for the "Hermansky-Pudlak syndrome" (albinism, visual problems, platelet defects with bleeding, lung disease, and often kidney and gastrointestinal disease).

Various health authorities and companies code differently, creating various consistency issues most evident in data exchange.

SPONSOR

One of the various terms used by the FDA and others for the company (or person) holding the marketing authorization (NDA) for a product. Synonyms include manufacturer (though this may not always be a true synonym, as the manufacturer may sell the drug to another company, who then holds the NDA and markets the drug), pharmaceutical company, etc.

SPONTANEOUS REPORTING SYSTEM

Also known as a pharmacovigilance system, spontaneous reporting scheme, and yellow card system. A methodology for spontaneous reporting by healthcare professionals, consumers, and patients of suspected adverse reactions seen with marketed medical products, and for the collection and evaluation of those reports by a pharmaceutical company or health authority with the aim of detecting signals and taking measures to reduce the risks. The first scheme was implemented in the UK in the wake of the thalidomide tragedy.

It is generally considered to represent passive surveillance, whereas structured studies used in pharmacoepidemiology represent active surveillance.

STANDARD OPERATING PROCEDURE

A written set of instructions detailing how a particular action or function is to be done.

Written formal SOPs, working documents, and guidances are obligatory in drug safety departments under Good Clinical Practices (GCP) requirements from the International Conference on Harmonization (ICH), the FDA, the European Medicines Agency (EMEA), and elsewhere. In addition, there may be manuals, guidances, and job aids that accompany the SOPs (e.g., a data entry manual). The SOPs govern the handling of safety data, report preparation, training, database and computer issues, and crisis management. It is not uncommon for a drug safety department to have 50 to 100 such SOPs and guidances. The creation, review (yearly, at least), maintenance, and updating of SOPs is a function that must be ensured in a safety department. SOPs and guidances must be version controlled so that everyone has access to them and is working from the latest versions. This may mean controlled distribution of paper copies or availability of SOPs online only (and not as paper copies).

STANDARDIZED CODING DICTIONARIES

See also Data Dictionaries, MedDRA, Uppsala Monitoring Centre, WHO Drug Dictionary.

As in any language or means of communication, if the speaker (sender) and receiver of the communication have not agreed upon what words to use and what the words mean, communication will be impossible.

In drug safety, the two key areas where terminology has been standardized are in AE/ADR terms and drug names.

AE/ADR terms: There have been many dictionaries and code lists developed over the years, including COSTART, WHO-ART, HARTS, and others. Through ICH a single agreed-upon AE coding dictionary, MedDRA, was developed. This has been widely adopted throughout the world and is now the main dictionary used for coding of AE terms. It is available in several languages and is controlled and "standardized" by a single organization (the MSSO). This major accomplishment has markedly improved global communication of AE reports.

Drug names: There is one major global drug dictionary currently in use: the WHO Drug Dictionary, which is maintained by the Uppsala Monitoring Centre (UMC) in Sweden. Because there is a time lag between the marketing of new drugs (or old drugs with new names) and their appearance in the Drug Dictionary (even though it is revised several times a year), many companies and health authorities use home-grown drug dictionaries or older versions of the WHO Drug Dictionary that they update and modify themselves. This makes communication more difficult among companies and health agencies.

STARTING THE REGULATORY CLOCK
See Clock Start Date.

STATISTICAL APPROACHES TO RISK EVALUATION
See Data Mining.

STEVENS-JOHNSON SYNDROME
In dermatovigilance, a severe form of erythema multiforme with bullae in the mouth, pharynx, and anogenital region. The eyes may also be affected. Often of drug origin. It is usually less severe than toxic epidermal necrosis (Lyell's syndrome), another bullous toxiderma that is often of drug origin.

STIMULATED REPORTING
The situation whereby a company or health authority requests practitioners (and rarely, patients) to report specific AEs (e.g., atrial fibrillation) or a class of AEs (e.g., any arrhythmias) seen with a drug or class of drugs.

This is usually done when there is a signal that needs to be investigated or when there is an insufficient number of cases to make an evaluation on risk management.

See also Solicited Report.

STORAGE OF SAFETY DATA AND DOCUMENTS
See Archiving.

STRUCTURED PRODUCT LABELING (SPL) INITIATIVE
From 2003 to 2006 the FDA issued new rules and guidances on the content, structure, and technology to be used for drug labeling. The regulations require that the content of labeling be submitted in a particular electronic form that the FDA can process, review, and archive.

It has been generally recognized that drug labeling in the United States is inconsistent, difficult to read, difficult to access, nonstandardized, and difficult to computerize in its present form. This forces patients and healthcare practitioners to use publications and websites that "digest" this information and present it in a more user-friendly format.

FDA has enacted these initiatives to manage the risks of drugs and to reduce medical errors. The first initiative was the development of structured product labeling (SPL) in which all labeling has three basic parts:

1. The header with general information about the label and product.
2. The sections with blocks of text (e.g., indications, contraindications, warnings, etc.).
3. The data elements with product-specific information (e.g., active ingredient, dosage form, how supplied, etc.).

In 2003 the FDA introduced the new requirements for SPL in which prescription and over-the-counter (OTC) drug labeling must be filed with the FDA using an XML-based format standard. This is an internationally accepted standard and allows for easy accessibility and transfer to other databases. Its use became obligatory as of October 2005.

The new rules on content do not apply to OTC products or to patient information. The first major change is that there will now be a "highlights" section. This section, which should run about 1/2 page in length, will include the most commonly used information in the label:

- The date of the approval of the original product
- A summary of any black box warning
- Recent major changes made within the last year regarding black boxes, indications and usage, dosage and administration, contraindications, and warnings and precautions
- Adverse reactions: the most frequent adverse reactions that are important for reasons other than frequency
- AE reporting contact information for both the FDA and the manufacturer
- Drug interactions
- Use in specific populations

There are also format and reordering changes in the labeling in addition to the highlights section. Risk information is consolidated with the AE section after the warnings and precautions section. Some information formerly in the precautions section (use in specific populations, drug interactions, and patient counseling information) is now in other sections. In addition, bold type is used in some sections, as well as more white space and minimum font sizes to make reading easier. This new rule applies to drugs approved after the rule went into effect as well as drugs approved in the five years before the effective date of the rule and older drugs for which there is a major change in the prescribing information. Manufacturers may apply this to older drugs too if they wish. Companies have between three and seven years to implement this for the older drugs depending on when (in the last five years) the drug was approved.

SUBJECT

A normal person exposed to a drug and presenting with an AE/ADR. This may be several contexts, including use of an OTC product, a young healthy woman taking a contraceptive, or a healthy volunteer participating in a clinical trial (such as phase I). The term subject in this context is distinct from patient. A patient is a diseased person taking a drug either in the postmarketing setting or during a clinical trial.

Authors' note: Many people use these terms synonymously and make no distinction between a subject and a patient.

SUBMITTING CASES TO REGULATORY AGENCIES

Individual case safety reports must be sent to health authorities in order to remain within regulatory compliance and to inform the agencies of important new AEs/ADRs. The usual mechanisms are by E2B (see Electronic Data Transfer), the post office ("snail mail"), fax or by courier.

When submitting a case the sender must ensure that the case is received. In E2B this is done by one or more electronic acknowledgements that are sent by the receiver to the sender noting receipt and then upload into the receiver's database. Postal mail should be sent certified, return receipt requested or Internet verification of delivery. Courier services usually have Internet-based methods to check on delivery (email notification, verification on their website, etc.).

SUICIDALITY

Suicidal (self-destructive) feelings, thoughts, or actions.

Authors' note: Paradoxically, suicidal thoughts or actions may rarely be associated with drugs aimed at preventing suicidality in depressed patients. In this sense, suicidality is considered a paradoxical ADR (see this term).

SUMMARY BRIDGING REPORT FOR PSUR

A summary bridging report integrates two or more PSURs to cover a specific time period for which a single report is requested. Thus two 6-month PSURs could be used to create a summary bridging report to cover the full year or ten 6-month reports to cover a 5-year PSUR. The bridging report does not contain new data but briefly summarizes the data in the shorter reports. The report should not contain line listings but may have summary tables.

SUMMARY OF PHARMACOVIGILANCE SYSTEM(S)

A document prepared by a company to be submitted to the health authority before an audit. It was primarily developed by the UK Health Agency (MHRA) but is used with adaptations for audits by other health agencies. It is a ~25-page document summarizing the company's drug safety functions:

Section 1: Contact details in regard to who covers PV and where. It identifies the Qualified Person.

Section 2: Company structure and operating model for pharmacovigilance

- Provides a brief company profile. Holding/parent company. Subsidiaries/world-wide presence. Company's therapeutic areas of expertise and product portfolio (marketed products and IMPs). Recent mergers or acquisitions (include relevance to/impact upon pharmacovigilance).
- Provides a succinct overview as to how pharmacovigilance is managed within the organisation i.e. the operating model.

Section 3: Pharmacovigilance System

- Provides a summary of the pharmacovigilance activities undertaken by the main pharmacovigilance site(s) in the UK and the global pharmacovigilance department(s).
- How the Company ensures that European legislative requirements are met:
  - A summary of the pharmacovigilance activities performed by other departments that interface with pharmacovigilance (e.g. Medical Information, Regulatory Affairs and Product Quality).
  - Process for spontaneous and clinical trial ADR management—from receipt to data entry, review and expedited reporting (if appropriate). It may be useful to provide flow diagrams(s) illustrating the information flow for safety reports of different origins and types.
  - Details of compliance monitoring activities that are performed.
  - Management and monitoring of clinical trial drug safety (including data reconciliation).

- Process for PSUR preparation and submission to competent authorities.
- Qualified Person for Pharmacovigilance—what pharmacovigilance activities is the QP routinely involved in?
- Processes for signal generation, trend evaluation and labelling changes.
- Risk Management Plans—has the Company produced any and for which products?

Section 4: Computerised systems used in Pharmacovigilance
Present Situation - global and local systems:

- Provides details of the computerised system(s) & database(s) used to collect, collate and evaluate information about suspected adverse reactions (e.g. spontaneously reported adverse drug reactions and solicited reports including clinical trial SAEs). Include:
  - Whether the system was developed commercially (and whether the system has been configured/customised following purchase) or in-house (bespoke).
  - Validation status (and where the validation documentation is located).
  - Version details.
  - Details of the group(s) responsible for maintenance and support of the system.
- Provides details of any computerised systems used by the UK pharmacovigilance department to capture/track UK ADR reports (including databases used to log medical information enquiries).
- Provides a summary of the legacy databases used over the last 5 years for pharmacovigilance.

Section 5: Quality Management System

- Does the Company intend to maintain the pharmacovigilance system in its current state for the next six months? If the answer is "no", provide a summary of the planned changes.
- Who is responsible for conducting audits of the Company's pharmacovigilance system? Provide a brief description. How long are audit reports retained and where are these stored?

Section 6: Training Records

- Briefly describes the UK training record system including the location of records, CVs and job descriptions for key personnel involved in pharmacovigilance activities.

Section 7: Archiving

- Provides a brief description of archiving activities for pharma-covigilance documents. If a contract archive company (ies) is/are used to store pharmacovigilance documents in the UK, provide the name(s) and address(es) of the archive facilities.

Multiple appendices are also required:

Organigrams of the local and headquarters organizations.
CV of the Qualified Person
A list of all products licensed in the UK with:
- Active ingredient(s).
- UK trade name.
- State if the product is not marketed in the UK.
- Method of approval (national, mutual recognition, cen-tralised).
- Reference Member State (for mutually recognised products).
- Indicate whether any of the products have black triangle sta-tus in the UK.
- Indicate the five products that generated the greatest number of ADR reports in the last year.

Studies
- A list of all ongoing phase I-III company sponsored clinical trials that have at least one site in the EU/EEA.
- A global list of all ongoing post-authorisation clinical studies, including interventional clinical studies (as defined in Directive 2001/20/EC) and non-interventional studies, for products licensed in the UK. Indicate on the list whether the trial is interventional or non-interventional and whether there are any sites in the EU/EEA.

Quality Management Systems
- Details of the global and local procedural document(s) de-scribing the content, format, approval and review procedures for all levels of procedural documentation (i.e. SOP on SOPs).
- A list of all the titles of all global, regional and local (UK) phar-macovigilance procedural documents (e.g. policies, SOPs and working instructions). Please order this list according to doc-ument scope i.e. global, regional or local.
- A list of all the titles of all other local (UK) procedural docu-ments (policies, SOPs, working instructions etc.) that relate to pharmacovigilance (i.e. those that are followed by depart-ments that interface with pharmacovigilance (e.g. Medical Information, Product Quality, Regulatory Affairs).

Regulatory Reporting Compliance Statistics (spontaneous reports only).

- For the last two years, a breakdown per month to include:
  - Total number of ADR reports (non-serious and serious) received by company (on a global basis).
  - Total number of ADR reports submitted to MHRA on an expedited basis.
  - Total number of late reports submitted to MHRA.
  - Number of late reports as a percentage of the total number of expedited submissions to MHRA.
- Compliance with expedited reporting requirements to MHRA (clinical trial reports only).

- For the last two years, please provide a breakdown per month to include:
  - Total number of SUSAR reports submitted to MHRA on an expedited basis.
  - Total number of late SUSAR reports submitted to MHRA.
  - Number of late reports as a percentage of the total number of expedited submissions to MHRA.
- Compliance with the requirement for PSURs to be submitted within 60 days of the data lock point
  - For PSURs submitted to the MHRA in the last two years, please provide the following information:
    - Product.
    - Data lock point.
    - Date submitted to MHRA.
    - If no PSURs have been submitted in the last two years, please provide information pertaining to the last five PSUR submissions to date.

Third Party Agreements with licensing partners (co-licensing, co-marketing, distribution, licensing-in licensing-out) and other service providers e.g. contract organisations providing a medical information or pharmacovigilance service

- A list of all local (UK) licensing agreements with third parties concerning marketed products and products not yet marketed/under development.
- A list of all global licensing agreements with third parties concerning marketed products and products not yet marketed/under development.
- Details of any activities/functions—those directly or indirectly related to pharmacovigilance—that are out-sourced in the UK (e.g. medical information, regulatory affairs, sales force, PSUR preparation, expedited reporting).

- Details of any pharmacovigilance activities—those directly or indirectly related to pharmacovigilance—that are out-sourced by the global pharmacovigilance department(s) e.g. perhaps the preparation of all PSURs has been out-sourced to company x, perhaps the global department in the USA deals with all medical information enquiries from the USA market and this function has been out-sourced to company y.

Product related safety issues

- Details of any products (licensed in the EEA) that have been withdrawn (from any global market) in the last five years due to safety reasons e.g. date of withdrawal, country of withdrawal, and nature of safety issue.
- Details of all Urgent Safety Restrictions, instigated by either the Company or a regulatory authority, in the last two years.

Documents—a copy of the relevant procedural document(s) relating to:

- Case processing of spontaneous adverse drug reactions reports.
- Case processing of clinical trial SAE reports.
- Follow-up of individual cases.
- Regulatory reporting of expedited reports to MHRA and EMEA.
- Monitoring of regulatory compliance with 7 and 15-day requirements.
- PSUR preparation and submission.
- Signal detection/trend analysis.
- Enquiry handling by medical information function in the UK.

Authors' note: This is a critical document and will be necessary for audits from the UK health authority and frequently in a similar form for other EU health authority audits. It should be prepared in advance and kept up to date periodically. See the website for further information on audits and the SPS: www.mhra.gov.uk/home/ idcplg?IdcService=GET_FILE&dID=21423&noSaveAs=1&Rendition= WEB

SUMMARY OF PRODUCT CHARACTERISTICS (SPC OR SmPC)

The official labeling for a product in the EU. See the Guideline on Summary of Product Characteristics October 2005 (http://ec. europa.eu/enterprise/pharmaceuticals/eudralex/vol-2/c/ spcguidrev1-oct2005.pdf).

The SPC sets out the agreed position of the medicinal product as distilled during the course of the assessment process. As such the content cannot be changed except with the approval of the originating competent authority. The SPC is the basis of information for health professionals on how to use the medicinal product safely and effectively.

The sections include:

1. Name of the medicinal product.
2. Qualitative and quantitative composition.
3. Pharmaceutical form.
4. Clinical particulars (e.g., indications, dose, formulation, contraindications, use in special populations, warnings and precautions, interactions, pregnancy and lactation, undesirable effects, overdose).
5. Pharmacological properties.
6. Pharmaceutical particulars (e.g., shelf life, excipients, container and storage information).
7. Marketing authorization holder.
8. Marketing authorization number(s).
9. Date of first authorization/renewal.
10. Date of revision of the text.
11. Dosimetry—for radiologic preparations.
12. Instructions for preparation of radiopharmaceuticals (if applicable).

SURROGATE MARKER

A laboratory test (or more rarely a sign or symptom) that is used as an indication of a disease or adverse event when the actual measurement or confirmation of the disease or AE is not possible. A surrogate marker may also be used to measure the extent or course of a known disease.

For example, the levels of the liver enzymes (AST, ALT) are surrogate markers for liver disease (e.g., drug-induced hepatitis) when one does not or cannot do a liver biopsy to make a more definitive diagnosis. The level of the enzymes may also be used to measure the progression of the hepatitis and sometimes its normalization after stopping the suspected drug.

Prolongation of the QT interval on the EKG may be used, in safety pharmacology carried out during preclinical development, as a surrogate (biomarker) for the more serious arrhythmia known as *torsades de pointes*.

In clinical trials where the endpoints are death (or duration of life), surrogate markers may be used if one is not able to run the study long enough to draw conclusions. For example, serum lipids may be measured in trials of statins or other lipid-lowering drugs when the clinically meaningful endpoints of the study are myocardial infarctions and cardiovascular death. It may not be possible to do a longitudinal study for, say, 20 or 30 years to ascertain whether the statins have produced these desirable effects. Thus measurement of serum lipids may serve as surrogate markers since there is a recognized correlation between elevated lipids and myocardial infarction.

In general, surrogate markers are never as good as direct measurement of the endpoint desired but in the real world, these may be the only measurements possible. Even so, the use of clinical outcomes is essential when a new product influences surrogate markers through a novel mechanism. For example, a drug that lowers blood glucose by a new mechanism may not necessarily protect from the complications of diabetes to the same extent as an older drug. A drug that modifies blood lipids may not automatically protect consumers against cardiac mortality.

SURVEILLANCE, DRUG

In drug safety, equivalent to pharmacovigilance.

In pharmacotherapy, surveillance of the patient's responsiveness, intolerance, and, in some situations, blood levels/activity, in order to adjust dosing or stop treatment.

SURVEY

In drug safety, an organized data collection of safety information on signals, labeled AEs, actual use of a product, compliance with RiskMAP requirements, and confusion over sound-alike or look-alike products. Usually (per the FDA) a written protocol with details on the methodology, including patient or healthcare professional recruitment and follow-up, projected sample size, and methods of data collection, management, and analysis. Validation should be done against medical or pharmacy records or through interviews with healthcare providers. Where possible, validated or piloted instruments should be used.

SUSAR

See Suspected Unexpected Serious Adverse Reaction.

SUSPECT DRUG

In an individual case safety report, the drug or drugs felt by the reporter and/or the manufacturer to be the most likely product(s) causing the AE/ADR in question. The suspicion may extend to a drug felt to be interacting with another (drug–drug interaction). The nonsuspect products are referred to as concomitant medications.

SUSPECTED ADVERSE REACTION (SAR; SUSPECTED ADR)

These expressions are redundant. An AE that is suspected of being due to a drug becomes an ADR, and the drug in question becomes a suspect drug. *See* Adverse Event. SAR may also, confusingly, mean serious adverse reaction.

SUSPECTED UNEXPECTED SERIOUS ADVERSE REACTION (SUSAR)

An adverse event that the reporter and/or manufacturer feels is most likely caused by one or more drugs, thus making the adverse event into an adverse drug reaction or suspected adverse drug reaction, and which does not appear in the official drug labeling (e.g., US package insert, SmPC, etc.).

SUSPENSION FROM THE MARKET

The cessation of selling or marketing of a drug. This is usually temporary and contrasts to a withdrawal, which may be permanent. It is similar to a recall (see this term). Temporary suspensions may become permanent (i.e., withdrawals).

SWEDISH MEDICAL BIRTH REGISTRY

A part of the Centre for Epidemiology at the National Board of Health and Welfare in Sweden. What makes this center of unique interest is that its aim is to collect prospective gestation and pregnancy data on all births in Sweden—between 85,000 and 120,000 per year. Data collected include information on previous gestation, smoking habits, medication, family situation, hospital, length of gestation, type of delivery, diagnoses of mother and child, operations, type of analgesia, sex, weight, length, size of head, birth conditions, place of residence, nationality, as well as outcome, delivery, and infant information.

See their website: http://www.sos.se/epc/english/Medical%20Birth%20Registry.htm. This is a major source of information on pregnancy, birth outcomes, and drug use.

This Centre, as well as the Canadian *Motherisk* Program in Toronto, is also known as a Teratovigilance Center.

SYSTEM ORGAN CLASS (SOC)

The fifth, highest, and least granular (specific) level in MedDRA, the main dictionary of adverse events. There are 26 SOCs. The next level down is the High Level Group Terms which are more granular. *See also* MedDRA.

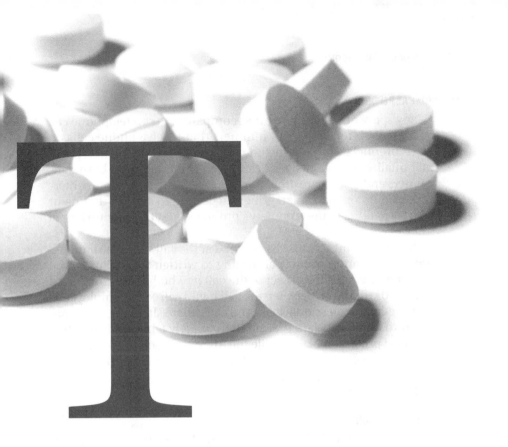

TAMPER-RESISTANT PACKING REGULATIONS (FDA)

Regulations issued in 1982 by the FDA to prevent poisonings such as deaths from cyanide placed in Tylenol® capsules. The Federal Anti-Tampering Act passed in 1983 makes it a crime to tamper with packaged consumer products.

TARGETED EDUCATION AND OUTREACH

In drug safety this refers to programs set up by sponsors to encourage patients to stay the course with their therapy and to educate on the best ways to handle any issues that might arise such as managing AEs/ADRs. Such AEs/ADRs, if noted in a sponsor-supported program, must be reported to the sponsor and handled as solicited AEs.

Authors' note: Advocacy groups believe that these coaching programs are a form of direct to consumer promotion aimed at increasing sales through prolonged patient compliance. Whether this is the case or not, they are useful when they increase the ADR reporting rate associated with the drug in question.

TELEPHONE AE REPORTS

Many sponsors run or hire other companies to run telephone call centers with toll-free (800) numbers that receive phone calls on their products. The calls include not just AEs/ADRs but also product quality complaints, requests for information from both consumers and healthcare professionals, etc. In addition, some centers will also do outward marketing, suggesting to a caller that he or she try another of the company's products (e.g., OTC or nutritional products).

It is important that all AEs received at the call center be handled rapidly and appropriately according to written SOPs. This is true whether the AE is the object of the call or whether it is uncovered during the dialogue between the caller and call center employee. If nonmedical professionals take the calls, there should be a mechanism to either escalate the call immediately ("hot transfer") to a medical professional to handle the AE or to obtain the basic information and contact information for a call-back from the medical professional at a later time.

See Call Center.

TEMPORAL ASSOCIATION

This refers to the timing of the onset of the AE after the use of the drug in question. A temporal association is very important in analyzing individual case safety reports and case series. In analyzing a possible drug cause of an AE, in almost all cases the drug must be used before the occurrence of the AE. (Interestingly, this is not always the case. *See* Anticipatory Nausea and Vomiting, a nocebo effect occurring before the first dose.) One must avoid the logical error known as "post hoc ergo propter hoc," which means "after this therefore because of this." Multiple other factors must also be analyzed such as the pharmacokinetics and dynamics of the drug, the nature of the AE, biologic plausibility, etc.

For example, if one takes an analgesic for a headache and the next day a cancer of the colon is diagnosed, it is not possible to ascribe the cancer (which takes years to develop) to the analgesic taken the day before. Similarly, if one takes a delayed release drug that requires a long period of time for absorption, it is hard to ascribe a type A reaction (pharmacologic) that occurs five minutes after dosing to the drug (unless it is an acute allergic reaction).

As is noted in CIOMS VI (2005), there is no definitive way to determine causality of a particular AE with only a temporal association.

TEMPORAL BIAS

See Secular Effect.

TEMPORAL WINDOW

In pharmacotherapy, the time frame limiting the administration modalities. For example, in treating a disease the critical temporal window for treatment may be within the first 24–48 hours after the appearance of symptoms. As a specific example, when treating myocardial infarctions, the critical time for thrombolytic treatment is within the first few hours; treatment after 12 hours is usually not beneficial.

In drug safety, the temporal window for the appearance of an ADR may be when the blood concentration of the drug and its key metabolites is above a certain level. This will be a function of the kinetics of the drug in that particular patient. In assessing causality, if the AE/ADR occurs outside the likely temporal window of that drug the likelihood of the AE/ADR being due to the drug is very low. For example, the likelihood of a pharmacologic AE occurring 12 hours after taking an analgesic with a half-life of one hour is very small.

With thalidomide exposure in utero, there is a temporal window (in days of pregnancy) for each type of congenital abnormality.

In causality assessment, the time to onset and time to offset must be biologically plausible.

TERATOGENICITY

The ability of a drug or other substance to cause birth defects/congenital malformations.

In the Animal

Preclinical animal studies of reproduction and development are required by regulation in most countries. Six segments can be distinguished:

- *Fertility:* From mating to conception.
- *Preembryonic period:* From conception to implantation.
- *Embryonic period:* From implantation to closure of the palate.
- *Fetal period:* From closure of the palate to birth.
- *Perinatal and postnatal periods:* From birth to the end of nursing.
- *Late effects:* From the end of nursing to the sexual maturity of the animal.

In the Human

The use of medications by a pregnant woman can cause several types of harmful consequences. The various types of toxicities should be distinguished: inhibition of fertility vs. abortive effects (abortifacients); neonatal toxicity before birth due to placental passage of the drug or its metabolites vs. medications taken during nursing and passed to the newborn in the breast milk.

- *Segmentation phase (blastogenesis):* During the 15 pre-embryonic days a medication can have a toxic or fatal effect on the blastocyte.
- *Embryonic period:* Teratogenicity is possible if the drug is taken (or persists in the tissues) during the 15th through the 90th day after conception (the first trimester). The period of organogenesis (days 15 to 56) represents the period of the greatest risk for malformations.
- *Fetal period:* Fetal toxicity is possible if the drug is consumed between the 90th day and birth. Both structural (bone, brain) and growth abnormalities can occur.

TERATOGENICITY AND FETAL TOXICITY LABELING

See Pregnancy Rating or Categories of Drugs.

TERATOLOGY INFORMATION SERVICES (TIS)

An umbrella organization for teratology agencies. This organization covers the United States, Canada, the United Kingdom, and Israel and serves as a clearinghouse for information and research on drug therapies. It often maintains (retrospective) teratology registries of reported birth defects from hospitals in its catchment area. See its website at http://www.otispregnancy.org/.

TERATOVIGILANCE

Narrow Definition

Surveillance of fertile, sexually active women with the goal of prevention of congenital malformations. This is done by studying malformations seen with the use of medications (or toxic substances) taken from conception to the end of the embryonic development period.

Broad Definition

Extended surveillance through the perinatal period. This includes fetal toxicity and neonatal toxicity until the end of weaning. Also called maternal and neonatal pharmacovigilance.

Authors' note: This subdomain of pharmacovigilance is quite technical and requires expertise in several fields, including embryology, epidemiology, genetics, neonatology, obstetrics, and pharmacology. Causality determination poses special problems. The use of a universal algorithm is not possible. A pharmacovigilance center wishing to develop a particular specialty in this domain must develop a clinical registry, which includes detailed prospective information on the mothers, fathers, and their offspring. Thousands to millions of records must be kept by a dedicated team of experts, with the ultimate goal of being able to answer the questions: "I took drug X while pregnant. What will happen to my baby?" and "Can I safely use drug Y during my pregnancy?" Although it may never be possible to give yes or no responses to these questions, it may ultimately be possible to respond with clear probabilities and recommendations backed by solid medical and scientific data. The responses to these questions will lead to irreversible decisions and lifelong consequences for mother, father, and child, the three "victims" of a birth defect.

TGA

See Therapeutic Goods Administration.

THALIDOMIDE

A major drug safety disaster in the early 1960s, when the NDA for thalidomide was valiantly opposed by Dr. Frances Kelsey at the FDA because of insufficient safety information despite strong pressure to approve it. Though never marketed in the United States, thalidomide was extensively used in over 50 countries as a sleep aid and as a treatment for morning sickness in pregnant women. By 1962 the terrible teratogenic aspect of the drug became known as over 10,000 babies were born with severe abnormalities, including badly deformed arms and legs (phocomelia). This led to legislation in the US that introduced the modern era of drug regulation. As a result of the legislation drug manufacturers now had to demonstrate to the FDA both safety and efficacy before marketing a new drug.

Thalidomide was reintroduced to the US market in the late 1990s (with extensive warnings about the teratogenicity) for multiple myeloma and erythema nodosum leprosum. Patients taking the drug must participate in a telephone survey and patient registry to prevent exposure during pregnancy.

THERAPEUTIC GOODS ADMINISTRATION (TGA)

The Australian health authority. See their website on pharmacovigilance: http://www.tga.gov.au/safety/monitoring.htm#pharmaco.

The New Zealand and Australian governments have agreed to establish a trans-Tasman therapeutic products agency. The joint agency will replace the Australian Therapeutic Goods Administration (TGA) and the New Zealand Medicines and Medical Devices Safety Authority (Medsafe). Preparations were stopped in mid-2007 when New Zealand announced it would not proceed for now.

THERAPEUTIC INDEX

Also known as the Therapeutic Ratio or Margin of Safety. It is a ratio formed by dividing the therapeutic dose by the toxic dose. Unlike the benefit/risk "ratio" or analysis there is a mathematical way to express the therapeutic index in some cases. This uses two data points found in animal testing: the LD_{50} (the dose that would kill half the population studied) divided by the ED_{50} (the effective dose in half the population studied). That is, $TI = LD_{50} / ED_{50}$. Ideally one wishes the TI to be very high—that is, the toxic dose is much greater than the effective dose. A ratio around 1 suggests a very narrow therapeutic range where the effective dose is very close to the toxic dose. Such drugs (e.g., lithium, digoxin, theophylline, coumadin) require very careful patient monitoring (e.g., blood levels where available) and dose level adjustment.

TIME TO DISAPPEARANCE

In drug safety this may be:

1) The time between the appearance of the AE/ADR and its disappearance, irrespective of suspect drug continuation; this should be called duration.
2) The time taken for the AE/ADR to disappear after the suspect drug is stopped; also known as time to offset. The disappearance itself, not the time taken, constitutes a positive dechallenge.

The term is also used in pharmacokinetics. For example, one may look at blood levels of a drug and calculate the time to disappearance of 50% (half-life) and then 100% of the drug in the blood.

TIME TO ONSET

The time interval between the taking of a drug and the beginning of an AE/ADR or the appearance of its first manifestation. It should be calculated by using the critical dose, e.g., the first dose in most instances or the last dose for a withdrawal reaction or for a rebound reaction or the first increase in dosage in a dose-related reaction.

TOME (THE)

Proposed new regulations printed in the *Federal Register* by the FDA in early 2003 but that have never been put into final effect (and may never be in their entirety). They represented a major change in the way drug safety would be handled in the US.

TORSADES DE POINTES

A type of polymorphic ventricular tachycardia with abnormal QRS complexes on the electrocardiogram that can vary from beat to beat. The ventricular rate is usually from 150–250 beats per minute. The major causes include drug therapy, familial long QT syndrome, and various cardiac and metabolic abnormalities. The underlying rhythm is characterized by a prolonged QT syndrome.

In the recent decade or so, much attention has been focused on drugs that can produce this potentially fatal ADR usually via prolongation of the QT interval.

TOXIC EPIDERMAL NECROLYSIS (TEN)

A type of bullous skin reaction also designated Lyell's syndrome. It is more severe than Stevens-Johnson syndrome and is often of drug origin. It is a medical emergency and treatment, similar to that of severely burned patients, is often required at a tertiary care medical center.

TOXICOLOGY, CLINICAL

The study of poisons in humans, of the noxious effects of environmental and household chemicals, but also of drugs and biologics, therapeutic or recreational, accidental or voluntary, taken acutely or chronically.

As the term notes it is "clinical," meaning that medical data are collected from observations or studies of humans. *See* Toxicology, Preclinical.

In medical parlance the word toxicology usually refers to acute or chronic intoxication (poisoning) with chemicals found in nature, absorbed from food, water, and air.

Poison control center directors are often called clinical toxicologists. Forensic medicine often resorts to the expertise of clinical toxicologists.

TOXICOLOGY, PRECLINICAL

The study of the noxious effects of chemicals, drugs, biologics, etc., in animals (in vivo) or tissues or cells in the laboratory (in vitro). This work may not be restricted to medicinals or products aimed at treating or preventing disease, but may also cover compounds found in the environment where the toxicity profile needs to be known.

TOXICOVIGILANCE

The surveillance of drug poisonings (overdoses), usually carried out by poison control centers managed by clinical toxicologists. The concept of toxicovigilance includes the active detection, validation, and follow-up of clinical adverse events related to toxic exposures in humans. These centers play a major role because poisoning databases are required to establish risk factors, incidence, and severity, as well as outcomes of corrective treatments.

Authors' note: Attribution of causality after a successful suicide with high blood levels of an antidepressant may be complex. Did the drug induce suicidality, or was the drug taken in overdose the cause of death? The answers are important to add valid information to the safety profile of the drug in question.

TRADITIONAL PERIODIC SAFETY REPORT (TPSR)

The term used by the FDA in the 2003 safety regulation rewrite (*see* the Tome) to describe the classic NDA periodic report submitted to the FDA for marketed drugs. This is in contrast to the Periodic Safety Update Report (PSUR).

See NDA Periodic Report and Periodic Safety Update Report.

TRAINING IN PHARMACOVIGILANCE

This is now obligatory for people working in the drug safety department and anyone who has dealings with adverse events including sales representatives, legal, regulatory, telephone operators, mailroom personnel, etc. One of the first things an auditor from the FDA or the EU will look for is the content and documentation of training of all personnel.

The level of training varies as a function of the job. A telephone operator need only be able to identify something as a complaint or "bad thing" and direct the call to the appropriate safety person to handle it. The clinical research and drug safety personnel, in contrast, will need far more extensive training.

Authors' note: There is very little formal pharmacovigilance training given to medical professionals. Only a few universities around the world include pharmacovigilance in their curricula. The leaders in the field seem to be the pharmacy schools. Regrettably, nurses and physicians rarely receive formal training. A few universities have programs that are aimed at drug safety specialists (postgraduates). Most medical schools offer only a few hours on drug safety during an entire medical course, an unacceptable situation for future prescribers; the same comment applies to continuing medical education. Some for-profit groups give short courses (a day to a week) in applied pharmacovigilance aimed at industry personnel. Obviously, there is a significant need for training medical personnel, prescribers, and the public, if we hope to decrease ADRs in the population.

TRANSIT SITE REACTION

An ADR occuring in a hollow viscus (e.g., the GI tract) and causing obstruction, ulceration, perforation, or hemorrhage. Causality assessment is often "very probable," or even "definite," when the drug is removed endoscopically from the esophagus or stomach.

TREATMENT EMERGENT AE

An AE/ADR that arises during the use of a drug during a clinical trial or from postmarketing reports.

TREATMENT IND PROGRAMS

See Compassionate Use Programs.

TRIAGE OF AEs

This term refers to the handling of an individual case safety report when it is first received in a company or health authority. The first receiver of an AE/ADR must be trained to recognize such a report and to forward the information to the appropriate person or department in the appropriate time frame (urgently for a serious AE). These functions require training by the drug safety department.

The next level of triage occurs in the drug safety department where the case must be determined to be serious or not, possibly expedited or not, and whether there is an urgent public health issue or not.

An urgent case may be a death or a very unusual case that will require immediate action (stopping of a study, recall or withdrawal, suspected tampering, etc.). Another urgency would be a serious case that appears to be an expedited report but which is, for whatever reason, received late in the drug safety department, leaving little time to prepare and send the case out.

Similarly, in the health authority, the safety personnel must examine the case to see whether or not there is a public health urgency.

TRIAL

See Clinical Study/Trial.

TRYPTOPHAN AND THE FDA

The FDA issued a nationwide recall in 1989 of all over-the-counter dietary supplements containing 100 milligrams or more of L-tryptophan, due to a clear link between the consumption of L-tryptophan tablets and its association with a US outbreak of eosinophilia myalgia syndrome (EMS), characterized by fatigue, shortness of breath, and other symptoms. By 1990 the Centers for Disease Control and Prevention confirm over 1,500 cases of EMS, including 38 deaths, and the FDA prohibits the importation of L-tryptophan. *See* Eosinophilia Myalgia Syndrome.

TWO BY TWO TABLE

Also called an ABCD table.

In epidemiology, a contingency table with four cells used to present the results of a structured study where:

a = exposed patients with a particular AE
b = exposed patients without the AE
c = unexposed patients with the AE
d = unexposed patients without the AE

	Patients with the AE (Cases)	Patients without the AE (Controls)
Exposed	a	b
Unexposed	c	d

IF THE DATA IS FROM A COHORT STUDY
The attributable risk is calculated as follows:

$$a/[a + b] - c/[c + d]$$

The relative risk is calculated as follows:

$$a/[a + b], c/[c + d]$$

IF THE DATA IS FROM A CASE-CONTROL STUDY
The attributable risk can be calculated. In addition the odds ratio can be calculated:

$$[a/c], [b/d] \text{ or } ad/bc$$

If the cases are rare—for example, under 2%—the odds ratio can be used as a statistically acceptable approximation of the relative risk, called the approximate relative risk.

TYPE A REACTION

A pharmacologically predictable dose-related ADR. It includes exaggeration of a desired pharmacological effect. Examples would include bruising or hematoma formation in patients using warfarin or other anticoagulants.

TYPE B REACTION

A "bizarre," pharmacologically unpredictable ADR not dose related. Also called idiosyncratic reactions. An example would be an allergic reaction to a drug.

TYPE C REACTION

An ADR arising from chronic use of a drug.

TYPE D REACTION

A delayed ADR, appearing long after exposure.

TYPE E REACTION

An end-of-dose ADR, such as rebound and withdrawal.

TYPE F REACTION

A failure of therapy (efficacy).

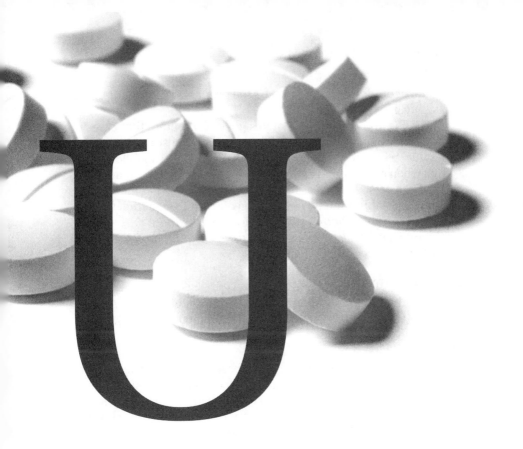

UMC

See Uppsala Monitoring Centre.

UNBLINDING

In drug safety this refers to the opening of the blinding code used in a clinical trial to prevent the patients and/or investigators from knowing which patients receive which treatment.

The issue is whether to open the blind on an individual patient if that patient has a serious AE that is unexpected and possibly related to the study drug, thereby becoming a 15-day (or if a death occurs, a 7-day) expedited report. The discussion is over the use to the sponsor and the health authority of receiving an expedited report where one does not know the whether the patient received the study drug or not.

This question was discussed in 1997 by the FDA, which stated that "sponsors should only break the blind for the subject in question. Sponsors should consult with the FDA review division responsible for their IND in situations in which the sponsor believes that breaking the blind would compromise their study (e.g. when a fatal or other serious outcome is the primary efficacy endpoint in a clinical investigation)."

The EU and the member states generally require that cases be unblinded before submission. For example, for postmarketing studies E2A, which the FDA also references and wishes to follow, notes that when possible and appropriate, the blind should be maintained for those persons, such as biometrics (statistics) personnel. In large companies this often turns out to be difficult to do in practice.

Authors' note: Some companies, especially those making ophthalmology products, do not like to use the word "blinded" and prefer to use the word "masked."

UNCOMMON (AE/ADR FREQUENCY)

Under the CIOMS III definition, uncommon refers to an AE/ADR that occurs from 0.1% to 1% of the time (1/1000 to 1/100).

UNCONTROLLED STUDY

Strictly speaking, a clinical study (observational or experimental) that has no comparison group or no control group. Also called a nonanalytical study. It is thus very hard to infer causality since the exposed population or sample cannot be compared explicitly with a control group. This applies both to efficacy and safety findings.

In a wider sense, it is a clinical trial without control measures for eliminating systematic errors (biases and confounders) and random errors (due to sampling variability). These measures may include a comparative group (stratification, randomization), double-blindness, compliance checks, uniformity of experimental conditions, and statistical analyses.

An observational study also needs proper control measures.

Authors' note: In practice, however, a small, open, uncontrolled trial (done, of course, under GCP with all patient protections in place) may be quite useful in testing a hypothesis where historical controls are clear. For example, if in past experience a disease is uniformly fatal and a new drug appears to save lives, it merits further exploration in a controlled trial.

UNDER-REPORTING

See Rate.

UNEXPECTED, UNEXPECTEDNESS

"For a pre-marketed product: Any adverse drug experience, the specificity or severity of which is not consistent with the current investigator's brochure; or, if an investigator brochure is not required or available, the specificity or severity of which is not consistent with the risk information described in the general investigational plan or elsewhere in the current application, as amended. For example, under this definition, cerebral thromboembolism and cerebral vasculitis would be unexpected (by virtue of greater specificity) if the investigator brochure only listed cerebral vascular accidents" (21CFR312.32(a)).

"For marketed products: Any adverse drug experience that is not listed in the current labeling (package insert or summary of product characteristics) for the drug product. This includes events that may be symptomatically and pathophysiologically related to an event listed in the labeling, but differ from the event because of greater severity or specificity. For example, under this definition, hepatic necrosis would be unexpected (by virtue of greater severity) if the labeling only referred to elevated hepatic enzymes or hepatitis" (21 CFR 314.80(a)). AEs that are "class related" (i.e., allegedly seen with all products in this class of drugs) and are mentioned in the labeling (package insert or summary of product characteristics) or investigator brochure, but are not specifically described as occurring with this product, are considered unexpected.

UNEXPECTED ADVERSE REACTION

Any adverse reaction, the nature, severity, or outcome of which is not consistent with the information labeled in the investigator brochure, the data sheet, the monograph, or the summary of product characteristics. Equivalent to unlabeled.

UNEXPECTED BENEFICIAL DRUG REACTION

The occasional observation of new and often unexpected beneficial effects represents an advantageous byproduct of pharmacovigilance after the launch of a new product, both for patients and for the manufacturer. Sometimes these effects are followed up with controlled clinical trials, the submission of a new NDA/HRD, and the addition of a new indication to the labeling. Sometimes—and perhaps even more satisfying—is the turning of an adverse event into a therapeutic benefit. For example, minoxidil produced abnormal hair growth in patients using the product for hypertension. The drug was studied in a different formulation and was relaunched as a topical product to promote hair growth.

UNLABELED

Unlabeled refers to the ADRs not contained in official product safety information for marketed products (e.g., Summary of Product Characteristics in the European Union or the Package Insert in the US). Unlabeled is different from unlisted, which refers to an ADR absent from the Core Safety Information (*see* Unlisted).

UNLIKELY

See Causality Determination.

One of the terms used in causality determination (e.g., related, probably related, possibly related, weakly related, unrelated, and unassessable). Unlikely suggests a small possibility that the AE is related to the drug but that the probability is low.

Authors' note: The use of such a broad and granular array of terms is very useful in the analysis of signals and in the creation of tables for investigator brochures, product labeling, and monographs, to give a feel for the certainty or lack thereof in regard to the AEs and the relationship to the drug in question.

However, for the drug safety group, which has to make a determination of whether a clinical trial case meets the three criteria (seriousness, expectedness, causality) for expedited reporting, the decision is a yes or no decision. That is, the drug safety group must make the choice between unrelated and related. There is no middle ground or gray zone for causality here.

Thus the drug safety group has to make a rapid decision on whether the case is clearly unrelated (absolutely, positively) and everything else (possibly, probably, unlikely, weakly, etc.). Some drug safety groups consider "unlikely related" to be unrelated and other groups consider it in the broad "related" category.

Whichever way is decided, it should be made clear to everyone what is done. Many drug safety officers believe that unless a case is clearly and absolutely unrelated, the causality should be, for reporting purposes, "related." To put it another way, the default causality for all cases is "possibly related" until there is evidence that the case is "unrelated." It is realized that this may not ultimately agree with the case analysis in the final clinical research study report where a more nuanced opinion may be recorded.

In short, there are two causality choices for regulatory reporting purposes in the world of drug safety: unrelated (thus making the case not reportable as an expedited case) and everything else.

UNLISTED

Unlisted refers to the ADRs not contained in the core safety information (CSI) for a marketed product or within the development CSI in the investigator's brochure. Unlisted is different from unlabeled (*see* Unlabeled), which refers to local or national drug labeling.

UNRELATED

A causality judgment, meaning the AE in question is not due to the drug. This is a positive, absolute, and unequivocal determination, meaning there is not even the small possibility that the AE might be related to the drug. *See* Causality Determination.

UNSOLICITED REPORT

Also called a spontaneous report.

An individual case safety report (AE/ADR) that is sent into the sponsor or health authority spontaneously and without being requested. These reports form the basis for the spontaneous reporting surveillance system for AEs/ADRs in place in most countries of the world. They are the constituents of the so-called passive surveillance system.

UNTOWARD EFFECT

This is a loosely defined term that has been used as a synonym for both adverse event and adverse drug reaction (the latter includes the suspicion of causality).

UPDATE REPORT

See PSUR.

UPPSALA MONITORING CENTRE (UMC)

The Uppsala Monitoring Centre has been one of the pioneering founders of the globalization of drug safety and pharmacovigilance activities by national drug agencies. See its website: www.who-umc.org/.

From their website: "The UMC is an independent centre responsible for the collection of data about adverse drug reactions from around the world, especially from countries that are members of the WHO, and the generation of signals of drugs which might possibly have problematic side-effects."

Vision and Goals

The vision is to support WHO's leadership in the field of world health by providing excellence in the science and concepts of all aspects of pharmacovigilance to prevent harm to humans from the effects of medicines to gather and share objective intelligence and opinion in the field of drug safety through open and transparent means of communication to support the promotion of the rational use of drugs, and the achievement of improved patient therapy and public health in global education and communications in benefit, harm, effectiveness and risk in medical therapy.

"We will achieve this by developing leading-edge systems and science for the identification and communication of safety hazards in drugs and other substances used in medicine carrying out research pushing forward the ethical, intellectual and scientific boundaries of theory and practice in pharmacovigilance pursuing active collaboration and communication with all stakeholders pursuing the goal of a single, global database for drug safety data.

And in particular we aim to ensure that effective, timely international collective effort will never miss a signal of a potential hazard ensure that all stakeholders evaluate and learn from decisions and actions through positive impact-assessment, follow-up and debate encourage the growth of pharmacovigilance activities around the world, in particular the establishment of new National Centres promote existing National Centres and other stakeholders in the field to contribute actively to the global vision of the WHO Programme to use and share available information openly and transparently to sponsor and support others in their pharmacovigilance activities to exploit fully the resources of the UMC, stimulate the development of coherent, harmonised systems worldwide for pharmacovigilance, through education, training, promoting and participating in international forums, the promotion of best practice and the publication of guidelines maintain and develop useful products, services and tools in pursuit of the vision and goals of the WHO Programme and the UMC."

The UMC has several products used by many in the field of drug safety including the WHO Drug Dictionary, WHO-ART Dictionary, the WHO Herbal Dictionary, and Vigibase.

See also Vigibase.

URTICARIA

Superficial vasodilatation and edema of the dermis with a red appearance that blanches with pressure and that can change site from day to day. It can evolve into angioedema. It is often pruritic (itchy). A medication etiology should always be considered in patients with urticaria. Drug-induced urticaria usually disappears rapidly after cessation of the causative agent (dechallenge).

US FOOD AND DRUG ADMINISTRATION.

See FDA.

USAN (US ADOPTED NAMES COUNCIL)

The US Adopted Names Council (USAN), which is officially sponsored by the American Medical Association, the US Pharmacopeial Convention, and the American Pharmacists Association, assigns generic names that are unique and nonproprietary for drugs. The USAN works closely with the International Nonproprietary Name (INN) Program of the World Health Organization (WHO), which assigns international "generic" names.

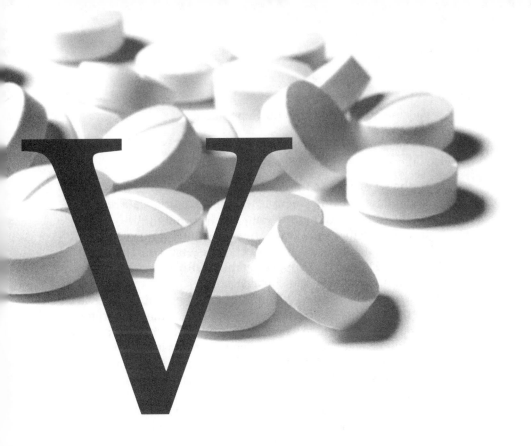

VACCINE ADVERSE EVENT REPORTING SYSTEM (VAERS)

The Vaccine Adverse Event Reporting System is a cooperative program for vaccine safety of the Centers for Disease Control and Prevention (CDC) and the Food and Drug Administration (FDA). VAERS is a postmarketing safety surveillance program, collecting information about adverse events (possible side effects) that occur after the administration of US licensed vaccines. http://vaers. hhs.gov/

VACCINOVIGILANCE

The postmarketing surveillance of adverse events that occur after the administration of vaccines in a population.

This function is usually the responsibility of a governmental agency separate from that handling drug vigilance (pharmacovigilance). Severe adverse reactions from vaccines are relatively uncommon. The FDA's VAERS system reports that 85% of its reports are minor while 15% are serious events, such as seizures, high fevers, life-threatening illnesses, or deaths. The true ratio is hard to know because all AEs are not reported.

VAERS

See Vaccine Adverse Event Reporting System.

VALIDATED REPORT

Five different meanings are in use:

(1) In the regulatory sense, a report from a consumer or patient, verified by a healthcare professional. The initial data received by the manufacturer or agency are followed up with a communication to the physician, nurse, hospital, pharmacist, etc., to ensure that the data are correct. Additional, complementary data is usually also supplied by the healthcare provider. This means that the case is medically valid.

(2) The reporter, the form, the product, and the AE are sufficiently identified. For example a report (phone, fax, email, letter) may be said to be validated when the identity of the reporter and/or the source of the report have been confirmed in order to avoid duplicate reports (different from follow-up reports, duplicates) and pranksters. This means that the case is well identified. The data are not fabricated.

(3) A report may be said to be valid when the evidence contained has been verified as being exact: suspect product identification and dose, precise description of adverse event, etc. Valid in this sense means accurate, i.e., the facts are true.

(4) A report may be said to be valid when confidence in causality is above zero. This situation occurs when causality has not been excluded by finding, for example, strong evidence of alternative etiologies; when there is enough information to raise the suspicion of a clinician, even if the suspicion is very slight. Valid in this sense means there is ground for suspicion of a causal link.

(5) A report may be called valid when the information is complete enough to permit causality assessment. In this sense validity equals completeness.

See Minimum Information for Reportability.

VALIDATION, DATA

See Data and Software Validation and Verification and Validated Report.

In drug safety, the processes put in place to ensure the integrity of the data.

VALIDATION AND VERIFICATION OF DATA AND SOFTWARE

In 2002 the FDA defined these concepts: "Software verification provides objective evidence that the design outputs of a particular phase of the software development life cycle meet all of the specified requirements for that phase." Validation is "confirmation by examination and provision of objective evidence that software specifications conform to user needs and intended uses, and that the particular requirements implemented through software can be consistently fulfilled."

Another definition would be that the informatics system in question has been correctly implemented, conforms to the specifications in the original requirements, and has been so ascertained by a third party not directly involved in its implementation or use.

For safety systems, this includes:

- 21CFR11 compliance
- Change control
- Acceptable to US, European Union, and other inspectors
- Complete audit trails
- Labeling functions
- The database should be able to store the AEs.

Authors' note: In practice this means any computer system that stores safety data and that is used for submission of data to health authorities should be designed, tested, and validated to ensure that the data entered is not changed or altered without proper change control and audit trails (tracking of who did what and when) and that what comes out of the system is a true representation of what was entered.

VARIABILITY IN AE CODING

See Coding and Splitters and Lumpers.

VENOUS THROMBOEMBOLISM

A blood clot in the veins (deep vein thrombosis) that breaks off and subsequently lodges in (and usually blocks off) vessels at a distant site. Earlier versions of oral contraceptives, for example, had been associated with unacceptable rates of leg vein thrombi embolizing to the lungs, sometimes with serious consequences.

VERSION CONTROL

The tracking of all changes to a document (AE report, CIOMS form, MedWatch form, SOP etc.) so that all additions, changes, subtractions, etc., are evident and transparent. Each change must be recorded and tracked so that the reason and source of the change is evident. This ensures that no inappropriate alterations are made to the document or electronic file and that all people using it are using the latest version. This is a requirement of Good Clinical

Practices and other "predicate rules." Version control is examined carefully by auditors from the FDA, the EMEA, etc.

VERY COMMON (ADR FREQUENCY)

Under the CIOMS III definition, very common refers to an AE/ADR that occurs 10% or more of the time. The denominator may represent the number of patients exposed, the number of prescriptions, the number of drug courses, etc.

VERY-LONG-TERM AEs

See Late-Occurring AEs.

VIDAL

The compendium of drug labeling in France; the counterpart of the US *Physicians' Desk Reference* and the *CPS* in Canada. See www.vidal.fr/ (website is in French).

VIGIBASE

Vigibase is a collection of international drug safety data maintained by the Uppsala Monitoring Center (UMC). The data is now available in a wide range of forms. The services range from advanced neural network analysis to basic case report retrieval. The Vigibase services will help find useful information about the safety profile of a company's products compared to its competitors.

Since 1978 the UMC has been the focal point of independent global pharmacovigilance. The Vigibase data resource is the largest and most comprehensive in the world, and is developed and maintained by the UMC on behalf of the World Health Organization. The data held is collected from 77 countries participating in the WHO Programme for International Drug Monitoring. Vigibase comprises more than 3.5 million case reports, to which around 50,000 new reports are added quarterly. All of these cases are available to anyone with a health professional degree-level education (physician, dentist, nurse, pharmacist). The case reports in the WHO database do not identify the patient or reporter nor do they contain narratives. Reference to the original case report is made through a national case identification number.

VOLUME 9A

The Rules Governing Medicinal Products in the European Union— Guidelines on Pharmacovigilance for Medicinal Products for Human Use. Issued 2007 and replacing the previous edition known as "Volume 9." This is the fundamental set of rules governing drug safety and pharmacovigilance in the European Union. The official version contains 233 pages. It can be found at http://ec.europa.eu/enterprise/pharmaceuticals/eudralex/vol-9/pdf/vol9A_2007-04.pdf/.

VOLUME OF AE REPORTING

The number of AE/ADR cases reported is enormous. The FDA received in 2004 about 400,000 AE reports and their database (AERS) contains over 3 million cases in total. Large pharmaceutical companies may also receive over 100,000 cases per year. These cases may generate, in one multinational company, over 250,000 expedited reports submitted to health authorities (the same reports submitted to multiple authorities as required by law and regulation).

The volume appears to be increasing by 5% to 10% per year overall, but by even greater numbers when new drugs are launched that are widely used. It was estimated at one point in the United Kingdom that only 10% of serious ADRs and 2% to 4% of nonserious ADRs that occur were reported (Rawlins, 1995), but lower figures have been observed in other settings; underreporting of unexpected serious ADRs is widespread.

Authors' note: The increasing volume of AEs and the accompanying need for storage facilities for the enormous amount of paper generated and personnel to process and analyze all of these reports is a major problem for the industry and health authorities. Neither companies nor health authorities can increase resources at the pace needed to handle all the cases. Although efficiencies are being introduced (E2B reporting, "paperless offices," etc.), there are still many issues to address to tackle this problem. Perhaps the biggest issue is to identify the cases that matter and that need to be looked at, as well as identifying the cases that do not even need to be collected (e.g., nonserious, expected AEs on OTC products on the market for more than 50 years, such as aspirin, except in the case of a previously unknown drug interaction). How this will play out in the future, with the public demanding safer drugs and more oversight of both companies and health authorities, remains to be seen.

VOLUNTARY REPORTING

See Spontaneous Reporting System.

VOLUNTARY WITHDRAWAL

Withdrawal of a drug from the market by the manufacturer due to:

- A change in the benefit:risk evaluation. This could be due to an internal company examination of the safety profile and the realization that the benefit:risk analysis is no longer favorable.

Other nonsafety related business reasons (dropping sales, loss of patent, etc.) may also cause a market withdrawal.

- Pressure from the health authorities.
- Pressure from various sources such as consumer groups (via petitions, adverse publicity, picketing, etc.), the media, lawsuits (individual or class action), etc. A "voluntary" withdrawal is not always "voluntary."

VOLUNTEER

A person who, of his or her own free will and without any coercion, agrees to participate in a clinical drug trial. Often these people stand to gain nothing in addition to what they would have received with normal medical treatment (e.g., patients randomized to conventional treatment—not the new drug) or even less (e.g., patients enrolled in a study who receive a new treatment that turns out to be inferior to the standard treatment).

Sometimes patients are compensated for participation in trials with small amounts of money (e.g., to cover transportation), but others receive larger sums for participation, such as in phase I trials.

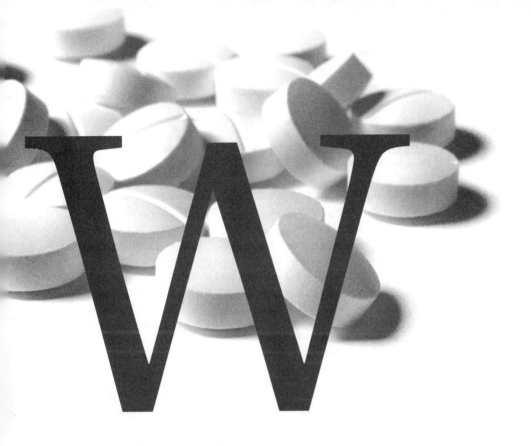

WAREHOUSE, DATA

See Data Warehouse.

WARNING AND PRECAUTIONS (IN LABELING)

This section of the US label should include clinically significant ADRs for which there is reasonable evidence of a causal association between the drug and the adverse reaction (a causal relationship need not have been established). This includes ADRs that are serious; that require discontinuation, dosage, or regimen adjustment; or that require addition of another drug; that could be prevented or managed with appropriate patient selection or avoidance of concomitant therapy; that significantly affect patient compliance; or if the product interferes with a laboratory test. Known or predicted drug interactions with serious or otherwise clinically significant outcomes should also be included.

The section may also include ADRs that are predicted to occur with a drug but have yet to be observed. Noteworthy ADRs occurring in unapproved indications should also be mentioned, along with a statement indicating that safety and effectiveness have not been established in that setting and that the use is not approved by FDA.

The section should provide:

- A description of the adverse reaction and outcome (e.g., clinical features and timing, seriousness of outcome).
- An estimate of risk or adverse reaction rate.
- A discussion of known risk factors for the adverse reaction (e.g., age, gender, race, comorbid conditions, dose, duration of use, coadministered drugs).
- A discussion of steps to take to reduce the risk of, decrease the likelihood of, shorten the duration of, or minimize the severity of an adverse reaction. These steps could include, for example, necessary evaluation prior to use, titration and other kinds of dose adjustment, monitoring during dose adjustment or prolonged use, avoidance of other drugs or substances, or special care during comorbid events (e.g., dehydration, infection).
- A discussion of how to treat, or otherwise manage, an adverse reaction that has occurred.

The information and advice provided in this section should be reasonably qualified, where appropriate, to convey whatever uncertainties may exist about judgments and conclusions made (e.g., concerning causality assessments, estimated adverse reaction rates, and value of proposed monitoring).

See the FDA website http://www.fda.gov/cder/guidance/5538dft.htm.

In the European Summary of Product Characteristics the warning section should note special warnings and precautions for use and, in the case of immunological medicinal products, any special precautions to be taken by persons handling such products and administering them to patients, together with any precautions to be taken by the patient.

See the website http://ec.europa.eu/enterprise/pharmaceuticals/eudralex/vol-1/consol_2004/human_code.pdf.

WARNING LETTER (FDA)

A written communication from the FDA to a company or individual noting that some of its actions are in significant violation of laws or regulations. It may be issued for other violations, such as quality (GMP) issues, incorrect or misleading advertising or promotional claims, marketing an unapproved new drug, and other violations. For drug safety matters, it is usually sent after an inspection by the FDA. Such letters are posted on the FDA's website: http://www.fda.gov/cder/warn/index.htm.

The FDA has stated that "the following violations are considered significant to warrant issuance of a Warning Letter:

1. Failure to submit ADE reports for serious and unexpected adverse drug experience events.
2. 15-day alert reports that are submitted as part of a periodic report and which were not otherwise submitted under separate cover as 15-day alert reports. This applies to foreign and domestic ADE information from scientific literature and post-marketing studies as well as spontaneous reports.
3. 15-day alert reports that are inaccurate and/or not complete.
4. 15-day alert reports that are not submitted on time.
5. The repeated or deliberate failure to maintain or submit periodic reports in accordance with the reporting requirements.
6. Failure to conduct a prompt and adequate follow-up investigation of the outcome of ADEs that are serious and unexpected.
7. Failure to maintain ADE records for marketed prescription drugs or to have written procedures for investigating ADEs for marketed prescription drugs without approved applications.
8. Failure to submit 15-day reports derived from a postmarketing study where there is a reasonable possibility that the drug caused the adverse drug experience."

The receipt of a warning letter is a very serious issue. It is addressed to senior management (sometimes the chief executive officer of the corporation) and requires a detailed written response within a short time (usually 15 days) indicating the corrective actions to be taken.

WEAKLY RELATED

A level in causality determination. Equivalent to "unlikely, doubtful." Also, the determination that an AE might be related to the drug in question but that the evidence is not strong.

WEBER EFFECT

Also called the "product life cycle effect." This term describes increased voluntary reporting after the initial launch of a new drug because voluntary AE reporting does not occur at a uniform rate. For as long as two years (or even more) after launch a larger number of spontaneously reported AEs/ADRs is expected, compared to the steady-state levels afterward. It is to be distinguished from Secular Effect (see this term).

WEBSITE AE REPORTS

An AE/ADR that is reported on a website maintained by a pharmaceutical company, health authority, or third party. In general, a pharmaceutical company is obliged to search for AEs/ADRs that might be reported on its own websites or those where it has control. Many companies design websites that do not allow the entry of data by the public (noninteractive websites) in order to avoid this issue. This is an accepted practice. There is, in general, no obligation for a company to scan the Internet to search out AEs/ADRs on other websites.

Once found, a website AE/ADR must be treated like any other AE/ADR with evaluation, follow-up, regulatory reporting, etc.

WHO ADVERSE REACTION TERMINOLOGY (WHO-ART)

A dictionary of terms used for coding AEs and ADRs developed and maintained by the Uppsala Monitoring Centre. It was in wide use for many years but has been largely replaced by MedDRA (*see* MedDRA). See the website http://www.umc-products.com/DynPage.aspx?id=4918.

WHO DRUG DICTIONARY ENHANCED (WHO DD)

A dictionary of drug names maintained by the Uppsala Monitoring Centre. It contains primarily prescription drugs but some OTC, biotech, and blood products; diagnostic substances; and contrast media listings as well. As of March 2007 the dictionary contained 185,463 unique names, 1,095,695 different medicinal products, and 9,814 different ingredients mentioned in these products.

The dictionary is hierarchical, using system organ classes and the chemical, pharmacologic, and therapeutic properties of each drug. A numerical code is also assigned to each drug. See their website: http://www.umc-products.com/DynPage.aspx?id=2829.

WITHDRAWAL

Regulatory

Withdrawal of a drug from the market. This refers to a voluntary or involuntary cessation of the selling or marketing of a product or particular lots or formulations of a product. It is often used (incorrectly) to mean both withdrawal and recall from the market (see the FDA's definition of these terms below).

The FDA defines market withdrawal as "a firm's removal or correction of a distributed product which involves a minor violation that would not be subject to legal action by the Food and Drug Administration or which involves no violation, e.g., normal stock rotation practices, routine equipment adjustments and repairs, etc." 21CFR7.3(j)

The FDA distinguishes between a withdrawal and a recall: "Recall means a firm's removal or correction of a marketed product that the Food and Drug Administration considers to be in violation of the laws it administers and against which the agency would initiate legal action, e.g., seizure. Recall does not include a market withdrawal or a stock recovery." 21CFR7.3(g) *See* Recall.

In clinical studies
The removal of a patient from a clinical study. Such patients are also referred to as "dropouts."

In such studies, patients are screened using inclusion and exclusion criteria and, if accepted, begin treatment in a clinical study. Most patients in most trials will complete the trial without incident. However, in some trials, patients will leave the trial for various reasons: death, adverse events, intercurrent illnesses, moving to a new residence far away, changes in personal circumstances, and being otherwise lost to follow-up. Up to 25% of patients do not complete their participation in long-term trials. It is important that they are included in the efficacy and safety analyses.

WITHDRAWAL EFFECT
Also called Drug Withdrawal Effect. Adverse events, signs, or symptoms that occur when a drug that has been taken for a length of time is stopped. They result from the physiological adaption to the drug's pharmacologic effects. Rebound effects and withdrawal effects are the two varieties that may occur when the drug is stopped: the underlying condition reappears (rebound effect) or new problems may emerge (withdrawal effect).

Rebound: Examples of the return of an underlying problem would include an increase in chest pain (angina pectoris) that might occur when beta blockers are withdrawn from cardiac patients or seizures that might occur in epilepsy patients when their anticonvulsants are withdrawn.

Withdrawal: Examples of new problems are seen in some individuals who stop using recreational drugs (drug abuse) and then experience hallucinations, cravings, unusual behavior, or even suicide.

In daily life drug withdrawal problems are very common. Heavy coffee drinkers who stop their intake may develop anxiety, nervousness, tremors, and headaches. In alcoholics, the sudden withdrawal of alcohol can lead to delirium tremens ("DTs"). In smokers, the sudden cessation of smoking may lead to nicotine withdrawal symptoms such as anxiety, irritability, concentration difficulty, headaches, and weight gain.

Particular attention must be paid to this issue in the medical setting when changes in medications are made. Before surgery, the treating physicians must decide which medications can safely be stopped and which cannot.

See also Rebound Effect.

WORLD MEDICAL ASSOCIATION (WMA)

An international organization of physicians founded in 1947. "The purpose of the WMA is to serve humanity by endeavoring to achieve the highest international standards in Medical Education, Medical Science, Medical Art and Medical Ethics, and Health Care for all people in the world." They are best known for establishing the Declaration of Helsinki in 1964, which the WMA has amended several times.

See their website: http://www.wma.net/e/index.htm.

See Declaration of Helsinki.

WORST PILLS, BEST PILLS

A book, newsletter, and website from Public Citizens Health Research Group (see this term), a consumer advocacy organization. They offer advice on medications, including those not to take under any circumstances, cheaper alternatives, drug interactions, etc. Their website is https://www.worstpills.org/bookpurchase.cfm?src=P5XWPWBK.

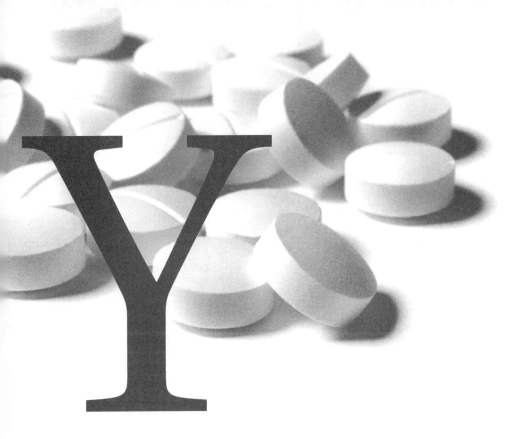

YELLOW CARD AND SCHEME

Name given to the reporting form color of the first national Spontaneous Reporting Scheme, which was founded in the UK by Bill Inman following the thalidomide disaster. The name is still used although printed forms are being replaced by electronic ones available on the Web, and the national forms are not yellow but usually white; even blue in Australia.

The Yellow Card Scheme is run by the MHRA and Commission on Human Medicines in the UK. The Scheme is used to collect information from health professionals and patients on suspected adverse drug reactions (ADRs).

Information is collected on prescription medicines, herbal remedies, over-the-counter medicines, and unlicensed medicines in cosmetic treatments.

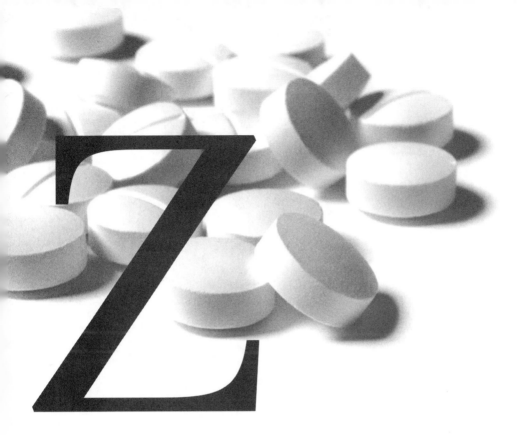

ZELNORM® (TEGASEROD MALEATE)

An example of a product that was removed from the U.S. market for safety reasons and then re-introduced to the market under a limited access treatment in the same year.

Appendix 1

Imputation Guide

A Practical Guide to Causality Assessment

PREVIOUS DOCUMENTATION

1. **Suspect product**
   - Is it recognized as being **capable** of causing the reaction, i.e. is the ADR mentioned in the medical literature, the official labeling, the manufacturer's files (see proposed scale below)?
   - Is the ADR **frequent** with this product?
   - Is the ADR pharmacologically **predictable?** (exaggeration of its pharmacologic effect, side effect)
   - Are present **predisposing** factors related to product **exposure**? (overdose, mode of administration, medication error)
2. **Adverse event**
   - Is it **often** drug-related? (e.g., aplastic anemia, bullous toxidermia, *torsades de pointes*, fixed-drug eruption, neuroleptic malignant syndrome, acute liver failure) Is it **often** related to the suspect drug? (e.g., statins and rhabdomyolysis, SSRIs and the serotoninergic syndrome, anti-HIVs and lipodystrophy, isotretinoin and congenital anomaly)

PATIENT'S HISTORY

3. **Prior events** specific to the ADR
   - Prior **exposure** to the suspect drug? If yes, was there a reaction? (prechallenge: n/a, positive, or negative)
   - Prior **occurrence** of the AE? If yes, in which circumstances?

4. **Pharmaceutical history**
   - **Concomitant medication?** Are there any other potential **suspects** apart from the suspect drug? Is there a potential for a drug–drug **interaction?**
5. **Medical history**
   - **Concomitant morbidity?** Does the indication for the suspect drug or other pathologies represent potential etiologic **alternatives** for the AE? Are **predisposing** factors present related to the patient's **condition?** (e.g., renal failure, allergy, age, sex, weight)

CLINICAL PRESENTATION

6. **Chronology**
   - **Time to onset,** since first dose, first dose augmentation, last dose, single dose. A short time to onset is often very suggestive but its length should be plausible with the dynamics and the kinetics of the suspect product.
   - **Duration** of AE before stopping or reducing the dosage or after a single dose
   - Course upon **dechallenge** (n/a, positive, or negative)
   - Course upon **rechallenge** (n/a, positive, or negative)
   - Response to **corrective** treatment
7. **Clinical features**
   - Are the nonchronologic clinical or laboratory **features** of the AE suggestive of a drug reaction? (e.g., drug-induced hepatitis, lupus-like syndrome)
   - Is the reaction **located in situ?** Site of application (skin), transit (esophagus), concentration (kidney), excretion (lithiasis)

Proposed scale for ranking the prior documentation concerning the AE and the suspect drug

Level 4 **Fully labeled**
Level 3 **Recognized but not yet fully labeled**
Level 2 **Anecdotal or predictable**
Level 1 **Unpublished and unpredictable**
Level 0 **Unreported worldwide** (from manufacturer's and UMC database)

Proposed scale for quantifying causality assessment

Level 4 **Definite** (>95% confidence in causality)
Level 3 **Probable** (50% to 95% confidence in causality)
Level 2 **Possible** (5% to 50% confidence in causality)

Level **1**   **Unlikely, doubtful** (<5% but >0% confidence in causality)

Level **0**   **Causality assessment impossible** (insufficient case data)

Level **-1**   **Causality ruled out** (after reviewing the case data)

For regulatory purposes in most jurisdictions, levels 1 to 4 are usually ranked as "possibly related" or having "a reasonable possibility."

In civil lawsuits, levels 3 and 4 may be deemed sufficient to infer causality ("more likely than not"). In criminal cases, even more than level 4 may be required, such as 99.9% confidence in causality.

Appendix 2

Reporting Rate Determinants

The reasons for the admittedly low rate of reporting of spontaneous AEs can be grouped into categories linked to (a) the clinician, (b) when the reporter him- or herself has the AE, (c) the manufacturer, (d) the AE/ADR itself, (e) the pharmacovigilance program, and (f) the suspect product.

FACTORS TIED TO THE CLINICIAN

Many factors can be described:

1. **Is the report reimbursed (i.e., paid for)?** The influence of being paid for each AE report has been studied in the setting of hospitals in Ireland. Reporting by physicians quadrupled when they were paid for the reports and returned to baseline when the reimbursements ceased.
2. **Reimbursement on a fee-for-service basis.** In Great Britain, where general practitioners are almost all paid a salary as employees of the National Health Service, the level of suspected ADR reporting is quite satisfactory. In North America, where physicians are reimbursed on a fee-for-service basis, for the most part, the reporting rate is lower while salaried, hospital-based pharmacists have a higher reporting rate and are, in fact, supplanting physicians as suspected ADR reporters.
3. **Lack of interest.** Inman used the polite term "lethargy" to summarize the lack of interest, time, remuneration, and other excuses for failure to report suspected ADRs.

4. **Uncertainty about causality.** The uncertainty that the clinician has regarding the drug's causality of the event plays a role. In a study of British physicians, it was found that the fear of ridicule and that a pharmacovigilance committee might feel that a report is unfounded as well as the lack of confidence in the role of the drug in producing the event were major inhibitory factors in suspected ADR reporting. Belton. *Brit J Clin Pharm* 1995;39:223.

5. **Awaiting a second case.** This refers to the phenomenon of multiple simultaneous published reports of an ADR. It is not unusual to see two or three cases of the same ADR published together by a single reporter. Why should a clinician refrain from publishing his first clinical observation until he has a second or third case in his practice? One answer may be that if there's no suspicion, there's no ADR report. It is only after the second case occurs that the clinician's threshold of suspicion is reached so that he is compelled to report. This phenomenon is an important source of delay in the publication or reporting of important signals, particularly when the second case occurs a year or two after the first. Another way to look at this is to say that the initial report is unlikely to be drug related and must be "validated" by a second case.

   Although the desire for scientific validation with a second case is very understandable, the clinician is requiring that the second case come from his own practice when it could, in fact, be seen and thus validated by a different observer somewhere else. The failure to report to the pharmacovigilance authorities (either the health agencies or the manufacturer) can delay the appropriate analysis and actions (e.g., a call for additional cases) of a serious signal.

6. **Belief in the innocence of the drug.** This refers to an exaggerated confidence in the safety of a drug. This is the incorrect belief that the phase III development of a drug reveals its entire safety profile. This may be a form of scientific naïvete believing that "only safe drugs are marketed" (to use the words of McGettigan). This credulity has many causes including the promotion of the drug, which may stress efficacy at the expense of safety issues.

7. **Fear of being sued.** This fear seems to be mainly found in the United States. In Ireland only 4.1% of those studied cited this reason (Feely. *BMJ* 90;300:22) whereas in France, of 507 physicians in private practice interviewed, only 1% were concerned about legal liability. Pierfitte. *Thérapie* 1995:50:171 (in French).

8. **Ambition.** Among specialists and academics in medical schools and university hospitals the desire to publish and enlarge one's curriculum vitae may come before the desire to notify the government health authority. This attitude is unfortunate because the author could use the date of notification to prove that he was the first to make the observation.

9. **Prescriber guilt.** There exists the entirely understandable sense in the eyes of the prescriber that he has given a patient a medication that has produced harm.

10. **The fear of appearing foolish.** The fear of being ridiculed for having sent to a pharmacovigilance unit "an effect that everybody is already aware of" and is of little or no signaling value was cited by Irish physicians in a study as a reason to hesitate about reporting a suspected ADR.

11. **Profession.** In 2004 the FDA's Office of Drug Safety noted the sources of reports were as follows:
    - Pharmacists, 37%
    - Unknown, 18%
    - Consumers, 17%
    - Physicians, 12%
    - Nurses, 11%
    - Dentists, 1%

12. **Fear of an attack on the freedom to prescribe medications as the clinician sees fit.** If the drug was used for an off-label (unapproved) indication, the prescriber may not wish to call attention to this.

13. **Loss of anonymity.** The reporter may not want to supply privileged patient details (even if anonymized) along with his or her name and address to governments and manufacturers.

14. **Religion.** Protestant countries seem to have a higher level of reporting than Catholic countries, even in countries that have large populations of both religions such as Belgium, Germany, and Ireland. The reporting rate in Protestant Denmark before 1986 was 1/3,850 inhabitants compared to 1/200,000 inhabitants in Catholic Italy giving a reporting ratio of 52:1. Griffin. *Intl Pharmacy J* 1987;1:145.

Even within the same city this effect persists: A study in Montreal showed that English-speaking Protestant parents report more AEs/ADRs seen in their children than French-speaking Catholic parents report in their children. It was noted in a telephone interview study that anglophone mothers reported 3.2 times more ADRs associated with antibiotic therapy in their children than francophone mothers. Before 1986, there were 10.9 times more

Protestants residing in Ontario than in Quebec, according to Statistics Canada, and 8.6 times more spontaneous reports came from Ontario than from Quebec. Kramer. *J Pediatr* 1985;106:305; Biron. *J Pediatr* 1987;110:665.

THE REPORTER HIMSELF AS THE PATIENT

Two situations are possible: (1) the healthcare professional is him or herself the patient and user of the drug, and (2) a nonmedical consumer has a suspected ADR and becomes the reporter of the event.

A medical professional has an AE. When the NSAID suproxofen was launched in the US, many physicians received samples of the product that they used themselves or distributed to their families. Forty percent of the initial reports of AEs were from healthcare professionals who "benefited" from the samples themselves. Rossi. *JAMA* 1988;259:1203. Many years ago, some of the victims of the congenital abnormalities produced by thalidomide occurred in the children of physicians whose wives used samples given to their husbands.

AE/ADR reports by nonmedical consumers. The Dutch have compared the suspected ADR reports received at the Dutch Centre of Pharmacovigilance from patients with those received from healthcare professionals regarding serotonin uptake inhibitor antidepressants. Two years after launch, patients had submitted 120 reports whereas clinicians had reported 89. The time lag between the first notification of the new ADR by a patient and the first notification of a new ADR by a medical professional also showed a difference. The patients were faster by a mean of 273 days. Egberts. *Brit Med J* 1996;313:530.

It is also noted that if consumers have access to toll-free (800) numbers for the manufacturers, the number of AE/ADR reports (including lack of efficacy) increases if the consumers are aware that the manufacturer will provide reimbursement or a discount for the same or another of the manufacturer's products (especially OTC products). Thus there is an indirect monetary incentive to report an AE/ADR.

THE MANUFACTURER

Time and effort involved in follow-up. In most countries the manufacturer is obliged by law or regulation to obtain follow-up information on AEs. Conscientious manufacturers will thus contact the reporter by phone, letter and/or fax requesting follow-up data including patient charts, laboratory reports, cardiograms etc. This costs the reporter significant time and effort and may be the reason a physician will think twice about reporting a case. Many manufacturers will also collect and report AEs/ADRs even when reporting is not obligatory as part of good medical and pharmacovigilance practices.

Loss of grants. The concern that an academic researcher or university hospital or medical school opinion leader might lose a grant or subsidy from a pharmaceutical company is a possible reason for reticence in reporting spontaneous suspected ADRs. This does not apply to AEs and ADRs in clinical trials where the safety and efficacy profiles of the drug are being actively sought. This issue does not seem to occur in reports to health agencies since there is rarely a question of financing or grants in these cases.

Attitude. The attitude of the company can be closed and defensive or open and accepting. Remarks of the type, "this is the first time we've heard of this kind of reaction . . . You are the only person in the country to have reported this" can be daunting and discouraging. This phenomenon, which was seen more in the past, seems to be receding with the need for safety monitoring now understood and accepted (even by the marketing departments of pharmaceutical companies).

THE REACTION

Several characteristics of the AE/ADR can play a role in underreporting:

1. **The severity.** A more severe AE/ADR is more likely to be reported. A British study suggests that if it is assumed that 5% of ADRs are serious in general medicine, then it is six times more likely that an ADR is reported if it is serious rather than innocuous [Mann]. The death rate of agranulocytosis is 10% in cohort studies [Heinpel], while the death rate of agranulocytoses in Great Britain is 30%. The seriousness increased the changes of its being reported by threefold. Of 507 French physicians surveyed, 81% of them were motivated to report the event by its seriousness. In an Irish study, 94.9% considered that the seriousness is an important determinant of reportability. Feely. *BMJ* 90;300:22 [Pierfitte]. Heinpel. *Med Toxicol* 1988;3:449. Mann. *PEDS* 1992;1:19 MCA/CSM. *Current Problems in Pharmacovigilance* 1993(Nov);19.

2. **The natural rarity of the AE/ADR.** The rarity, in addition to the severity, of the event raises its visibility. When zimeldine was followed for the Guillain-Barré syndrome (very rare and serious, sometimes fatal), this was relatively easy to classify as a signal. The initial series of cases were studied in depth and the drug was withdrawn from the market. Phocomelia produced by thalidomide is easier to recognize as an ADR than a dry cough produced by angiotensin-converting enzyme inhibitors.

3. **Visibility on the skin.** Cutaneous reactions are reported more often, all things being equal, than noncutaneous reactions, particularly when the reporter is not a physician.

4. **Rapidity of appearance (short lag period).** Suspicion increases with the brevity of the lag between ingestion of the drug and appearance of the adverse event. This suggests that an increase in reporting rates will follow.

THE PHARMACOVIGILANCE PROGRAM

What is pharmacovigilance? In general, very few physicians and healthcare professionals are aware of the nature of drug development, the (relatively small) number of patients exposed to the drug in phases II and III, and the need for ongoing AE/ADR reporting after marketing to flesh out the safety profile of a product. Few medical schools around the world include pharmacovigilance in their curricula or, if they do, it is done in a cursory manner. If the medical community is barely aware of pharmacovigilance, the lay community is even less so. Most consumers feel a drug is "safe and effective" or it would not be on the market.

THE SUSPECT PRODUCT

Two characteristics of the product itself can play a role in the reporting rates:

The pharmacologic class. Traditionally oncologists do not report serious and unexpected adverse reactions related to chemotherapy to pharmacovigilance agencies. Rather they discuss them amongst themselves. It is presumed that the severity of the indication (cancer) makes the severity of the ADRs less unacceptable. It is also felt by the oncologists that all patients in chemotherapy will have ADRs and that, except for the very unusual or very severe one (out of proportion to what they have seen in the past), it is too time-consuming and of little value to report ADRs.

The commercial age of the product. It is during the first 2 or more years or less after launch that active AE/ADR reporting is seen to peak. This has been well documented and has been called the Weber Effect (see this term). In terms of stimulus to AE/ADR reporting, seriousness of the event is the most important factor followed by the newness of the drug. It is presumed that the clinicians feel that the signaling value in these cases is greater than in older drugs.

Appendix 3

Rule of Threes

An expression relating to statistical power proposed by Hanley, "If nothing goes wrong, is everything alright?" *JAMA* 1983;249:1743. If no case of an AE is seen in N patients exposed to a drug, it can be concluded with [1-alpha] confidence that the incidence of this AE does not exceed 3/N if alpha = 0.05. For example, if 300 patients are given a new NSAID and there are no cases of fatal gastrointestinal bleeding, it can be said with 95% confidence (1–0.05) that the true incidence does not exceed 3/300 or 1/100.

From this it follows that, at the 95% confidence level, in order to say that the incidence of this AE is less than or equal to 1/10,000, it is necessary to have 30,000 exposed patients without observing the AE.

Thus it is not really possible to prove the negative concept that the incidence of an AE is zero ("This AE does not occur."). Since absolute safety cannot be proven, we must content ourselves with relative safety within certain limits.

The number three is derived from Poisson's law, which permits the calculation of the upper end of the confidence interval when the observed number of AEs is zero. The natural logarithm (ln) of the negative value of alpha can be calculated:

- For an 80% confidence interval (CI) or a 20% risk of error, ln $(-0.2) = 1.6$
- For a 90% CI or a 10% risk of error, ln $(-0.1) = 2.3$
- For a 95% CI or a 5% risk of error, ln $(-0.05) = 3$
- For a 99% CI or a 1% risk of error, ln $(-0.01) = 4.6$

From this it follows that, continuing the example above, to obtain a 99% confidence that the incidence of an AE is $< 1/10,000$ it would be necessary to have no cases of the AE in 46,000 patients.

Appendix 4

SUSPECT ADVERSE REACTION REPORT	

I. REACTION INFORMATION

1. PATIENT INITIALS (first, last)	1a. COUNTRY	2. DATE OF BIRTH			2a. AGE Years	3. SEX	4-6 REACTION ONSET			8-12 CHECK ALL APPROPRIATE TO ADVERSE REACTION
		Day	Month	Year			Day	Month	Year	

7 + 13 DESCRIBE REACTION(S) (including relevant tests/lab data)

☐ PATIENT DIED

☐ INVOLVED OR PROLONGED INPATIENT HOSPITALISATION

☐ INVOLVED PERSISTENCE OR SIGNIFICANT DISABILITY OR INCAPACITY

☐ LIFE THREATENING

II. SUSPECT DRUG(S) INFORMATION

14. SUSPECT DRUG(S) (include generic name)		20 DID REACTION ABATE AFTER STOPPING DRUG? ☐ YES ☐ NO ☐ NA
15. DAILY DOSE(S)	16. ROUTE(S) OF ADMINISTRATION	21. DID REACTION REAPPEAR AFTER REINTRO-DUCTION? ☐ YES ☐ NO ☐ NA
17. INDICATION(S) FOR USE		
18. THERAPY DATES (from/to)	19. THERAPY DURATION	

III. CONCOMITANT DRUG(S) AND HISTORY

22. CONCOMITANT DRUG(S) AND DATES OF ADMINISTRATION (exclude those used to treat reaction)

23. OTHER RELEVANT HISTORY (e.g. diagnostics, allergics, pregnancy with last month of period, etc.)

IV. MANUFACTURER INFORMATION

24a. NAME AND ADDRESS OF MANUFACTURER		
	24b. MFR CONTROL NO.	
24c. DATE RECEIVED BY MANUFACTURER	24d. REPORT SOURCE ☐ STUDY ☐ LITERATURE ☐ HEALTH PROFESSIONAL	
DATE OF THIS REPORT	25a. REPORT TYPE ☐ INITIAL ☐ FOLLOWUP	

Appendix 5

Form Approved: OMB No. 0910-0291, Expires: 10/31/08
See OMB statement on reverse.

U.S. Department of Health and Human Services
Food and Drug Administration

For use by user-facilities,
importers, distributors and manufacturers
for MANDATORY reporting

Mfr Report #

UF/Importer Report #

MEDWATCH

FORM FDA 3500A (10/05)

Page ____ of ____

FDA Use Only

A. PATIENT INFORMATION	C. SUSPECT PRODUCT(S)

A. PATIENT INFORMATION

1. Patient Identifier

2. Age at Time of Event:
or _____
Date
In confidence   of Birth:

3. Sex
☐ Female
☐ Male

4. Weight
_____ lbs
or
_____ kgs

B. ADVERSE EVENT OR PRODUCT PROBLEM

1. ☐ Adverse Event   and/or   ☐ Product Problem *(e.g., defects/malfunctions)*

2. Outcomes Attributed to Adverse Event
(Check all that apply)
☐ Death: _____ *(mm/dd/yyyy)*
☐ Life-threatening
☐ Hospitalization - initial or prolonged
☐ Required Intervention to Prevent Permanent Impairment/Damage (Devices)
☐ Disability or Permanent Damage
☐ Congenital Anomaly/Birth Defect
☐ Other Serious (Important Medical Events)

3. Date of Event *(mm/dd/yyyy)*

4. Date of This Report *(mm/dd/yyyy)*

5. Describe Event or Problem

6. Relevant Tests/Laboratory Data, Including Dates

7. Other Relevant History, Including Preexisting Medical Conditions *(e.g., allergies, race, pregnancy, smoking and alcohol use, hepatic/renal dysfunction, etc.)*

PLEASE TYPE OR USE BLACK INK

C. SUSPECT PRODUCT(S)

1. Name *(Give labeled strength & mfr/labeler)*
#1 _____
#2 _____

2. Dose, Frequency & Route Used
#1 _____
#2 _____

3. Therapy Dates *(If unknown, give duration) from/to (or best estimate)*
#1 _____
#2 _____

4. Diagnosis for Use *(Indication)*
#1 _____
#2 _____

5. Event Abated After Use Stopped or Dose Reduced?
#1 ☐ Yes ☐ No ☐ Doesn't Apply
#2 ☐ Yes ☐ No ☐ Doesn't Apply

6. Lot #
#1
#2

7. Exp. Date
#1
#2

8. Event Reappeared After Reintroduction?
#1 ☐ Yes ☐ No ☐ Doesn't Apply
#2 ☐ Yes ☐ No ☐ Doesn't Apply

9. NDC# or Unique ID

10. Concomitant Medical Products and Therapy Dates *(Exclude treatment of event)*

D. SUSPECT MEDICAL DEVICE

1. Brand Name

2. Common Device Name

3. Manufacturer Name, City and State

4. Model #
Catalog #
Serial #

Lot #
Expiration Date *(mm/dd/yyyy)*
Other #

5. Operator of Device
☐ Health Professional
☐ Lay User/Patient
☐ Other:

6. If Implanted, Give Date *(mm/dd/yyyy)*

7. If Explanted, Give Date *(mm/dd/yyyy)*

8. Is this a Single-use Device that was Reprocessed and Reused on a Patient?
☐ Yes   ☐ No

9. If Yes to Item No. 8, Enter Name and Address of Reprocessor

10. Device Available for Evaluation? *(Do not send to FDA)*
☐ Yes   ☐ No   ☐ Returned to Manufacturer on: _____ *(mm/dd/yyyy)*

11. Concomitant Medical Products and Therapy Dates *(Exclude treatment of event)*

E. INITIAL REPORTER

1. Name and Address

Phone #

2. Health Professional?
☐ Yes ☐ No

3. Occupation

4. Initial Reporter Also Sent Report to FDA
☐ Yes ☐ No ☐ Unk.

Submission of a report does not constitute an admission that medical personnel, user facility, importer, distributor, manufacturer or product caused or contributed to the event.

MEDWATCH

FORM FDA 3500A (10/05) *(continued)*   Page ____ of ____

FDA USE ONLY

F. FOR USE BY USER FACILITY/IMPORTER *(Devices Only)*

1. Check One
☐ User Facility   ☐ Importer

2. UF/Importer Report Number

3. User Facility or Importer Name/Address

4. Contact Person

5. Phone Number

6. Date User Facility or Importer Became Aware of Event *(mm/dd/yyyy)*

7. Type of Report
☐ Initial
☐ Follow-up #

8. Date of This Report *(mm/dd/yyyy)*

9. Approximate Age of Device

10. Event Problem Codes *(Refer to coding manual)*
Patient Code _____ - _____ - _____
Device Code _____ - _____ - _____

11. Report Sent to FDA?
☐ Yes ____ *(mm/dd/yyyy)*
☐ No

12. Location Where Event Occurred
☐ Hospital
☐ Home
☐ Nursing Home
☐ Outpatient Treatment Facility
☐ Other: ____ *(Specify)*
☐ Outpatient Diagnostic Facility
☐ Ambulatory Surgical Facility

13. Report Sent to Manufacturer?
☐ Yes ____ *(mm/dd/yyyy)*
☐ No

14. Manufacturer Name/Address

G. ALL MANUFACTURERS

1. Contact Office - Name/Address *(and Manufacturing Site for Devices)*

2. Phone Number

3. Report Source *(Check all that apply)*
☐ Foreign
☐ Study
☐ Literature
☐ Consumer
☐ Health Professional
☐ User Facility
☐ Company Representative
☐ Distributor
☐ Other:

4. Date Received by Manufacturer *(mm/dd/yyyy)*

5.
(A)NDA # ____
IND # ____
STN # ____
PMA/ 510(k) # ____
Combination Product ☐ Yes
Pre-1938 ☐ Yes
OTC Product ☐ Yes

6. If IND, Give Protocol #

7. Type of Report *(Check all that apply)*
☐ 5-day   ☐ 30-day
☐ 7-day   ☐ Periodic
☐ 10-day   ☐ Initial
☐ 15-day   ☐ Follow-up # ____

9. Manufacturer Report Number

8. Adverse Event Term(s)

H. DEVICE MANUFACTURERS ONLY

1. Type of Reportable Event
☐ Death
☐ Serious Injury
☐ Malfunction
☐ Other:

2. If Follow-up, What Type?
☐ Correction
☐ Additional Information
☐ Response to FDA Request
☐ Device Evaluation

3. Device Evaluated by Manufacturer?
☐ Not Returned to Manufacturer
☐ Yes ☐ Evaluation Summary Attached
☐ No *(Attach page to explain why not)* or provide code:

4. Device Manufacture Date *(mm/yyyy)*

5. Labeled for Single Use?
☐ Yes   ☐ No

6. Evaluation Codes *(Refer to coding manual)*
Method _____ - _____ - _____ - _____
Results _____ - _____ - _____ - _____
Conclusions _____ - _____ - _____ - _____

7. If Remedial Action Initiated, Check Type
☐ Recall   ☐ Notification
☐ Repair   ☐ Inspection
☐ Replace   ☐ Patient Monitoring
☐ Relabeling   ☐ Modification/ Adjustment
☐ Other: ____

8. Usage of Device
☐ Initial Use of Device
☐ Reuse
☐ Unknown

9. If action reported to FDA under 21 USC 360i(f), list correction/ removal reporting number:

10. ☐ Additional Manufacturer Narrative   and / or   **11.** ☐ Corrected Data

---

The public reporting burden for this collection of information has been estimated to average 66 minutes per response, including the time for reviewing instructions, searching existing data sources, gathering and maintaining the data needed, and completing and reviewing the collection of information. Send comments regarding this burden estimate or any other aspect of this collection of information, including suggestions for reducing this burden to:

Department of Health and Human Services
Food and Drug Administration - MedWatch
10903 New Hampshire Avenue
Building 22, Mail Stop 4447
Silver Spring, MD 20993-0002
Please DO NOT RETURN this form to this address.

OMB Statement:
"An agency may not conduct or sponsor, and a person is not required to respond to, a collection of information unless it displays a currently valid OMB control number."